DSM-5®
Self-Exam
Questions

Test Questions for the
Diagnostic Criteria

DSM-5® Self-Exam Questions

Test Questions for the Diagnostic Criteria

Edited by

Philip R. Muskin, M.D.

Professor of Psychiatry,
Columbia University Medical Center;
Chief of Service, Consultation-Liaison Psychiatry,
NY–Presbyterian Hospital/Columbia University Medical Center,
New York, New York

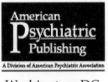

American Psychiatric Publishing
A Division of American Psychiatric Association

Washington, DC
London, England

If you would like to buy between 25 and 99 copies of this or any other American Psychiatric Publishing title, you are eligible for a 20% discount; please contact Customer Service at appi@psych.org or 800-368-5777. If you wish to buy 100 or more copies of the same title, please e-mail us at bulksales@psych.org for a price quote.

Copyright © 2014 American Psychiatric Association

ALL RIGHTS RESERVED

Manufactured in the United States of America on acid-free paper

18 17 16 15 14   5 4 3 2 1

ISBN 978-1-58562-467-6

First Edition

Typeset in Adobe's Palatino and Helvetica.

American Psychiatric Publishing,
a Division of American Psychiatric Association
1000 Wilson Boulevard
Arlington, VA 22209-3901
www.appi.org

Contents

Part II: Answer Guide

Contributors

Lawrence Amsel, M.D., M.P.H.
Assistant Professor of Clinical Psychiatry, Columbia University College of Physicians and Surgeons, New York, New York

Elizabeth L. Auchincloss, M.D.
Vice-Chair, Graduate Medical Education, Department of Psychiatry, Weill Cornell Medical College; Senior Associate Director, Columbia University Center for Psychoanalytic Training and Research, New York, New York

Robert J. Boland, M.D.
Professor of Psychiatry and Human Behavior; Associate Director, Residency Training, Alpert School of Medicine, Brown University, Providence, Rhode Island

Joyce T. Chen, M.D.
Public Psychiatry Postdoctoral Clinical Fellow, Department of Psychiatry, New York State Psychiatric Institute/Columbia University Medical Center, New York, New York

Christina Kitt Garza, M.D.
Instructor in Psychiatry, NY-Presbyterian Hospital/Columbia University Medical Center, New York, New York

Philip R. Muskin, M.D.
Professor of Psychiatry, Columbia University Medical Center; Chief of Service, Consultation-Liaison Psychiatry at NY-Presbyterian Hospital/Columbia University Medical Center, New York, New York

Michelle B. Riba, M.D., M.S.
Professor and Associate Chair for Integrated Medical and Psychiatric Services, Department of Psychiatry; Associate Director, University of Michigan Comprehensive Depression Center; Director, PsychOncology Program, University of Michigan Comprehensive Cancer Center; Associate Director, Michigan Institute for Clinical and Health Research, Ann Arbor, Michigan

Julie K. Schulman, M.D.
Assistant Professor of Clinical Psychiatry, Columbia University College of Physicians and Surgeons; Consultation-Liaison Psychiatry at NY–Presbyterian Hospital/Columbia University Medical Center, New York, New York

Peter A. Shapiro, M.D.
Professor of Psychiatry, Columbia University Medical Center; Associate Director, Consultation-Liaison Psychiatry Service, and Director, Fellowship Training Program in Psychosomatic Medicine, NY–Presbyterian Hospital/Columbia University Medical Center, New York, New York

Jonathan A. Slater, M.D.
Clinical Professor of Psychiatry (in Pediatrics), Columbia University College of Physicians and Surgeons; Director, Consultation and Emergency Service, Morgan Stanley Children's Hospital of New York, NY–Presbyterian Hospital/Columbia University Medical Center, New York, New York

Disclosure of Interests

The contributors have declared all forms of support received within the 12 months prior to manuscript submittal that may represent a competing interest in relation to their work published in this volume, as follows:

Philip R. Muskin, M.D.   *Speakers Bureau:* Otsuka.

The following contributors stated that they had no competing interests during the year preceding manuscript submission: Lawrence Amsel, M.D., M.P.H.; Elizabeth L. Auchincloss, M.D.; Robert J. Boland, M.D.; Joyce T. Chen, M.D.; Christina Kitt Garza, M.D.; Michelle B. Riba, M.D., M.S.; Julie K. Schulman, M.D.; Peter A. Shapiro, M.D.; Jonathan A. Slater, M.D.

Preface

This self-examination guide is a companion to, not a replacement for, a thorough reading of DSM-5. The most recent edition of the diagnostic manual brings a new set of diagnoses while retaining many familiar diagnoses. There are new approaches to diagnosis in DSM-5. Our framework in preparing this self-examination guide was to challenge the reader, hopefully engagingly, to learn about the new diagnoses, to understand the changes from DSM-IV, and to self-educate about new approaches to the diagnostic endeavor. Some questions will seem obvious or easy and some questions will be quite difficult. As you work through the book, let it guide you to diagnostic sections where you would like to learn more as well as reassure you about those areas in which you are already well versed. The contributors took on a daunting task—i.e., to write a book about a book that was itself being written. The contributors to this book are a group of clinicians and educators who undertook the task of learning about DSM-5 in order to help others self-educate. There is no commentary or politics about diagnosis in this study guide. The contributors have graciously donated the proceeds from this book to a charitable foundation.

Philip R. Muskin, M.D.
New York, New York

PART I

Questions

DSM-5 Introduction

I.1   DSM-IV employed a multiaxial diagnostic system. Which of the following statements best describes the multiaxial system in DSM-5?

A. There is a different multiaxial system in DSM-5.
B. The multiaxial system in DSM-IV has been retained in DSM-5.
C. DSM-5 has moved to a nonaxial documentation of diagnosis.
D. Axis I (Clinical Disorders) and Axis II (Personality Disorders) have been retained in DSM-5.
E. Axis IV (Psychosocial and Environmental Problems) and Axis V (Global Assessment of Functioning) have been retained in DSM-5.

I.2   True or False: The Global Assessment of Functioning (GAF) Scale (DSM-IV Axis V) remains a separate category that should be coded in DSM-5.

A. True.
B. False.

I.3   To enhance diagnostic specificity, DSM-5 replaced the previous "not otherwise specified" (NOS) designation with two options for clinical use: Other Specified [disorder] and Unspecified [disorder]. Which of the following statements about use of the Unspecified designation is *true?*

A. The Unspecified designation is used when the clinician chooses not to specify the reason that criteria for a specific disorder were not met.
B. The Unspecified designation is used when there is no recognized Other Specified disorder (e.g., recurrent brief depression, sexual aversion).
C. The Unspecified designation is used when the individual has fewer than three symptoms of any of the recognized disorders within the diagnostic class.
D. The Unspecified designation is used when the individual presents with symptomatology of disorders in two or more diagnostic classes.
E. The Unspecified designation is used when the clinician believes the condition is of a temporary nature.

CHAPTER 1

Neurodevelopmental Disorders

1.1 Which of the following is *not* required for a DSM-5 diagnosis of intellectual disability (intellectual developmental disorder)?

A. Full-scale IQ below 70.
B. Deficits in intellectual functions confirmed by clinical assessment.
C. Deficits in adaptive functioning that result in failure to meet developmental and sociocultural standards for personal independence and social responsibility.
D. Symptom onset during the developmental period.
E. Deficits in intellectual functions confirmed by individualized, standardized intelligence testing.

1.2 A 7-year-old boy in second grade displays significant delays in his ability to reason, solve problems, and learn from his experiences. He has been slow to develop reading, writing, and mathematics skills in school. All through development, these skills lagged behind peers, although he is making slow progress. These deficits significantly impair his ability to play in an age-appropriate manner with peers and to begin to acquire independent skills at home. He requires ongoing assistance with basic skills (dressing, feeding, and bathing himself; doing any type of schoolwork) on a daily basis. Which of the following diagnoses best fits this presentation?

A. Childhood-onset major neurocognitive disorder.
B. Specific learning disorder.
C. Intellectual disability (intellectual developmental disorder).
D. Communication disorder.
E. Autism spectrum disorder.

1.3 A 7-year-old boy in second grade displays significant delays in his ability to reason, solve problems, and learn from his experiences. He has been slow to develop reading, writing, and mathematics skills in school. All through development, these skills lagged behind peers, although he is making slow progress. These deficits significantly impair his ability to play in an age-appropriate manner with peers and to begin to acquire independent skills at home. He requires ongoing assistance with basic skills (dressing, feeding, and bathing himself; doing any type of schoolwork) on a daily basis. What is the appropriate severity rating for this patient's current presentation?

A. Mild.
B. Moderate.
C. Severe.
D. Profound.
E. Cannot be determined without an IQ score.

1.4 Which of the following statements about intellectual disability (intellectual developmental disorder) is *false?*

A. Individuals with intellectual disability have deficits in general mental abilities and impairment in everyday adaptive functioning compared with age- and gender-matched peers from the same linguistic and sociocultural group.
B. For individuals with intellectual disability, the full-scale IQ score is a valid assessment of overall mental abilities and adaptive functioning, even if subtest scores are highly discrepant.
C. Individuals with intellectual disability may have difficulty in managing their behavior, emotions, and interpersonal relationships and in maintaining motivation in the learning process.
D. Intellectual disability is generally associated with an IQ that is 2 standard deviations from the population mean, which equates to an IQ score of about 70 or below (±5 points).
E. Assessment procedures for intellectual disability must take into account factors that may limit performance, such as sociocultural background, native language, associated communication/language disorder, and motor or sensory handicap.

1.5 Which of the following statements about the diagnosis of intellectual disability (intellectual developmental disorder) is *false?*

A. An individual with an IQ of less than 70 would receive the diagnosis if there were no significant deficits in adaptive functioning.
B. An individual with an IQ above 75 would not meet diagnostic criteria even if there were impairments in adaptive functioning.
C. In forensic assessment, severe deficits in adaptive functioning might allow for a diagnosis with an IQ above 75.
D. Adaptive functioning must take into account the three domains of conceptual, social, and practical functioning.
E. The specifiers mild, moderate, severe, and profound are based on IQ scores.

1.6 Which of the following is *not* a diagnostic feature of intellectual disability (intellectual developmental disorder)?

A. A full-scale IQ of less than 70.
B. Inability to perform complex daily living tasks (e.g., money management, medical decision making) without support.

C. Gullibility, with naiveté in social situations and a tendency to be easily led by others.

D. Lack of age-appropriate communication skills for social and interpersonal functioning.

E. All of the above are diagnostic features of intellectual disability.

1.7   Which of the following statements about adaptive functioning in the diagnosis of intellectual disability (intellectual developmental disorder) is *true?*

A. Adaptive functioning is based on an individual's IQ score.

B. "Deficits in adaptive functioning" refers to problems with motor coordination.

C. At least two domains of adaptive functioning must be impaired to meet Criterion B for the diagnosis of intellectual disability.

D. Adaptive functioning in intellectual disability tends to improve over time, although the threshold of cognitive capacities and associated developmental disorders can limit it.

E. Individuals diagnosed with intellectual disability in childhood will typically continue to meet criteria in adulthood even if their adaptive functioning improves.

1.8   Which of the following statements about development of and risk factors for intellectual disability (intellectual developmental disorder) is *true?*

A. Intellectual developmental disorder should not be diagnosed in the presence of a known genetic syndrome, such as Lesch-Nyhan or Prader-Willi syndrome.

B. Etiologies are confined to perinatal and postnatal factors and exclude prenatal events.

C. In severe acquired forms of intellectual developmental disorder, onset may be abrupt following an illness (e.g., meningitis) or head trauma occurring during the developmental period.

D. When intellectual disability results from a loss of previously acquired cognitive skills, as in severe traumatic brain injury (TBI), only the TBI diagnosis is assigned.

E. Prenatal, perinatal, and postnatal etiologies of intellectual developmental disorder are demonstrable in approximately 33% of cases.

1.9   Which of the following statements about the developmental course of intellectual disability (intellectual developmental disorder) is *true?*

A. Delayed motor, language, and social milestones are not identifiable until after the first 2 years of life.

B. Intellectual disability caused by an illness (e.g., encephalitis) or by head trauma occurring during the developmental period would be diagnosed as a neurocognitive disorder, not as intellectual disability (intellectual developmental disorder).

C. Intellectual disability is always nonprogressive.

D. Major neurocognitive disorder may co-occur with intellectual developmental disorder.

E. Even if early and ongoing interventions throughout childhood and adulthood lead to improved adaptive and intellectual functioning, the diagnosis of intellectual disability would continue to apply.

1.10 The DSM-5 diagnosis of intellectual developmental disorder includes severity specifiers—Mild, Moderate, Severe, and Profound—with which to indicate the level of supports required in various domains of adaptive functioning. Which of the following features would *not* be characteristic of an individual with a "Severe" level of impairment?

A. The individual generally has little understanding of written language or of concepts involving numbers, quantity, time, and money.

B. The individual's spoken language is quite limited in terms of vocabulary and grammar.

C. The individual requires support for all activities of daily living, including meals, dressing, bathing, and toileting.

D. In adulthood, the individual may be able to sustain competitive employment in a job that does not emphasize conceptual skills.

E. The individual cannot make responsible decisions regarding the well-being of self or others.

1.11 A 10-year-old boy with a history of dyslexia, who is otherwise developmentally normal, is in a skateboarding accident in which he experiences severe traumatic brain injury. This results in significant global intellectual impairment (with a persistent reading deficit that is more pronounced than his other newly acquired but stable deficits, along with a full-scale IQ of 75). There is mild impairment in his adaptive functioning such that he requires support in some areas of functioning. He is also displaying anxious and depressive symptoms in response to his accident and hospitalization. What is the *least likely* diagnosis?

A. Intellectual disability (intellectual developmental disorder).

B. Traumatic brain injury.

C. Specific learning disorder.

D. Major neurocognitive disorder due to traumatic brain injury.

E. Adjustment disorder.

1.12 In which of the following situations would a diagnosis of global developmental delay be *inappropriate?*

A. The patient is a child who is too young to fully manifest specific symptoms or to complete requisite assessments.

B. The patient, a 7-year-old boy, has a full-scale IQ of 65 and severe impairment in adaptive functioning.
C. The patient's scores on psychometric tests suggest intellectual disability (intellectual developmental disorder), but there is insufficient information about the patient's adaptive functional skills.
D. The patient's impaired adaptive functioning suggests intellectual developmental disorder, but there is insufficient information about the level of cognitive impairment measured by standardized instruments.
E. The patient's cognitive and adaptive impairments suggest intellectual developmental disorder, but there is insufficient information about age at onset of the condition.

1.13 Which of the following statements about global developmental delay is *true?*

A. The diagnosis is typically made in children younger than 5 years of age.
B. The etiology can usually be determined.
C. The prevalence is estimated to be between 0.5% and 2%.
D. The condition is progressive.
E. The condition does not generally occur with other neurodevelopmental disorders.

1.14 A 3½-year-old girl with a history of lead exposure and a seizure disorder demonstrates substantial delays across multiple domains of functioning, including communication, learning, attention, and motor development, which limit her ability to interact with same-age peers and require substantial support in all activities of daily living at home. Unfortunately, her mother is an extremely poor historian, and the child has received no formal psychological or learning evaluation to date. She is about to be evaluated for readiness to attend preschool. What is the most appropriate diagnosis?

A. Major neurocognitive disorder.
B. Developmental coordination disorder.
C. Autism spectrum disorder.
D. Global developmental delay.
E. Specific learning disorder.

1.15 A 5-year-old boy has difficulty making friends and problems with initiating and sustaining back-and-forth conversation; reading social cues; and sharing his feelings with others. He makes good eye contact, has normal speech intonation, displays facial gestures, and has a range of affect that generally seems appropriate to the situation. He demonstrates an interest in trains that seems abnormal in intensity and focus, and he engages in little imaginative or symbolic play. Which of the following diagnostic requirements for autism spectrum disorder are *not* met in this case?

A. Deficits in social-emotional reciprocity.

B. Deficits in nonverbal communicative behaviors used for social interaction.

C. Deficits in developing and maintaining relationships.

D. Restricted, repetitive patterns of behavior, interests, or activities as manifested by symptoms in two of the specified four categories.

E. Symptoms with onset in early childhood that cause clinically significant impairment.

1.16   Which of the following statements about the development and course of autism spectrum disorder (ASD) is *false?*

A. Symptoms of ASD are typically recognized during the second year of life (12–24 months of age).

B. Symptoms of ASD are usually not noticeable until 5–6 years of age or later.

C. First symptoms frequently involve delayed language development, often accompanied by lack of social interest or unusual social interactions.

D. ASD is not a degenerative disorder, and it is typical for learning and compensation to continue throughout life.

E. Because many normally developing young children have strong preferences and enjoy repetition, distinguishing restricted and repetitive behaviors that are diagnostic of ASD can be difficult in preschoolers.

1.17   Which of the following was a criterion symptom for autistic disorder in DSM-IV that was eliminated from the diagnostic criteria for autism spectrum disorder in DSM-5?

A. Stereotyped or restricted patterns of interest.

B. Stereotyped and repetitive motor mannerisms.

C. Inflexible adherence to routines.

D. Persistent preoccupation with parts of objects.

E. None of the above.

1.18   A 7-year-old girl presents with a history of normal language skills (vocabulary and grammar intact) but is unable to use language in a socially pragmatic manner to share ideas and feelings. She has never made good eye contact, and she has difficulty reading social cues. Consequently, she has had difficulty making friends, which is further complicated by her being somewhat obsessed with cartoon characters, which she repetitively scripts. She tends to excessively smell objects. Because she insists on wearing the same shirt and shorts every day, regardless of the season, getting dressed is a difficult activity. These symptoms date from early childhood and cause significant impairment in her functioning. What diagnosis best fits this child's presentation?

A. Asperger's disorder.

B. Autism spectrum disorder.

C. Pervasive developmental disorder not otherwise specified (NOS).

D. Social (pragmatic) communication disorder.

E. Rett syndrome.

1.19 A 15-year-old boy has a long history of nonverbal communication deficits. As an infant he was unable to follow someone else directing his attention by pointing. As a toddler he was not interested in sharing events, feelings, or games with his parents. From school age into adolescence, his speech was odd in tonality and phrasing, and his body language was awkward. What do these symptoms represent?

A. Stereotypies.

B. Restricted range of interests.

C. Developmental regression.

D. Prodromal schizophreniform symptoms.

E. Deficits in nonverbal communicative behaviors.

1.20 A 10-year-old boy demonstrates hand-flapping and finger flicking, and he repetitively flips coins and lines up his trucks. He tends to "echo" the last several words of a question posed to him before answering, mixes up his pronouns (refers to himself in the second person), tends to repeat phrases in a perseverative fashion, and is quite fixated on routines related to dress, eating, travel, and play. He spends hours in his garage playing with his father's tools. What do these behaviors represent?

A. Restricted, repetitive patterns of behaviors, interests, or activities characteristic of autism spectrum disorder.

B. Symptoms of obsessive-compulsive disorder.

C. Prototypical manifestations of obsessive-compulsive personality.

D. Symptoms of pediatric acute-onset neuropsychiatric syndrome (PANS).

E. Complex tics.

1.21 A 25-year-old man presents with long-standing nonverbal communication deficits, inability to have a back-and-forth conversation or share interests in an appropriate fashion, and a complete lack of interest in having relationships with others. His speech reflects awkward phrasing and intonation and is mechanical in nature. He has a history of sequential fixations and obsessions with various games and objects throughout childhood; however, this is not currently a major issue for him. This patient meets criteria for autism spectrum disorder; true or false?

A. True.

B. False.

1.22 A 9-year-old girl presents with a history of intellectual impairment, a structural language impairment, nonverbal communication deficits, disinterest in peers, and inability to use language in a social manner. She has extreme food and tactile sensitivities. She is obsessed with one particular computer game that she plays for hours each day, and she scripts and imitates the characters in this game. She is clumsy, has an odd gait, and walks on her tiptoes. In the past year she has developed a seizure disorder and has begun to bang her wrists against the wall repetitively, causing bruising. On the other hand, she plays several musical instruments in an extremely precocious manner. Which feature of this child's clinical presentation fulfills a criterion symptom for DSM-5 autism spectrum disorder?

A. Motor abnormalities.
B. Seizures.
C. Structural language impairment.
D. Intellectual impairment.
E. Nonverbal communicative deficits.

1.23   An 11-year-old girl with autism spectrum disorder displays no spoken language and is minimally responsive to overtures from others. She can be somewhat inflexible, which interferes with her ability to travel, do schoolwork, and be managed in the home; she has some difficulty transitioning; and she has trouble organizing and planning activities. These problems can usually be managed with incentives and reinforcers. What severity levels should be specified in the DSM-5 diagnosis?

A. Level 3 (requiring very substantial support) for social communication, and level 1 (requiring support) for restricted, repetitive behaviors.
B. Level 1 (requiring support) for social communication, and level 3 (requiring very substantial support) for restricted, repetitive behaviors.
C. Level 1 (requiring support) for social communication, and level 2 (requiring substantial support) for restricted, repetitive behaviors.
D. Level 3 (requiring very substantial support) for social communication, and level 1 (requiring support) for restricted, repetitive behaviors.
E. Level 2 (requiring substantial support) for social communication, and level 1 (requiring support) for restricted, repetitive behaviors.

1.24   Which of the following is *not* a specifier included in the diagnostic criteria for autism spectrum disorder?

A. With or without accompanying intellectual impairment.
B. With or without associated dementia.
C. With or without accompanying language impairment.
D. Associated with a known medical or genetic condition or environmental factor.
E. Associated with another neurodevelopmental, mental, or behavioral disorder.

1.25   Which of the following is *not* characteristic of the developmental course of children diagnosed with autism spectrum disorder?

A. Behavioral features manifest before 3 years of age.
B. The full symptom pattern does not appear until age 2–3 years.
C. Developmental plateaus or regression in social-communicative behavior is frequently reported by parents.
D. Regression across multiple domains occurs after age 2–3 years.
E. First symptoms often include delayed language development, lack of social interest or unusual social behavior, odd play, and unusual communication patterns.

1.26   A 5-year-old girl has some mild food aversions. She enjoys having the same book read to her at night but does not become terribly upset if her mother asks her to choose a different book. She occasionally spins around excitedly when her favorite show is on. She generally likes her toys neatly arranged in bins but is only mildly upset when her sister leaves them on the floor. These behaviors should be considered suspicious for an autism spectrum disorder; true or false?

A. True.
B. False.

1.27   Which of the following is *not* representative of the typical developmental course for autism spectrum disorder?

A. Lack of degenerative course.
B. Behavioral deterioration during adolescence.
C. Continued learning and compensation throughout life.
D. Marked presence of symptoms in early childhood and early school years, with developmental gains in later childhood in areas such as social interaction.
E. Good psychosocial functioning in adulthood, as indexed by independent living and gainful employment.

1.28   A 21-year-old man, not previously diagnosed with a developmental disorder, presents for evaluation after taking a leave from college for psychological reasons. He makes little eye contact, does not appear to pick up on social cues, has become disinterested in friends, spends hours each day on the computer surfing the Internet and playing games, and has become so sensitive to smells that he keeps multiple air fresheners in all locations of the home. He reports that he has had long-standing friendships dating from childhood and high school (corroborated by his parents). He reports making many friends in his fraternity at college. His parents report good social and communication skills in childhood, although he was quite shy and was somewhat inflexible and ritualistic at home. What is the *least likely* diagnosis?

A. Depression.

B. Schizophreniform disorder or schizophrenia.

C. Autism spectrum disorder.

D. Obsessive-compulsive disorder.

E. Social anxiety disorder (social phobia).

1.29 Which of the following characteristics is generally *not* associated with autism spectrum disorder?

A. Anxiety, depression, and isolation as an adult.

B. Catatonia.

C. Poor psychosocial functioning.

D. Insistence on routines and aversion to change.

E. Successful adaptation in regular school settings.

1.30 Which of the following disorders is generally *not* comorbid with autism spectrum disorder (ASD)?

A. Attention-deficit/hyperactivity disorder (ADHD).

B. Rett syndrome.

C. Selective mutism.

D. Intellectual disability (intellectual developmental disorder).

E. Stereotypic movement disorder.

1.31 Which of the following is *not* a criterion for the DSM-5 diagnosis of attention-deficit/hyperactivity disorder (ADHD)?

A. Onset of several inattentive or hyperactive-impulsive symptoms prior to age 12 years.

B. Manifestation of several inattentive or hyperactive-impulsive symptoms in two or more settings (e.g., at home, school, or work; with friends or relatives; in other activities).

C. Persistence of symptoms for at least 12 months.

D. Clear evidence that symptoms interfere with, or reduce the quality of, social, academic, or occupational functioning.

E. Inability to explain symptoms as a manifestation of another mental disorder (e.g., mood disorder, anxiety disorder, dissociative disorder, personality disorder, substance intoxication or withdrawal).

1.32 The parents of a 15-year-old female tenth grader believe that she should be doing better in high school, given how bright she seems and the fact that she received mostly A's through eighth grade. Her papers are handed in late, and she makes careless mistakes on examinations. They have her tested, and the WAIS-IV results are as follows: Verbal IQ, 125; Perceptual Reasoning Index, 122; Full-Scale IQ, 123; Working Memory Index, 55th percentile; Processing Speed Index, 50th percentile. Weaknesses in executive function are noted. During a psychiatric evaluation, she reports a long history of failing to give close attention to details, difficulty sustaining attention while in class or doing homework, failing to finish chores and tasks, and significant difficulties with time management, planning, and organization. She is forgetful, often loses things, and is easily distracted. She has no history of restlessness or impulsivity, and she is well liked by her peers. What is the most likely diagnosis?

A. Adjustment disorder with anxiety.
B. Specific learning disorder.
C. Attention-deficit/hyperactivity disorder, predominantly inattentive.
D. Developmental coordination disorder.
E. Major depressive disorder.

1.33 A 7-year-old boy is having behavioral and social difficulties in his second-grade class. Although he seems to be able to attend and is doing "well" from an academic standpoint (though seemingly not what he is capable of), he is constantly interrupting, fidgeting, talking excessively, and getting out of his seat. He has friends, but he sometimes annoys his peers because of his difficulty sharing and taking turns and the fact that he is constantly talking over them. Although he seeks out play dates, his friends tire of him because he wants to play sports nonstop. At home, he can barely stay in his seat for a meal and is unable to play quietly. Although he shows remorse when the consequences of his behavior are pointed out to him, he can become angry in response and seems nevertheless unable to inhibit himself. What is the most likely diagnosis?

A. Bipolar disorder.
B. Autism spectrum disorder.
C. Generalized anxiety disorder.
D. Attention-deficit/hyperactivity disorder, predominantly hyperactive/impulsive.
E. Specific learning disorder.

1.34 A 37-year-old Wall Street trader schedules a visit after his 8-year-old son is diagnosed with attention-deficit/hyperactivity disorder (ADHD), combined inattentive and hyperactive. Although he does not currently note motor restlessness like his son, he recalls being that way when he was a boy, along with being quite inattentive, being impulsive, talking excessively, interrupting, and having problems waiting his turn. He was an underachiever in high school and college, when he inconsistently did his work and had difficulty following rules. Nevertheless, he never failed any classes, and he was never evaluated by a psychologist or psychiatrist. He works about 60–80 hours a week and often gets insufficient sleep. He tends to make impulsive business decisions, can be impatient and short-tempered, and notes that his mind tends to wander both in one-on-one interactions with associates and his wife and during business meetings, for which he is often late; he is forgetful and disorganized. Nevertheless, he tends to perform fairly well and is quite successful, although he can occasionally feel overwhelmed and demoralized. What is the most likely diagnosis?

A. Major depressive disorder.
B. Generalized anxiety disorder.
C. Specific learning disorder.
D. ADHD, in partial remission.
E. Oppositional defiant disorder.

1.35   A 5-year-old hyperactive, impulsive, and inattentive boy presents with hyper-telorism, highly arched palate, and low-set ears. He is uncoordinated and clumsy, he has no sense of time, and his toys and clothes are constantly strewn all over the house. He has recently developed what appears to be a motor tic involving blinking. He enjoys playing with peers, who tend to like him, al-though he seems to willfully defy all requests from his parents and kindergar-ten teacher, which does not seem to be due simply to inattention. He is delayed in beginning to learn how to read. What is the *least likely* diagnosis?

A. Autism spectrum disorder.
B. Developmental coordination disorder.
C. Oppositional defiant disorder (ODD).
D. Specific learning disorder.
E. Attention-deficit/hyperactivity disorder (ADHD).

1.36   What is the prevalence of attention-deficit/hyperactivity disorder (ADHD) in children?

A. 8%.
B. 10%.
C. 2%.
D. 0.5%.
E. 5%.

1.37   What is the prevalence of attention-deficit/hyperactivity disorder (ADHD) in adults?

A. 8%.
B. 10%.
C. 2.5%.
D. 0.5%.
E. 5%.

1.38   What is the gender ratio of attention-deficit/hyperactivity disorder (ADHD) in children?

A. Male:female ratio of 2:1.
B. Male:female ratio of 1:1.

C. Male:female ratio of 3:2.
D. Male:female ratio of 5:1.
E. Male:female ratio of 1:2.

1.39   Which of the following is a biological finding in individuals with attention-deficit/hyperactivity disorder (ADHD)?

A. Decreased slow-wave activity on electroencephalograms.
B. Reduced total brain volume on magnetic resonance imaging.
C. Early posterior to anterior cortical maturation.
D. Reduced thalamic volume.
E. Both B and C.

1.40   Which of the following is *not* associated with attention-deficit/hyperactivity disorder (ADHD)?

A. Reduced school performance.
B. Poorer occupational performance and attendance.
C. Higher probability of unemployment.
D. Elevated interpersonal conflict.
E. Reduced risk of substance use disorders.

1.41   Which of the following is *not* associated with attention-deficit/hyperactivity disorder (ADHD)?

A. Social rejection.
B. Increased risk of developing conduct disorder in childhood and antisocial personality disorder in adulthood.
C. Increased risk of Alzheimer's disease.
D. Increased frequency of traffic accidents and violations.
E. Increased risk of accidental injury.

1.42   A 15-year-old boy has developed concentration problems in school that have been associated with a significant decline in grades. When interviewed, he explains that his mind is occupied with worrying about his mother, who has a serious autoimmune disease. As his grades falter, he becomes increasingly demoralized and sad, and he notices that his energy level drops, further compromising his ability to pay attention in school. At the same time, he complains of feeling restless and unable to sleep. What is the most likely diagnosis?

A. Bipolar disorder.
B. Specific learning disorder.
C. Attention-deficit/hyperactivity disorder (ADHD).
D. Adjustment disorder with mixed anxiety and depressed mood.
E. Separation anxiety disorder.

1.43   A 5-year-old boy is consistently moody, irritable, and intolerant of frustration. In addition, he is pervasively and chronically restless, impulsive, and inattentive. Which diagnosis best fits his clinical picture?

A. Attention-deficit/hyperactivity disorder (ADHD).
B. ADHD and disruptive mood dysregulation disorder (DMDD).
C. Bipolar disorder.
D. Oppositional defiant disorder (ODD).
E. Major depressive disorder (MDD).

1.44   Which of the following statements about comorbidity in attention-deficit/hyperactivity disorder (ADHD) is *true*?

A. Oppositional defiant disorder co-occurs with ADHD in about half of children with the combined presentation and about a quarter of those with the predominantly inattentive presentation.
B. Most children with disruptive mood dysregulation disorder do not also meet criteria for ADHD.
C. Fifteen percent of adults with ADHD have some type of anxiety disorder.
D. Intermittent explosive disorder occurs in about 5% of adults with ADHD.
E. Specific learning disorder very seldom co-occurs with ADHD.

1.45   Specific learning disorder is defined by persistent difficulties in learning academic skills, with onset during the developmental period. Which of the following statements about this disorder is *true*?

A. It is part of a more general learning impairment as manifested in intellectual disability (intellectual developmental disorder).
B. It can usually be attributed to a sensory, physical, or neurological disorder.
C. It involves pervasive and wide-ranging deficits across multiple domains of information processing.
D. It can be caused by external factors such as economic disadvantage or lack of education.
E. It replaces the DSM-IV diagnoses of reading disorder, mathematics disorder, disorder of written expression, and learning disorder not otherwise specified.

1.46   In distinction to DSM-IV, DSM-5 classifies all learning disorders under the diagnosis of specific learning disorder, along with the requirement to "specify all academic domains and subskills that are impaired" at the time of assessment. Which of the following statements about specific learning disorder is *false*?

A. There are persistent difficulties in the acquisition of reading, writing, arithmetic, or mathematical reasoning skills during the formal years of schooling.

B. Current skills in one or more of these academic areas are well below the average range for the individual's age, gender, cultural group, and level of education.

C. There usually is a discrepancy of more than 2 standard deviations (SD) between achievement and IQ.

D. The learning difficulties significantly interfere with academic achievement, occupational performance, or activities of daily living that require these academic skills.

E. The learning difficulties cannot be acquired later in life.

1.47 Which of the following statements about the diagnosis of specific learning disorder is *false?*

A. Specific learning disorder is distinct from learning problems associated with a neurodegenerative cognitive disorder.

B. If intellectual disability (intellectual developmental disorder) is present, the learning difficulties must be in excess of those expected.

C. An uneven profile of abilities is typical in specific learning disorder.

D. Attentional difficulties and motor clumsiness that are subthreshold for attention-deficit/hyperactivity disorder or developmental coordination disorder are frequently associated with specific learning disorder.

E. There are four formal subtypes of specific learning disorder.

1.48 Which of the following statements about prevalence rates for specific learning disorder is *false?*

A. Prevalence rates range from 5% to 15% among school-age children across languages and cultures.

B. Prevalence in adults is approximately 4%.

C. Specific learning disorder is equally common among males and females.

D. Prevalence rates vary according to the range of ages in the sample, selection criteria, severity of specific learning disorder, and academic domains investigated.

E. Gender ratios cannot be attributed to factors such as ascertainment bias, definitional or measurement variation, language, race, or socioeconomic status.

1.49 Which of the following statements about comorbidity in specific learning disorder is *true?*

A. Attention-deficit/hyperactivity disorder (ADHD) does not co-occur with specific learning disorder more frequently than would be expected by chance.

B. Speech sound disorder and specific language impairments are not commonly comorbid with specific learning disorder.

C. Identified clusters of co-occurrences include severe reading disorders; fine motor problems and handwriting problems; and problems with arithmetic, reading, and gross motor planning.

D. The co-occurrence of specific learning disorder and specific language impairments has been shown in up to 20% of children with language problems.

E. Co-occurring disorders generally do not influence the course or treatment of specific learning disorder.

1.50　Which of the following statements about developmental coordination disorder (DCD) is *true?*

A. Some children with DCD show additional (usually suppressed) motor activity, such as choreiform movements of unsupported limbs or mirror movements.

B. The prevalence of DCD in children ages 5–11 years is 1%–3%.

C. In early adulthood, there is improvement in learning new tasks involving complex/automatic motor skills, including driving and using tools.

D. DCD has no association with prenatal exposure to alcohol or with low birth weight or preterm birth.

E. Impairments in underlying neurodevelopmental processes have not been found to primarily affect visuomotor skills.

1.51　Which of the following statements about developmental coordination disorder (DCD) is *true?*

A. The disorder is usually not diagnosed before the age of 7 years.

B. Symptoms have usually improved significantly at 1-year follow-up.

C. In most cases, symptoms are no longer evident by adolescence.

D. DCD has no clear relationship with prenatal alcohol exposure, preterm birth, or low birth weight.

E. Cerebellar dysfunction is hypothesized to play a role in DCD.

1.52　Which of the following is *not* a criterion for the DSM-5 diagnosis of stereotypic movement disorder?

A. Motor behaviors are present that are repetitive, seemingly driven, and apparently purposeless.

B. Onset of the behaviors is in the early developmental period.

C. The behaviors result in self-inflicted bodily injury that requires medical treatment.

D. The behaviors are not attributable to the physiological effects of a substance or neurological condition or better explained by another neurodevelopmental or mental disorder.

E. The behaviors interfere with social, academic, or other activities.

1.53 Which of the following statements about the developmental course of stereo-typic movement disorder is *false?*

A. The presence of stereotypic movements may indicate an undetected neuro-developmental problem, especially in children ages 1–3 years.
B. Among typically developing children, the repetitive movements may be stopped when attention is directed to them or when the child is distracted from performing them.
C. In some children, the stereotypic movements would result in self-injury if protective measures were not used.
D. Whereas simple stereotypic movements (e.g., rocking) are common in young typically developing children, complex stereotypic movements are much less common (approximately 3%–4%).
E. Stereotypic movements typically begin within the first year of life.

1.54 Which of the following is a DSM-5 diagnostic criterion for Tourette's disorder?

A. Tics occur throughout a period of more than 1 year, and during this period there was never a tic-free period of more than 3 consecutive months.
B. Onset is before age 5 years.
C. The tics may wax and wane in frequency but have persisted for more than 1 year since first tic onset.
D. Motor tics must precede vocal tics.
E. The tics may occur many times a day for at least 4 weeks, but no longer than 12 consecutive months.

1.55 At her child's third office visit, the mother of an 8-year-old boy with a 6-month history of excessive eye blinking and intermittent chirping says that she has noticed the development of grunting sounds since he started school this term. What is the most likely diagnosis?

A. Tourette's disorder.
B. Provisional tic disorder.
C. Temporary tic disorder.
D. Persistent (chronic) vocal tic disorder.
E. Transient tic disorder, recurrent.

1.56 A 5-year-old girl is referred to your care with a DSM-IV diagnosis of chronic motor or vocal tic disorder. Under DSM-5, she would meet criteria for persistent (chronic) motor or vocal tic disorder. Which of the following statements about her new diagnosis under DSM-5 is *false?*

A. She may have single or multiple motor or vocal tics, but not both.
B. Her tics must persist for more than 1 year since first tic onset without a tic-free period for 3 consecutive months to meet diagnostic criteria.

C. Her tics may wax and wane in frequency but have persisted for more than 1 year since first tic onset.

D. She has never met criteria for Tourette's disorder.

E. A specifier may be added to the diagnosis of persistent (chronic) motor or vocal tic disorder to indicate whether the girl has motor or vocal tics.

1.57 A highly functional 20-year-old college student with a history of anxiety symptoms and attention-deficit/hyperactivity disorder, for which she is prescribed lisdexamfetamine (Vyvanse), tells her psychiatrist that she has been researching the side effects of her medication for one of her class projects. In addition, she says that for the past week she has been feeling stressed by her schoolwork, and her friends have been asking her why she intermittently bobs her head up and down multiple times a day. What is the most likely diagnosis?

A. Provisional tic disorder.

B. Unspecified tic disorder.

C. Unspecified anxiety disorder.

D. Obsessive-compulsive personality disorder.

E. Unspecified stimulant-induced disorder.

1.58 Which of the following is *not* a DSM-5 diagnostic criterion for language disorder?

A. Persistent difficulties in the acquisition and use of language across modalities due to deficits in comprehension or production.

B. Language abilities that are substantially and quantifiably below those expected for age.

C. Symptom onset in the early developmental period.

D. Inability to attribute difficulties to hearing or other sensory impairment, motor dysfunction, or another medical or neurological condition.

E. Failure to meet criteria for mixed receptive-expressive language disorder or a pervasive developmental disorder.

1.59 Which of the following statements about speech sound disorder is *true?*

A. Speech sound production must be present by age 2 years.

B. "Failure to use developmentally expected speech sounds" is assessed by comparison of a child with his or her peers of the same age and dialect.

C. The difficulties in speech sound production need not result in functional impairment to meet diagnostic criteria.

D. Symptom onset is in the early developmental period.

E. Both A and C are true.

1.60 A mother brings her 4-year-old son to you for an evaluation with concerns that her son has struggled with speech articulation since very young. He has not sustained any head injuries, is otherwise healthy, and has a normal IQ. His preschool teacher reports that she does not always understand what he is saying and that other children tease him by calling him a "baby" due to his difficulty with communication. He does not have trouble relating to other people or understanding nonverbal social cues. What is the most likely diagnosis?

A. Selective mutism.
B. Global developmental delay.
C. Speech sound disorder.
D. Avoidant personality disorder.
E. Unspecified anxiety disorder.

1.61　A 6-year-old boy is failing school and continues to struggle significantly with grammar, sentence construction, and vocabulary. When he speaks, he also interjects "and" in between all his words. His teacher reports that he requires more verbal redirection than other students in order to stay on task. He is generally quiet and does not cause trouble otherwise. Which of the following diagnoses would be on your differential?

A. Language disorder.
B. Expressive language disorder.
C. Childhood-onset fluency disorder.
D. Attention-deficit/hyperactivity disorder (ADHD).
E. A and D.

1.62　Which of the following types of disturbance in normal speech fluency/time patterning included in the DSM-IV criteria for stuttering was omitted in the DSM-5 criteria for childhood-onset fluency disorder (stuttering)?

A. Sound prolongation.
B. Circumlocution.
C. Interjections.
D. Words produced with an excess of physical tension.
E. Sound and syllable repetitions.

1.63　A 14-year-old boy in regular education tells you that he thinks a girl in class likes him. His mother is surprised to hear this, because she reports that, since a young age, he has often struggled with making inferences or understanding nuances from what other people say. The teacher has also noticed that he sometimes misses nonverbal cues. He tends to get along better with adults, perhaps because they are not as likely to be put off by his overly formal speech. When he makes jokes, his peers do not always find the humor appropriate. Although he enjoys spending time with his best friend, he can be talkative and struggles with taking turns in conversation. What is the most likely diagnosis?

A. Social (pragmatic) communication disorder.
B. Asperger's disorder.
C. Autism spectrum disorder.

D. Social anxiety disorder.

E. Language disorder.

1.64 A 15-year-old boy with a prior diagnosis of Tourette's disorder is referred to your care. His mother tells you that during middle school he was teased for having vocal and motor tics. Since starting ninth grade, his tics have become less frequent. Currently, only mild motor tics remain. What is the appropriate DSM-5 diagnosis?

A. Tourette's disorder.

B. Persistent (chronic) motor tic disorder.

C. Provisional tic disorder.

D. Unspecified tic disorder.

E. Persistent (chronic) vocal tic disorder.

1.65 Tics typically present for the first time during which developmental stage?

A. Infancy.

B. Prepuberty.

C. Latency.

D. Adolescence.

E. Adulthood.

1.66 A 7-year-old boy who has speech delays presents with long-standing, repetitive hand waving, arm flapping, and finger wiggling. His mother reports that she first noticed these symptoms when he was a toddler and wonders whether they are tics. She says that he tends to flap more when he is engrossed in activities, such as while watching his favorite television program, but will stop when called or distracted. Based on the mother's report, which of the following conditions would be highest on your list of possible diagnoses?

A. Provisional tic disorder.

B. Persistent (chronic) motor or vocal tic disorder.

C. Chorea.

D. Dystonia.

E. Motor stereotypies.

1.67 Assessment of co-occurring conditions is important for understanding the overall functional consequence of tics on an individual. Which of the following conditions has been associated with tic disorders?

A. Attention-deficit/hyperactivity disorder (ADHD).

B. Obsessive-compulsive and related disorders.

C. Other movement disorders.

D. Depressive disorders.

E. All of the above.

1.68 By what age should most children have acquired adequate speech and language ability to understand and follow social rules of verbal and nonverbal communication, follow rules for conversation and storytelling, and change language according to the needs of the listener or situation?

A. Ages 2–3 years.
B. Ages 3–4 years.
C. Ages 4–5 years.
D. Ages 5–6 years.
E. Ages 6–7 years.

1.69 Having a family history of which of the following psychiatric disorders increases an individual's risk of social (pragmatic) communication disorder?

A. Social anxiety disorder (social phobia).
B. Autism spectrum disorder.
C. Attention-deficit/hyperactivity disorder (ADHD).
D. Specific learning disorder.
E. Either B or D.

1.70 A 6-year-old boy with a history of mild language delay is brought to your office by his mother, who is concerned that he is being teased in school because he misinterprets nonverbal cues and speaks in overly formal language with his peers. She tells you that her son was in an early intervention program, but his written and spoken language is now at grade level. The boy does not have a history of repetitive movements, sensory issues, or ritualized behaviors. Although he prefers constancy, he adapts fairly well to new situations. Additionally, he has a long-standing interest in trains and cars and is able to recite for you all the car models he memorized from a book on the history of transportation. Which of the following disorders would be a primary consideration in the differential diagnosis?

A. Social (pragmatic) communication disorder.
B. Autism spectrum disorder.
C. Global developmental delay.
D. Language disorder.
E. A and B.

1.71 Below what age is it difficult to distinguish a language disorder from normal developmental variations?

A. Age 2 years.
B. Age 3 years.
C. Age 4 years.
D. Age 5 years.
E. Age 6 years.

1.72　Which of the following psychiatric diagnoses is strongly associated with language disorder?

A. Attention-deficit/hyperactivity disorder.
B. Developmental coordination disorder.
C. Autism spectrum disorder.
D. Social (pragmatic) communication disorder.
E. All of the above.

1.73　Which of the following statements about the development of speech as it applies to speech sound disorder is *false?*

A. Most children with speech sound disorder respond well to treatment.
B. Speech sound production should be mostly intelligible by age 3 years.
C. Most speech sounds should be pronounced clearly and accurately according to age and community norms before age 10 years.
D. Lisping may or may not be associated with speech sound disorder.
E. It is abnormal for children to shorten words when they are learning to talk.

1.74　Which of the following would likely *not* be an important condition to rule out in the differential diagnosis of speech sound disorder?

A. Normal variations in speech.
B. Hearing or other sensory impairment.
C. Dysarthria.
D. Depression.
E. Selective mutism.

1.75　Which of the following statements about the development of childhood-onset fluency disorder (stuttering) is *true?*

A. Stuttering occurs by age 6 for 80%–90% of affected individuals.
B. Stuttering always begin abruptly and is noticeable to everyone.
C. Stress and anxiety do not exacerbate disfluency.
D. Motor movements are not associated with this disorder.
E. None of the above.

CHAPTER 2

Schizophrenia Spectrum and Other Psychotic Disorders

2.1   Criterion A for schizoaffective disorder requires an uninterrupted period of illness during which Criterion A for schizophrenia is met. Which of the following additional symptoms must be present to fulfill diagnostic criteria for schizoaffective disorder?

   A. An anxiety episode—either panic or general anxiety.
   B. Rapid eye movement (REM) sleep behavior disorder.
   C. A major depressive or manic episode.
   D. Hypomania.
   E. Cyclothymia.

2.2   There is a requirement for a major depressive episode or a manic episode to be part of the symptom picture for a DSM-5 diagnosis of schizoaffective disorder. In order to separate schizoaffective disorder from depressive or bipolar disorder with psychotic features, which of the following symptoms must be present for at least 2 weeks in the absence of a major mood episode at some point during the lifetime duration of the illness?

   A. Delusions or hallucinations.
   B. Delusions or paranoia.
   C. Regressed behavior.
   D. Projective identification.
   E. Binge eating.

2.3   A 27-year-old unmarried truck driver has a 5-year history of active and residual symptoms of schizophrenia. He develops symptoms of depression, including depressed mood and anhedonia, that last 4 months and resolve with treatment but do not meet criteria for major depression. Which diagnosis best fits this clinical presentation?

   A. Schizoaffective disorder.
   B. Unspecified schizophrenia spectrum and other psychotic disorder.
   C. Unspecified depressive disorder.

D. Schizophrenia and unspecified depressive disorder.

E. Unspecified bipolar and related disorder.

2.4 How common is schizoaffective disorder relative to schizophrenia?

A. Much more common.

B. Twice as common.

C. Equally common.

D. One-half as common.

E. One-third as common.

2.5 A 30-year-old single woman reports having experienced auditory and perse-cutory delusions for 2 months, followed by a full major depressive episode with sad mood, anhedonia, and suicidal ideation lasting 3 months. Although the depressive episode resolves with pharmacotherapy and psychotherapy, the psychotic symptoms persist for another month before resolving. What di-agnosis best fits this clinical picture?

A. Brief psychotic disorder.

B. Schizoaffective disorder.

C. Major depressive disorder.

D. Major depressive disorder with psychotic features.

E. Bipolar I disorder, current episode manic, with mixed features.

2.6 Which of the following statements about the incidence of schizoaffective disor-der is *true?*

A. The incidence is equal in women and men.

B. The incidence is higher in men.

C. The incidence is higher in women.

D. The incidence rates are unknown.

E. The incidence rates vary based on seasonality of birth.

2.7 Substance/medication-induced psychotic disorder cannot be diagnosed if the disturbance is better explained by an independent psychotic disorder that is not induced by a substance/medication. Which of the following psychotic symptom presentations would *not* be evidence of an independent psychotic disorder?

A. Psychotic symptoms that precede the onset of severe intoxication or acute withdrawal.

B. Psychotic symptoms that meet full criteria for a psychotic disorder and that persist for a substantial period after cessation of severe intoxication or acute withdrawal.

C. Psychotic symptoms that are substantially in excess of what would be ex-pected given the type or amount of the substance used or the duration of use.

D. Psychotic symptoms that occur during a period of sustained substance abstinence.

E. Psychotic symptoms that occur during a medical admission for substance withdrawal.

2.8   A 55-year-old man with a known history of alcohol dependence and schizophrenia is brought to the emergency department because of frank delusions and visual hallucinations. Which of the following would *not* be a diagnostic possibility for inclusion in the differential diagnosis?

A. Schizophrenia.
B. Substance/medication-induced psychotic disorder.
C. Alcohol dependence.
D. Psychotic disorder due to another medical condition.
E. Borderline personality disorder with psychotic features.

2.9   Which of the following sets of specifiers is included in the DSM-5 diagnostic criteria for substance/medication-induced psychotic disorder?

A. "With onset before intoxication" and "With onset before withdrawal."
B. "With onset during intoxication" and "With onset during withdrawal."
C. "With good prognostic features" and "Without good prognostic features."
D. "With onset prior to substance use" and "With onset after substance use."
E. "With catatonia" and 'Without catatonia."

2.10   A 65-year-old man with systemic lupus erythematosus who is being treated with corticosteroids witnesses a serious motor vehicle accident. He begins to have disorganized speech, which lasts for several days before resolving. What diagnosis best fits this clinical picture?

A. Schizophrenia.
B. Psychotic disorder associated with systemic lupus erythematosus.
C. Steroid-induced psychosis.
D. Brief psychotic disorder, with marked stressor.
E. Schizoaffective disorder.

2.11   Which of the following psychotic symptom presentations would *not* be appropriately diagnosed as "other specified schizophrenia spectrum and other psychotic disorder"?

A. Psychotic symptoms that have lasted for less than 1 month but have not yet remitted, so that the criteria for brief psychotic disorder are not met.
B. Persistent auditory hallucinations occurring in the absence of any other features.
C. Postpartum psychosis that does not meet criteria for a depressive or bipolar disorder with psychotic features, brief psychotic disorder, psychotic disor-

der due to another medical condition, or substance/medication-induced psychotic disorder.

D. Psychotic symptoms that are temporally related to use of a substance.

E. Persistent delusions with periods of overlapping mood episodes that are present for a substantial portion of the delusional disturbance.

2.12 Which of the following patient presentations would *not* be classified as psychotic for the purpose of diagnosing schizophrenia?

A. A patient is hearing a voice that tells him he is a special person.

B. A patient believes he is being followed by a secret police organization that is focused exclusively on him.

C. A patient has a flashback to a war experience that feels like it is happening again.

D. A patient cannot organize his thoughts and stops responding in the middle of an interview.

E. A patient presents wearing an automobile tire around his waist and gives no explanation.

2.13 In which of the following disorders can psychotic symptoms occur?

A. Bipolar and depressive disorders.

B. Substance use disorders.

C. Posttraumatic stress disorder.

D. Other medical conditions.

E. All of the above.

2.14 A 32-year-old man presents to the emergency department distressed and agitated. He reports that his sister has been killed in a car accident on a trip to South America. When asked how he found out, he says that he and his sister were very close and he "just knows it." After putting him on the phone with his sister, who was comfortably staying with friends while on her trip, the man expressed relief that she was alive. Which of the following descriptions best fits this presentation?

A. He had a delusional belief, because he believed it was true without good warrant.

B. He did not have a delusional belief, because it changed in light of new evidence.

C. He had a grandiose delusion, because he believed he could know things happening far away.

D. He had a nihilistic delusion, because it involved an untrue, imagined catastrophe.

E. He did not have a delusion, because in some cultures people believe they can know things about family members outside of ordinary communications.

2.15   Which of the following is *not* a commonly recognized type of delusion?

A. Persecutory.
B. Erotomanic.
C. Alien abduction.
D. Somatic.
E. Grandiose.

2.16   A 64-year-old man who had been a widower for 3 months presents to the emergency department on the advice of his primary care physician after he reports to the doctor that he hears his deceased wife's voice calling his name when he looks through old photos, and sometimes as he is trying to fall asleep. His primary care physician tells him he is having a psychotic episode and needs to get a psychiatric evaluation. Which of the following statements correctly explains why these experiences are not considered to be psychotic?

A. The voice he hears is from a family member.
B. The experience occurs as he is falling asleep.
C. He can invoke her voice with certain activities.
D. The voice calls his name.
E. Both B and C.

2.17   A 19-year-old college student is brought by ambulance to the emergency department. His college dorm supervisor, who called the ambulance, reports that the student was isolating himself, was pacing in his room, and was not responding to questions. In the emergency department, the patient gets down in a crouching position and begins making barking noises at seemingly random times. His urine toxicology report is negative, and all labs are within normal limits. What is the best description of these symptoms?

A. An animal delusion—the patient believes he is a dog.
B. Intermittent explosive rage.
C. A paranoid stance leading to self-protective aggression.
D. Catatonic behavior.
E. Formal thought disorder.

2.18   Which of the following does *not* represent a negative symptom of schizophrenia?

A. Affective flattening.
B. Decreased motivation.
C. Impoverished thought processes.
D. Sadness over loss of functionality.
E. Social disinterest.

2.19 Schizophrenia spectrum and other psychotic disorders are defined by abnormalities in one or more of five domains, four of which are also considered psychotic symptoms. Which of the following is *not* considered a psychotic symptom?

A. Delusions.
B. Hallucinations.
C. Disorganized thinking.
D. Disorganized or abnormal motor behavior.
E. Avolition.

2.20 What is the most common type of delusion?

A. Somatic delusion of distorted body appearance.
B. Grandiose delusion.
C. Thought insertion.
D. Persecutory delusion.
E. Former life regression.

2.21 Label each of the following beliefs as a bizarre delusion, a nonbizarre delusion, or a nondelusion.

A. A 25-year-old law student believes he has uncovered the truth about JFK's assassination and that CIA agents have been dispatched to follow him and monitor his Internet communications.
B. A 45-year-old homeless man presents to the psychiatric emergency room complaining of a skin rash. Upon removal of his clothes, it is seen that most of his body is wrapped in aluminum foil. The man explains that he is protecting himself from the electromagnetic ray guns that are constantly targeting him.
C. A 47-year-old unemployed plumber believes he has been elected to the House of Representatives. When the Capitol police evict him and bring him to the emergency department, he says that they are Tea Party activists who are merely impersonating police officers.
D. A 35-year-old high school physics teacher presents to your office with insomnia and tells you that he has discovered and memorized the formula for cold fusion energy, only to have the formula removed from his memory by telepathic aliens.
E. An 18-year-old recent immigrant from Eastern Europe believes that wearing certain colors will ward off the "evil eye" and prevent catastrophes that would otherwise occur.

2.22 Which of the following presentations would *not* be classified as disorganized behavior for the purpose of diagnosing schizophrenia spectrum and other psychotic disorders?

A. Masturbating in public.
B. Wearing slacks on one's head.
C. Responding verbally to auditory hallucinations in a conversational mode.
D. Crouching on all fours and barking.
E. Turning to face 180 degrees away from the interviewer when answering questions.

2.23 Which of the following statements about catatonic motor behaviors is *false*?

A. Catatonic motor behavior is a type of grossly disorganized behavior that has historically been associated with schizophrenia spectrum and other psychotic disorders.
B. Catatonic motor behaviors may occur in many mental disorders (such as mood disorders) and in other medical conditions.
C. A behavior is considered catatonic only if it involves motoric slowing or rigidity, such as mutism, posturing, or waxy flexibility.
D. Catatonia can be diagnosed independently of another psychiatric disorder.
E. Catatonic behaviors involve markedly reduced reactivity to the environment.

2.24 Which of the following statements about negative symptoms of schizophrenia is *false*?

A. Negative symptoms are easily distinguished from medication side effects such as sedation.
B. Negative symptoms include diminished emotional expression.
C. Negative symptoms can be difficult to distinguish from medication side effects such as sedation.
D. Negative symptoms include reduced peer or social interaction.
E. Negative symptoms include decreased motivation for goal-directed activities.

2.25 Which of the following statements correctly describes a way in which schizoaffective disorder may be differentiated from bipolar disorder?

A. Schizoaffective disorder involves only depressive episodes, never manic or hypomanic episodes.
B. In bipolar disorder, psychotic symptoms do not last longer than 1 month.
C. In bipolar disorder, psychotic symptoms are always cotemporal with mood symptoms.
D. Schizoaffective disorder never includes full-blown episodes of major depression.
E. In bipolar disorder, psychotic symptoms are always mood congruent.

2.26 Which of the following symptom combinations, if present for 1 month, would meet Criterion A for schizophrenia?

A. Prominent auditory and visual hallucinations.
B. Grossly disorganized behavior and avolition.
C. Disorganized speech and diminished emotional expression.
D. Paranoid and grandiose delusions.
E. Avolition and diminished emotional expression.

2.27 Which of the following statements about violent or suicidal behavior in schizophrenia is *false?*

A. About 5%–6% of individuals with schizophrenia die by suicide.
B. Persons with schizophrenia frequently assault strangers in a random fashion.
C. Compared with the general population, persons with schizophrenia are more frequently victims of violence.
D. Command hallucinations to harm oneself sometimes precede suicidal behaviors.
E. Youth, male gender, and substance abuse are factors that increase the risk for suicide among persons with schizophrenia.

2.28 Which of the following statements about childhood-onset schizophrenia is *true?*

A. Childhood-onset schizophrenia tends to resemble poor-outcome adult schizophrenia, with gradual onset and prominent negative symptoms.
B. Disorganized speech patterns in childhood are usually indicative of schizophrenia.
C. Because of the childhood capacity for imagination, delusions and hallucinations in childhood-onset schizophrenia are more elaborate than those in adult-onset schizophrenia.
D. In a child presenting with disorganized behavior, schizophrenia should be ruled out before other childhood diagnoses are considered.
E. Visual hallucinations are extremely rare in childhood-onset schizophrenia.

2.29 Which of the following statements about gender differences in schizophrenia is *true?*

A. Women with schizophrenia tend to have fewer psychotic symptoms than do men over the course of the illness.
B. A first onset of schizophrenia after age 40 is more likely in women than in men.
C. Psychotic symptoms in women tend to burn out with age to a greater extent than they do in men.

D. Negative symptoms and affective flattening are more frequently observed in women with schizophrenia than in men with the disorder.

E. The overall incidence of schizophrenia is higher in women than it is in men.

2.30 A 19-year-old female college student is brought to the emergency department by her family over her objections. Three months ago, she suddenly started feeling "odd," and she came home from college because she could not concentrate. Two weeks after she came home, she began hearing voices telling her that she is "a sinner" and must repent. Although never a religious person, she now believes she must repent, but she does not know how, and feels confused. She is managing her activities of daily living despite the ongoing auditory hallucinations and delusions, and she is affectively reactive on examination. Which diagnosis best fits this presentation?

A. Schizophreniform disorder, with good prognostic features, provisional.

B. Schizophreniform disorder, without good prognostic features, provisional.

C. Schizophreniform disorder, with good prognostic features.

D. Schizophreniform disorder, without good prognostic features.

E. Unspecified schizophrenia spectrum and other psychotic disorder.

2.31 A 24-year-old male college student is brought to the emergency department by the college health service team. A few weeks ago he was involved in a car accident in which one of his friends was critically injured and died in his arms. The man has not come out of his room or showered for the last 2 weeks. He has eaten only minimally, claimed that aliens have targeted him for abduction, and asserted that he could hear their radio transmissions. Nothing seems to convince him that this abduction will not happen or that the transmissions are not real. Which of the following diagnoses (and justifications) is most appropriate for this man?

A. Brief psychotic disorder with a marked stressor, because the symptoms began after the tragic car accident.

B. Brief psychotic disorder without a marked stressor, because the content of the psychosis is unrelated to the accident.

C. Unspecified schizophrenia spectrum and other psychotic disorder, because more information is needed.

D. Schizophreniform disorder, because there are psychotic symptoms but not yet a full-blown schizophrenia picture.

E. Delusional disorder, because the central symptom is a delusion of persecution.

CHAPTER 3

Bipolar and Related Disorders

3.1   Which of the following statements accurately describes a change in DSM-5 from the DSM-IV criteria for bipolar disorders?

A. Diagnostic criteria for bipolar disorders now include both changes in mood and changes in activity or energy.
B. Diagnostic criteria for bipolar I disorder, mixed type, now require a patient to simultaneously meet full criteria for both mania and major depressive episode.
C. Subsyndromal hypomania has been removed from the allowed conditions under *other specified bipolar and related disorder.*
D. There is now a stipulation that manic or hypomanic episodes cannot be associated with recent administration of a drug known to cause similar symptoms.
E. The clinical symptoms associated with hypomanic episodes have been substantially changed.

3.2   A 32-year-old man reports 1 week of feeling unusually irritable. During this time, he has increased energy and activity, sleeps less, and finds it difficult to sit still. He also is more talkative than usual and is easily distractible, to the point of finding it difficult to complete his work assignments. A physical examination and laboratory workup are negative for any medical cause of his symptoms and he takes no medications. What diagnosis best fits this clinical picture?

A. Manic episode.
B. Hypomanic episode.
C. Bipolar I disorder, with mixed features.
D. Major depressive episode.
E. Cyclothymic disorder.

3.3   A 42-year-old man reports 1 week of increased activity associated with an elevated mood, a decreased need for sleep, and inflated self-esteem. Although the man does not object to his current state ("I'm getting a lot of work done!"), he is concerned because he recalls a similar episode 10 years ago during which he began to make imprudent business decisions. A physical examination and laboratory work are unrevealing for any medical cause of his symptoms. He had taken fluoxetine for a depressive episode but self-discontinued it 3 months ago because he felt that his mood was stable. Which diagnosis best fits this clinical picture?

A. Bipolar I disorder.
B. Bipolar II disorder.
C. Cyclothymic disorder.
D. Other specified bipolar disorder and related disorder.
E. Substance/medication-induced bipolar disorder.

3.4 Approximately what percentage of individuals who experience a single manic episode will go on to have recurrent mood episodes?

A. 90%.
B. 50%.
C. 25%.
D. 10%.
E. 1%.

3.5 Which of the following factors is most predictive of incomplete recovery between mood episodes in bipolar I disorder?

A. Being widowed.
B. Living in a higher-income country.
C. Being divorced.
D. Having a family history of bipolar disorder.
E. Having a mood episode accompanied by mood-incongruent psychotic symptoms.

3.6 Which of the following is more common in men with bipolar I disorder than in women with the disorder?

A. Rapid cycling.
B. Alcohol abuse.
C. Eating disorders.
D. Anxiety disorders.
E. Mixed-state symptoms.

3.7 A patient with a history of bipolar I disorder presents with a new-onset manic episode and is successfully treated with medication adjustment. He notes chronic depressive symptoms that, on reflection, long preceded his manic episodes. He describes these symptoms as "feeling down," having decreased energy, and more often than not having no motivation. He denies other depressive symptoms but feels that these alone have been sufficient to negatively affect his marriage. Which diagnosis best fits this presentation?

A. Other specified bipolar and related disorder.

B. Bipolar I disorder, current or most recent episode depressed.

C. Cyclothymic disorder.

D. Bipolar I disorder and persistent depressive disorder (dysthymia).

E. Bipolar II disorder.

3.8   In which of the following ways do manic episodes differ from attention-deficit/hyperactivity disorder (ADHD)?

A. Manic episodes are more strongly associated with poor judgment.

B. Manic episodes are more likely to involve excessive activity.

C. Manic episodes have clearer symptomatic onsets and offsets.

D. Manic episodes are more likely to show a chronic course.

E. Manic episodes first appear at an earlier age.

3.9   A patient with a history of bipolar disorder reports experiencing 1 week of elevated and expansive mood. Evidence of which of the following would suggest that the patient is experiencing a hypomanic, rather than manic, episode?

A. Irritability.

B. Decreased need for sleep.

C. Increased productivity at work.

D. Psychotic symptoms.

E. Good insight into the illness.

3.10   A 25-year-old graduate student presents to a psychiatrist complaining of feeling down and "not enjoying anything." Her symptoms began about a month ago, along with insomnia and poor appetite. She has little interest in activities and is having difficulty attending to her schoolwork. She recalls a similar episode 1 year ago that lasted about 2 months before improving without treatment. She also reports several episodes of increased energy in the past 2 years; these episodes usually last 1–2 weeks, during which time she is very productive, feels more social and outgoing, and tends to sleep less, although she feels energetic during the day. Friends tell her that she speaks more rapidly during these episodes but that they do not see it as off-putting and in fact think she seems more outgoing and clever. She has no medical problems and does not take any medications or abuse drugs or alcohol. What is the most likely diagnosis?

A. Bipolar I disorder, current episode depressed.

B. Bipolar II disorder, current episode depressed.

C. Bipolar I disorder, current episode unspecified.

D. Cyclothymic disorder.

E. Major depressive disorder.

3.11 How do the depressive episodes associated with bipolar II disorder differ from those associated with bipolar I disorder?

A. They are less frequent than those associated with bipolar I disorder.
B. They are lengthier than those associated with bipolar I disorder.
C. They are less disabling than those associated with bipolar I disorder.
D. They are less severe than those associated with bipolar I disorder.
E. They are rarely a reason for the patient to seek treatment.

3.12 How does the course of bipolar II disorder differ from the course of bipolar I disorder?

A. It is more chronic than the course of bipolar I disorder.
B. It is less episodic than the course of bipolar I disorder.
C. It involves longer asymptomatic periods than the course of bipolar I disorder.
D. It involves shorter symptomatic episodes than the course of bipolar I disorder.
E. It involves a much lower number of lifetime mood episodes than the course of bipolar I disorder.

3.13 Which of the following features confers a worse prognosis for a patient with bipolar II disorder?

A. Younger age.
B. Higher educational level.
C. Rapid-cycling pattern.
D. "Married" marital status.
E. Less severe depressive episodes.

3.14 The course of bipolar II disorder would likely be worse for individuals who have an onset of the disorder at which of the following ages?

A. Age 10 years.
B. Age 20 years.
C. Age 40 years.
D. Age 70 years.
E. None of the above; there is no association between onset age and course.

3.15 Which of the following statements about postpartum hypomania is *true*?

A. It tends to occur in the late postpartum period.
B. It occurs in less than 1% of postpartum women.
C. It is a risk factor for postpartum depression.
D. It is easily distinguished from the normal adjustments to childbirth.
E. It is more common in multiparous women.

3.16   For an adolescent who presents with distractibility, which of the following additional features would suggest an association with bipolar II disorder rather than attention-deficit/hyperactivity disorder (ADHD)?

A. Rapid speech noted on examination.
B. A report of less need for sleep.
C. Complaints of racing thoughts.
D. Evidence that the symptoms are episodic.
E. Evidence that the symptoms represent the individual's baseline behavior.

3.17   A 50-year-old man with a history of a prior depressive episode is given an antidepressant by his family doctor to help with his depressive symptoms. Two weeks later, his doctor contacts you for a consultation because the patient now is euphoric, has increased energy, racing thoughts, psychomotor agitation, poor concentration and attention, pressured speech, and a decreased need to sleep. These symptoms began with the initiation of the patient's new medication. The patient stopped the medication after 2 days, as he no longer felt depressed; however, the symptoms have continued ever since. What is the patient's diagnosis?

A. Substance/medication-induced bipolar and related disorder.
B. Bipolar I disorder.
C. Bipolar II disorder.
D. Cyclothymic disorder.
E. Major depressive disorder.

3.18   In which of the following aspects does cyclothymic disorder differ from bipolar I disorder?

A. Duration.
B. Severity.
C. Age at onset.
D. Pervasiveness.
E. All of the above.

CHAPTER 4

Depressive Disorders

4.1   How does DSM-5 differ from DSM-IV in its classification of mood disorders?

A. There is no difference between the two editions.
B. DSM-IV separated mood disorders into different sections; DSM-5 consolidates mood disorders into one section.
C. DSM-IV included all mood disorders in a single section; DSM-5 places depressive and bipolar mood disorders in separate sections.
D. DSM-IV placed mood and anxiety disorders in separate sections; DSM-5 consolidates mood and anxiety disorders within a single section.
E. DSM-IV placed mood disorders with psychotic features in the same section as other mood disorders; DSM-5 places mood disorders with psychosis in a separate section.

4.2   How does DSM-5 differ from DSM-IV in its classification of premenstrual dysphoric disorder (PMDD)?

A. PMDD was in the Appendix in DSM-IV and remains in this location in DSM-5.
B. PMDD was not included in DSM-IV but is in the Appendix of DSM-5.
C. PMDD is no longer considered a valid psychiatric diagnosis.
D. PMDD is included in the "Depressive Disorders" chapter of DSM-5 but was not included in the "Mood Disorders" chapter of DSM-IV.
E. PMDD is included in DSM-5 but the name of the diagnosis has been changed.

4.3   What DSM-5 diagnostic provision is made for depressive symptoms following the death of a loved one?

A. Depressive symptoms lasting less than 2 months after the loss of a loved one are excluded from receiving a diagnosis of major depressive episode.
B. To qualify for a diagnosis of major depressive episode, the depression must start no less than 12 weeks following the loss.
C. To qualify for a diagnosis of major depressive episode, the depressive symptoms in such individuals must include suicidal ideation.
D. Depressive symptoms following the loss of a loved one are not excluded from receiving a major depressive episode diagnosis if the symptoms otherwise fulfill the diagnostic criteria.

E. Depressive symptoms following the loss of a loved one are excluded from receiving a major depressive episode diagnosis; however, a proposed diagnostic category for postbereavement depression is included in "Conditions for Further Study" (DSM-5 Appendix) pending further research.

4.4 Which of the following statements about how grief differs from a major depressive episode (MDE) is *false?*

A. In grief the predominant affect is feelings of emptiness and loss, while in MDE it is persistent depressed mood and the inability to anticipate happiness or pleasure.

B. The pain of grief may be accompanied by positive emotions and humor that are uncharacteristic of the pervasive unhappiness and misery characteristic of MDE.

C. The thought content associated with grief generally features a preoccupation with thoughts and memories of the deceased, rather than the self-critical or pessimistic ruminations seen in MDE.

D. In grief, feelings of worthlessness and self-loathing are common; in MDE, self-esteem is generally preserved.

E. If a bereaved individual thinks about death and dying, such thoughts are generally focused on the deceased and possibly about "joining" the deceased, whereas in MDE such thoughts are focused on ending one's own life because of feeling worthless, undeserving of life, or unable to cope with the pain of depression.

4.5 How do individuals with substance/medication-induced depressive disorder differ from individuals with major depressive disorder who do not have a substance use disorder?

A. They are more likely to be female.

B. They are more likely to have graduate school education.

C. They are more likely to be male.

D. They are more likely to be white.

E. They are less likely to report suicidal thoughts/attempts.

4.6 A 50-year-old man presents with persistently depressed mood for several weeks that interferes with his ability to work. He has insomnia and fatigue, feels guilty, has thoughts he would be better off dead, and has thought about how he could die without anyone knowing it was a suicide. His wife informs you that he requests sex several times a day and that she thinks he may be going to "massage parlors" regularly, both of which are changes from his typical behavior. He has told her he has ideas for a "better Internet," and he has invested thousands of dollars in software programs that he cannot use. She notes that he complains of fatigue but sleeps only 1 or 2 hours each night and seems to have tremendous energy during the day. Which diagnosis best fits this patient?

A. Manic episode.
B. Hypomanic episode.
C. Major depressive episode.
D. Major depressive episode, with mixed features.
E. Major depressive episode, with atypical features.

4.7   A 45-year-old man with classic features of schizophrenia has always experi-
       enced co-occurring symptoms of depression—including feeling "down in the
       dumps," having a poor appetite, feeling hopeless, and suffering from insom-
       nia—during his episodes of active psychosis. These depressive symptoms oc-
       curred only during his psychotic episodes and only during the 2-year period
       when the patient was experiencing active symptoms of schizophrenia. After
       his psychotic episodes were successfully controlled by medication, no further
       symptoms of depression were present. The patient has never met full criteria
       for major depressive disorder at any time. What is the appropriate DSM-5 di-
       agnosis?

A. Schizophrenia.
B. Schizoaffective disorder.
C. Persistent depressive disorder (dysthymia).
D. Schizophrenia and persistent depressive disorder (dysthymia).
E. Unspecified schizophrenia spectrum and other psychotic disorder.

4.8   What are the new depressive disorder diagnoses in DSM-5?

A. Subsyndromal depressive disorder, premenstrual dysphoric disorder, and
   mixed anxiety and depressive disorder.
B. Disruptive mood dysregulation disorder, premenstrual dysphoric disorder,
   and persistent depressive disorder (dysthymia).
C. Disruptive mood dysregulation disorder, premenstrual dysphoric disorder,
   and subsyndromal depressive disorder.
D. Disruptive mood dysregulation disorder, postmenopausal dysphoric disorder, and persistent depressive disorder (dysthymia).
E. Mixed anxiety and depressive disorder, bereavement-induced major depressive disorder, and postmenopausal dysphoric disorder.

4.9   A depressed patient reports that he experiences no pleasure from his normally
       enjoyable activities. Which of the following additional symptoms would be re-
       quired for this patient to qualify for a diagnosis of major depressive disorder
       with melancholic features?

A. Despondency, depression that is worse in the morning, and inability to fall
   asleep.
B. Depression that is worse in the evening, psychomotor agitation, and significant weight loss.

C. Inappropriate guilt, depression that is worse in the morning, and early-morning awakening.

D. Significant weight gain, depression that is worse in the evening, and excessive guilt.

E. Despondency, significant weight gain, and psychomotor retardation.

4.10 A 39-year-old woman reports that she became quite depressed in the winter last year when her company closed for the season, but she felt completely normal in the spring. She recalls experiencing several other episodes of depression over the past 5 years (for which she cannot identify a seasonal pattern) that would have met criteria for major depressive disorder. Which of the following correctly summarizes this patient's eligibility for a diagnosis of "major depressive disorder, with seasonal pattern"?

A. She does *not* qualify for this diagnosis: the episode must start in the fall, and the patient must have no episodes that do not have a seasonal pattern.

B. She *does* qualify for this diagnosis: the single episode described started in the winter and ended in the spring.

C. She does *not* qualify for this diagnosis: the patient must have had two episodes with a seasonal relationship in the past 2 years and no nonseasonal episodes during that period.

D. She *does* qualify for this diagnosis: the symptoms described are related to psychosocial stressors.

E. She *does* qualify for this diagnosis: the symptoms are not related to bipolar I or bipolar II disorder.

4.11 Which of the following statements about the prevalence of major depressive disorder in the United States is *true?*

A. The 12-month prevalence is 17%.

B. Females and males have equal prevalence at all ages.

C. Females have increased prevalence at all ages.

D. The prevalence in 18- to 29-year-olds is three times higher than that in 60-year-olds.

E. The prevalence in 60-year-olds is three times higher than that in 18- to 29-year-olds.

4.12 Which of the following statements about the heritability of major depressive disorder (MDD) is *true?*

A. Nearly 100% of people with genetic liability can be accounted for by the personality trait of dogmatism.

B. The heritability is approximately 40%, and the personality trait of neuroticism accounts for a substantial portion of this genetic liability.

C. Less than 10% of people with genetic liability can be accounted for by the personality trait of perfectionism.

D. Nearly 50% of people with genetic liability can be accounted for by the personality trait of aggressiveness.
E. The heritability of MDD depends on whether the individual's mother or father had MDD.

4.13 Which of the following statements about diagnostic markers for major depressive disorder (MDD) is *true?*

A. No laboratory test has demonstrated sufficient sensitivity and specificity to be used as a diagnostic tool for MDD.
B. Several diagnostic laboratory tests exist, but no commercial enterprise will offer them to the public.
C. Diagnostic laboratory tests have been withheld for fear that people testing positive for MDD may attempt suicide.
D. Tests that exist are adequate diagnostically but are not covered by health insurance.
E. Only functional magnetic resonance imaging (fMRI) provides absolute diagnostic reliability for MDD.

4.14 Which of the following statements about gender differences in suicide risk and suicide rates in major depressive disorder (MDD) is *true?*

A. The risk of suicide attempts and completions is higher for women.
B. The risk of suicide attempts and completions is higher for men.
C. The risk of suicide attempts and completions is equal for men and women.
D. The disparity in suicide rate by gender is much greater in individuals with MDD than in the general population.
E. The risk of suicide attempts is higher for women, but the risk of suicide completions is lower.

4.15 A 12-year-old boy begins to have new episodes of temper outbursts that are out of proportion to the situation. Which of the following is *not* a diagnostic possibility for this patient?

A. Disruptive mood dysregulation disorder.
B. Bipolar disorder.
C. Oppositional defiant disorder.
D. Conduct disorder.
E. Attention-deficit/hyperactivity disorder.

4.16 Which of the following features distinguishes disruptive mood dysregulation disorder (DMDD) from bipolar disorder in children?

A. Age at onset.
B. Gender of the child.
C. Irritability.

D. Chronicity.

E. Severity.

4.17 Children with disruptive mood dysregulation disorder are most likely to develop which of the following disorders in adulthood?

A. Bipolar I disorder.

B. Schizophrenia.

C. Bipolar II disorder.

D. Borderline personality disorder.

E. Unipolar depressive disorders.

4.18 An irritable 8-year-old child has a history of temper outbursts both at home and at school. What characteristic mood feature must be also present to qualify him for a diagnosis of disruptive mood dysregulation disorder?

A. The child's mood between outbursts is typically euthymic.

B. The child's mood between outbursts is typically hypomanic.

C. The child's mood between outbursts is typically depressed.

D. The child's mood between outbursts is typically irritable or angry.

E. The mood symptoms and temper outbursts must not have persisted for more than 6 months.

4.19 Children with disruptive mood dysregulation disorder (DMDD) often meet criteria for what additional DSM-5 diagnosis?

A. Pediatric bipolar disorder.

B. Oppositional defiant disorder.

C. Schizophrenia.

D. Intermittent explosive disorder.

E. Major depressive disorder.

4.20 The diagnostic criteria for disruptive mood dysregulation disorder (DMDD) state that the diagnosis should not be made for the first time before age 6 years or after 18 years (Criterion G). Which of the following statements best describes the rationale for this age range restriction?

A. Validity of the diagnosis has been established only in the age group 7–18 years.

B. The restriction represents an attempt to differentiate DMDD from bipolar disorder.

C. The restriction is based on existing genetic data.

D. The restriction represents an attempt to differentiate DMDD from intermittent explosive disorder.

E. The restriction represents an attempt to differentiate DMDD from autism spectrum disorder.

4.21 A 9-year-old boy is brought in for evaluation because of explosive outbursts when he is frustrated with schoolwork. The parents report that their son is well behaved and pleasant at other times. Which diagnosis best fits this clinical picture?

A. Disruptive mood dysregulation disorder.
B. Pediatric bipolar disorder.
C. Intermittent explosive disorder.
D. Major depressive disorder.
E. Persistent depressive disorder (dysthymia).

4.22 A 14-year-old boy describes himself as feeling "down" all of the time for the past year. He remembers feeling better while he was at camp for 4 weeks during the summer; however, the depressed mood returned when he came home. He reports poor concentration, feelings of hopelessness, and low self-esteem but denies suicidal ideation or changes in his appetite or sleep. What is the most likely diagnosis?

A. Major depressive disorder.
B. Disruptive mood dysregulation disorder.
C. Depressive episodes with short-duration hypomania.
D. Persistent depressive disorder (dysthymia), with early onset.
E. Schizoaffective disorder.

4.23 A 30-year-old woman reports 2 years of persistently depressed mood, accompanied by loss of pleasure in all activities, ruminations that she would be better off dead, feelings of guilt about "bad things" she has done, and thoughts about quitting work because of her inability to make decisions. Although she has never been treated for depression, she feels so distressed at times that she wonders if she should be hospitalized. She experiences an increased need for sleep but still feels fatigued during the day. Her overeating has led to a 12-kg weight gain. She denies drug or alcohol use, and her medical workup is completely normal, including laboratory tests for vitamins. The consultation was prompted by her worsened mood for the past several weeks. What is the most appropriate diagnosis?

A. Major depressive disorder (MDD).
B. Persistent depressive disorder (dysthymia), with persistent major depressive episode.
C. Cyclothymia.
D. Bipolar II disorder.
E. MDD, with melancholic features.

4.24 A 45-year-old woman with multiple sclerosis was treated with interferon beta-1a a year ago, which resolved her physical symptoms. She now presents with depressed mood (experienced daily for the past several months), middle insomnia (of recent onset), poor appetite, trouble concentrating, and lack of interest in sex. Although she has no physical symptoms, she is frequently absent from work. She denies any active plans to commit suicide but admits that she often thinks about it, as her mood has worsened. What is the most likely diagnosis?

A. Major depressive disorder.
B. Persistent depressive disorder (dysthymia).
C. Depressive disorder due to another medical condition.
D. Substance/medication-induced depressive disorder.
E. Persistent depressive disorder (dysthymia) and multiple sclerosis.

4.25 An 18-year-old college student, recently arrived in the United States from Beijing, complains to her gynecologist of irritability, problems with her roommates, increased appetite, feeling bloated, and feeling depressed for 3–4 days prior to the onset of menses. She reports that these symptoms have been present since she reached menarche at age 12 (although she has never kept a mood log). The gynecologist calls you for a consultation about the correct diagnosis, because she is as yet unfamiliar with the new DSM-5 diagnostic criteria. What is your response?

A. The patient has premenstrual syndrome because she does not meet criteria for premenstrual dysphoric disorder.
B. The patient would qualify for a provisional diagnosis of premenstrual dysphoric disorder; however, the diagnosis does not exist in DSM-5.
C. The patient would qualify for a provisional diagnosis of premenstrual dysphoric disorder.
D. The patient would qualify for a provisional diagnosis of premenstrual dysphoric disorder if the diagnosis had been validated in Asian women.
E. The patient has no DSM-5 diagnosis.

4.26 What is the appropriate method of confirming a diagnosis of premenstrual dysphoric disorder?

A. Laboratory tests.
B. Family history.
C. Neuropsychological testing.
D. Two or more months of prospective symptom ratings on validated scales.
E. One month of scoring high on the Daily Rating of Severity of Problems or 1 month of scoring high on the Visual Analogue Scales for Premenstrual Mood Symptoms.

4.27 A 29-year-old woman complains of sad mood every month in anticipation of her very painful menses. The pain begins with the start of her flow and continues for several days. She does not experience pain during other times of the month. She has tried a variety of treatments, none of which have given her relief. What is the appropriate diagnosis?

A. Premenstrual dysphoric disorder.
B. Premenstrual syndrome.
C. Dysmenorrhea.
D. Factitious disorder.
E. Persistent depressive disorder (dysthymia).

4.28 Which of the following symptoms must be present for a woman to meet criteria for premenstrual dysphoric disorder?

A. Marked affective lability.
B. Decreased interest in usual activities.
C. Physical symptoms such as breast tenderness.
D. Marked change in appetite.
E. A sense of feeling overwhelmed or out of control.

4.29 A 23-year-old woman reports that during every menstrual cycle she experiences breast swelling, bloating, hypersomnia, an increased craving for sweets, poor concentration, and a feeling that she cannot handle her normal responsibilities. She notes that she also feels somewhat more sensitive emotionally and may become tearful when hearing a sad story. She takes no oral medication but does use a drospirenone/ethinyl estradiol patch. What diagnosis best fits this clinical picture?

A. Premenstrual dysphoric disorder (PMDD).
B. Dysthymia.
C. Dysmenorrhea.
D. Premenstrual syndrome.
E. Substance/medication-induced depressive disorder.

4.30 A 31-year-old woman with no history of mood symptoms reports that she experiences distressing mood lability and irritability starting about 4 days before the onset of menses. She feels "on edge," cannot concentrate, has little enjoyment from any of her activities, and experiences bloating and swelling of her breasts. The patient reports that these symptoms started 6 months ago when she began taking oral contraceptives for the first time. If she stops the oral contraceptives and her symptoms remit, what would the diagnosis be?

A. Premenstrual dysphoric disorder.
B. Dysthymia.
C. Major depressive episode.
D. Substance/medication-induced depressive disorder.
E. Premenstrual syndrome.

4.31   A 45-year-old man is admitted to the hospital with profound hypothyroidism. He is depressed but does not meet full criteria for major depressive disorder (MDD), the diagnosis given to him by his internist. The patient has no prior history of a mood disorder, and all of the depressive symptoms are temporally related to the hypothyroidism. Based on this information, you determine that a change in diagnosis—to depressive disorder due to another medical condition—is warranted, as well as a specifier to indicate that full criteria for MDD are not met. How would the full diagnosis be recorded?

A. Hypothyroidism would be coded on Axis III in DSM-5.
B. There is no special coding procedure in DSM-5.
C. Hypothyroidism would be recorded as the name of the "other medical condition" in the DSM-5 diagnosis.
D. Medical disorders are not coded as part of a mental disorder diagnosis in DSM-5.
E. A revision to DSM-5 is planned to deal with this issue.

CHAPTER 5

Anxiety Disorders

5.1   Which of the following disorders is included in the "Anxiety Disorders" chapter of DSM-5?

    A. Obsessive-compulsive disorder.
    B. Posttraumatic stress disorder.
    C. Acute stress disorder.
    D. Panic disorder with agoraphobia.
    E. Separation anxiety disorder.

5.2   A 9-year-old boy cannot go to sleep without having a parent in his room. While falling asleep, he frequently awakens to check that a parent is still there. One parent usually stays until the boy falls asleep. If he wakes up alone during the night, he starts to panic and gets up to find his parents. He also reports frequent nightmares in which he or his parents are harmed. He occasionally calls out that he saw a strange figure peering into his dark room. The parents usually wake in the morning to find the boy asleep on the floor of their room. They once tried to leave him with a relative so they could go on a vacation; however, he became so distressed in anticipation of this that they canceled their plans. What is the most likely diagnosis?

    A. Specific phobia.
    B. Nightmare disorder.
    C. Delusional disorder.
    D. Separation anxiety disorder.
    E. Agoraphobia.

5.3   Which of the following is considered a culture-specific symptom of panic attacks?

    A. Derealization.
    B. Headaches.
    C. Fear of going crazy.
    D. Shortness of breath.
    E. Heat sensations.

5.4　Which of the following statements best describes how panic attacks differ from panic disorder?

A. Panic attacks require fewer symptoms for a definitive diagnosis.
B. Panic attacks are discrete, occur suddenly, and are usually less severe.
C. Panic attacks are invariably unexpected.
D. Panic attacks represent a syndrome that can occur with a variety of other disorders.
E. Panic attacks cannot be secondary to a medical condition.

5.5　The determination of whether a panic attack is expected or unexpected is ultimately best made by which of the following?

A. Careful clinical judgment.
B. Whether the patient associates it with external stress.
C. The presence or absence of nocturnal panic attacks.
D. Ruling out possible culture-specific syndromes.
E. 24-Hour electroencephalographic monitoring.

5.6　A 50-year-old man reports episodes in which he suddenly and unexpectedly awakens from sleep feeling a surge of intense fear that peaks within minutes. During this time, he feels short of breath and has heart palpitations, sweating, and nausea. His medical history is significant only for hypertension, which is well controlled with hydrochlorothiazide. As a result of these symptoms, he has begun to have anticipatory anxiety associated with going to sleep. What is the most likely explanation for his symptoms?

A. Anxiety disorder due to another medical condition (hypertension).
B. Substance/medication-induced anxiety disorder.
C. Panic disorder.
D. Sleep terrors.
E. Panic attacks.

5.7　A 32-year-old woman reports sudden, unexpected episodes of intense anxiety, accompanied by headaches, a rapid pulse, nausea, and shortness of breath. During the episodes she fears that she is dying, and she has presented several times to emergency departments. Each time she has been told that she is medically healthy; she is usually reassured for a time, but on the occurrence of a new episode she again becomes concerned that she has some severe medical problem. She was given lorazepam once but disliked the sedating effect and has not taken it again. She abstains from all medications and alcohol in an attempt to minimize potential causes for her attacks. What is the most likely explanation for her symptoms?

A. Panic disorder.
B. Somatic symptom disorder.
C. Anxiety due to another medical condition.

D. Illness anxiety disorder.

E. Specific phobia.

5.8   A 65-year-old woman reports being housebound despite feeling physically healthy. Several years ago, she fell while shopping; although she sustained no injuries, the situation was so upsetting that she became extremely nervous when she had to leave her house unaccompanied. Because she has no children and few friends whom she can ask to accompany her, she is very distressed that she has few opportunities to venture outside her home. What is the most likely diagnosis?

A. Specific phobia, situational type.

B. Social anxiety disorder (social phobia).

C. Posttraumatic stress disorder.

D. Agoraphobia.

E. Adjustment disorder.

5.9   A 32-year-old man has regularly experienced panic attacks when out of his home alone and when on the bus. He now avoids leaving home for fear of experiencing these attacks. What is the most appropriate diagnosis?

A. Panic disorder with agoraphobia.

B. Agoraphobia with panic attacks.

C. Specific phobia, situational type.

D. Two separate disorders: panic disorder and agoraphobia.

E. Delusional disorder.

5.10   A 35-year-old man is in danger of losing his job because it requires frequent long-range traveling and for the past year he has avoided flying. Two years earlier he was on a particularly turbulent flight, and although he was not in any real danger, he was convinced that the pilot minimized the risk and that the plane almost crashed. He flew again 1 month later and, despite having a smooth flight, the anticipation of turbulence was so distressing that he experienced a panic attack during the flight; he has not flown since. What is the most appropriate diagnosis?

A. Agoraphobia.

B. Acute stress disorder.

C. Specific phobia, situational type.

D. Social anxiety disorder (social phobia).

E. Panic disorder.

5.11   Which of the following types of specific phobia is most likely to be associated with vasovagal fainting?

A. Animal type.

B. Natural environment type.

C. Blood-injection-injury type.

D. Situational type.

E. Other (e.g.,. in children, loud sounds or costumed characters).

5.12 Which of the following most accurately describes people with specific phobias?

A. The average individual with a phobia has fears of only one object or situation.

B. The fear is usually quite mild in intensity.

C. Fewer than 10% of people fear more than one object or situation.

D. The fear occurs almost every time the person encounters the object or situation.

E. The fear is exactly the same in intensity each time the object or situation is encountered.

5.13 Although onset of a specific phobia can occur at any age, specific phobia most typically develops during which age period?

A. Childhood.

B. Late adolescence to early adulthood.

C. Middle age.

D. Old age.

E. Any age.

5.14 In social anxiety disorder (social phobia), the object of an individual's fear is the potential for which of the following?

A. Social or occupational impairment.

B. Harm to self or others.

C. Embarrassment.

D. Separation from objects of attachment.

E. Incapacitating symptoms.

5.15 When called on at school, a 7-year-old boy will only nod or write in response. The family of the child is surprised to hear this from the teacher, because the boy speaks normally when at home with his parents. The child has achieved appropriate developmental milestones, and a medical evaluation indicates that he is healthy. The boy is unable to give any explanation for his behavior, but the parents are concerned that it will affect his school performance. What diagnosis best fits this child's symptoms?

A. Separation anxiety disorder.

B. Autism spectrum disorder.

C. Agoraphobia.

D. Selective mutism.

E. Communication disorder.

5.16   Social anxiety disorder (social phobia) differs from normative shyness in that the disorder leads to which of the following?

A. Social or occupational dysfunction.
B. Marked social reticence.
C. Avoidance of social situations.
D. Derealization or depersonalization.
E. Pervasive social deficits with poor insight.

5.17   In addition to feeling restless or "keyed up," individuals with generalized anxiety disorder are most likely to experience which of the following symptoms?

A. Panic attacks.
B. Obsessions.
C. Muscle tension.
D. Multiple somatic complaints.
E. Social anxiety.

5.18   Which of the following characteristics of generalized anxiety disorder is especially common in children who have the disorder?

A. Complaining of physical aches and pains.
B. Excessively preparing for activities.
C. Avoiding activities that may provoke anxiety.
D. Seeking frequent reassurance from others.
E. Delaying or procrastinating before activities.

5.19   What is the primary difference in the clinical expression of generalized anxiety disorder across age groups?

A. Content of worry.
B. Degree of worry.
C. Patterns of comorbidity.
D. Predominance of cognitive versus somatic symptoms.
E. Severity of impairment.

5.20   In what aspect of generalized anxiety disorder do men and women most commonly differ?

A. Course.
B. Symptom profile.
C. Degree of impairment.
D. Patterns of comorbidity.
E. Age at onset.

5.21   Which of the following is more suggestive of anxiety that is not pathological than of anxiety that qualifies for a diagnosis of generalized anxiety disorder?

   A. Anxiety and worry that interferes significantly with functioning.
   B. Anxiety and worry that lasts for months to years.
   C. Anxiety and worry in response to a clear precipitant.
   D. Anxiety and worry focused on a wide range of life circumstances.
   E. Anxiety and worry accompanied by physical symptoms.

5.22   A 26-year-old man is brought to the emergency department suffering from a sudden, severe surge of panic. He has no history of panic disorder, but he reports taking several doses of an over-the-counter cold medication earlier that day. Which of the following clinical features, if present in this case, would help to confirm a diagnosis of substance/medication-induced anxiety disorder?

   A. Symptoms that are mild and do not impair functioning.
   B. Symptoms that persist for a long time after substance/medication use.
   C. Symptoms that are in excess of what would be expected for the substance/medication.
   D. Presence of a delirium or gross confusion.
   E. Lack of any history of anxiety disorder or panic symptoms.

5.23   In which of the following circumstances would a diagnosis of substance/medication-induced anxiety disorder be appropriate for an individual who stopped taking benzodiazepines the previous day?

   A. Significant anxiety symptoms are present.
   B. Anxiety is present that is clearly related to the withdrawal state.
   C. Anxiety is present that is sufficiently severe to warrant independent clinical attention.
   D. Anxiety is present only during bouts of delirium.
   E. Never: the diagnosis of substance withdrawal would supersede the anxiety disorder diagnosis.

5.24   A 60-year-old man has just been diagnosed with congestive heart failure. He is intensely anxious and reports feeling as if he cannot breathe, which causes him to panic. Which of the following features, if present in this case, would tend to support a diagnosis of anxiety disorder due to another medical condition rather than adjustment disorder with anxiety?

   A. The patient says that he is relieved to know his diagnosis.
   B. The patient has no anxiety-associated physical symptoms.
   C. The patient is focused on the reasons he has a cardiac disorder.
   D. The patient is delirious.
   E. The patient is extremely concerned that he will not be able to return to work.

CHAPTER 6

Obsessive-Compulsive and Related Disorders

6.1 Which of the following statements about compulsive behaviors in obsessive-compulsive disorder (OCD) is *true?*

A. Compulsions in OCD are best understood as a form of addictive behavior.
B. Compulsive behaviors in OCD are aimed at reducing the distress triggered by obsessions.
C. Examples of compulsive behaviors include paraphilias (sexual compulsions), gambling, and substance use.
D. Compulsions involve repetitive and persistent thoughts (e.g., of contamination), images (e.g., of violent or horrific scenes), or urges (e.g., to stab someone).
E. Compulsive behaviors in OCD are typically goal directed, fulfilling a realistic purpose.

6.2 A 52-year-old man with raw, chapped hands is referred to a psychiatrist by his primary care doctor. The man reports that he washes his hands repeatedly, spending up to 4 hours a day, using abrasive cleansers and scalding hot water. Although he admits that his hands are uncomfortable, he is entirely convinced that unless he washes in this manner he will become gravely ill. A medical workup is unrevealing, and the man takes no medications. What is the most appropriate diagnosis?

A. Delusional disorder, somatic type.
B. Illness anxiety disorder.
C. Obsessive-compulsive disorder, with absent insight.
D. Obsessive-compulsive personality disorder.
E. Generalized anxiety disorder.

6.3 Men with obsessive-compulsive disorder (OCD) differ from women with the disorder in which of the following ways?

A. Men tend to get OCD later in life.
B. Men are more likely to have comorbid tics.
C. Men are more likely to be obsessed with cleaning.
D. Men are more likely to spontaneously recover.
E. Men have much higher rates of OCD.

6.4 A 63-year-old woman has been saving financial documents and records for many years, placing papers in piles throughout her apartment to the point where it has become unsafe. She acknowledges that the piles are a concern; however, she says that the papers include important documents and she is afraid to throw them away. She recalls several instances in which her taxes were audited and she needed certain documents to avoid a penalty. She is concerned because her landlord is threatening to evict her unless she removes the piles of papers. What is the most likely diagnosis?

A. Obsessive-compulsive disorder.
B. Hoarding disorder.
C. Delusional disorder.
D. Nonpathological collecting behavior.
E. Dementia (major neurocognitive disorder).

6.5 Although gambling can seem compulsive, gambling disorder is not considered a type of obsessive-compulsive disorder (OCD) for which of the following reasons?

A. A person with gambling disorder derives direct pleasure from the behavior.
B. Individuals with gambling disorder have poorer insight into their irrational behavior.
C. Gambling disorder is better conceived of as a personality trait.
D. The repetitive behavior associated with gambling is meant to avoid anxiety.
E. In gambling disorder, individuals have control over their repetitive behaviors.

6.6 In addition to preoccupations with a perceived body flaw, which of the following behaviors would be most suggestive of a diagnosis of body dysmorphic disorder (BDD)?

A. Repetitive mirror checking in response to the preoccupation.
B. Consulting a psychiatrist because of the distress caused by the preoccupation.
C. Losing an unhealthy amount of weight in order to improve one's appearance.
D. Having a related preoccupation with having or acquiring a disfiguring illness.
E. Experiencing discomfort with one's primary or secondary sex characteristics.

6.7 A 25-year-old man is concerned that he looks "weak" and "puny" despite the fact that to neutral observers he appears very muscular. When confronted about his belief he believes he is being humored and that people are in fact making fun of his small size behind his back. He has tried a number of strategies to increase muscle mass, including exercising excessively and using anabolic steroids; however, he remains dissatisfied with his appearance. What is the most likely diagnosis?

A. Delusional disorder, somatic type.
B. Narcissistic personality disorder.
C. Body identity integrity disorder.
D. Body dysmorphic disorder, with muscle dysmorphia.
E. *Koro*.

6.8   A 19-year-old woman is referred to a psychiatrist by her internist after she admits to him that she recurrently pulls hair from her eyebrows to the point that she has scarring and there is little or no eyebrow hair left. She states that her natural eyebrows are "bushy" and "repulsive" and that she "looks like a caveman." A photograph of the woman before she began pulling her eyebrow hair shows a normal-looking teenager. What is the most appropriate diagnosis?

A. Trichotillomania (hair-pulling disorder).
B. Body dysmorphic disorder.
C. Delusional disorder, somatic type.
D. Normal age-appropriate appearance concerns.
E. Obsessive-compulsive disorder.

6.9   A 48-year-old man presents to a psychiatrist, stating that he was pressured by his wife to seek help. He explains that he likes to collect wine, and he does not see a problem with this; he claims that many of the wines are quite valuable and a potential investment. On further questioning, he admits that he rarely drinks the wines, because it "never seems the right time." He has never sold or given away any wine because he finds it hard to part with the bottles. He has had to use increasing portions of his house for storage of the wine, which, along with the financial hardship, is his wife's primary concern. He admits that many of the wine bottles have probably spoiled because he cannot afford to properly store the wine and the bottles have sat for years on shelves. What is the most appropriate diagnosis?

A. Normal collecting behavior.
B. Hoarding disorder, excessive acquisition type.
C. Obsessive-compulsive disorder.
D. Delusional disorder.
E. Narcissistic personality disorder.

6.10   Which of the following statements about risk and prognostic factors in hoarding disorder is *true?*

A. About 10% of individuals who hoard report having a relative who also hoards.
B. Approximately half of the variability in hoarding behavior is due to genetic factors.

C. Separation insecurity is a prominent temperamental feature of individuals with hoarding disorder and their first-degree relatives.

D. Hoarding disorder has been associated with high rates of childhood neglect and abuse.

E. Stressful or traumatic life events play no role in the onset or exacerbation of hoarding disorder.

6.11 Which of the following statements about the course of hoarding disorder is *true*?

A. Hoarding behavior tends to wax and wane in severity throughout an individual's life.

B. Hoarding behavior peaks in young adulthood and subsequently lessens in severity.

C. Hoarding behavior tends to become more severe with increasing age.

D. Hoarding disorder begins in childhood, is chronic, and tends not to change in severity.

E. Hoarding disorder has a worse course when it begins in later adulthood or old age.

6.12 What is the most common site of hair pulling in trichotillomania?

A. Scalp.

B. Axillary area.

C. Facial area.

D. Pubic area.

E. Perirectal area.

6.13 Although microscopic examination of hair can aid the diagnosis of trichotillomania (hair-pulling disorder), such examination is rarely performed, for which of the following reasons?

A. Patients generally admit to the hair pulling.

B. The effects on hair are easily observed macroscopically.

C. Patients generally have a long medical history of the disorder.

D. Patients rarely consent to the examination.

E. Microscopic examination is prohibitively expensive.

6.14 A 25-year-old man is referred to a psychiatrist by his primary care doctor after mentioning to the doctor that he routinely spends a lot of time pulling out facial hair with tweezers, even after carefully shaving. On evaluation, he admits to frequent pulling of his facial hair, consuming significant amount of time; he explains that he becomes anxious when looking at himself because his moustache, hairline, and sideburns are asymmetrical. He pulls out hairs in an effort to make them more symmetrical, but is rarely satisfied with the results. He finds this very upsetting but cannot resist the urge to try and "fix" his facial hair. What is the most appropriate diagnosis?

A. Trichotillomania (hair-pulling disorder).
B. Body dysmorphic disorder (BDD).
C. Delusional disorder, somatic type.
D. Normal age-appropriate appearance concerns.
E. Obsessive-compulsive disorder (OCD).

6.15 To fulfill diagnostic criteria for excoriation (skin-picking) disorder, the picking must be severe enough to result in which of the following?

A. Itching.
B. Skin lesions.
C. An infection.
D. Medical attention.
E. Permanent deformity.

6.16 Which of the following statements about the course of excoriation (skin-picking) disorder is *true?*

A. Skin-picking behavior tends to wax and wane in severity throughout an individual's life.
B. Skin-picking behavior peaks in young adulthood and subsequently lessens in severity.
C. Excoriation disorder tends to become more severe with increasing age.
D. Skin-picking behavior begins in childhood, is chronic, and tends not to change in severity.
E. Excoriation disorder has a worse course when it begins in later adulthood or old age.

6.17 In excoriation (skin-picking) disorder, which of the following is the most typical motivation for the skin-picking behavior?

A. Inflicting pain that brings relief by reaffirming one's ability to feel.
B. Appearance concerns.
C. Symmetry concerns.
D. Boredom.
E. Fear of infection.

6.18 A 55-year-old retail worker believes that he has "chronic halitosis" and fears that his bad breath is "scaring away shoppers." He is in danger of losing his job because he so frequently absents himself from the sales floor to brush his teeth and use mouthwash. He constantly chews mint gum, even though his employer has asked him not to. His coworkers regularly reassure him that his breath is fine, but he is convinced that they are just being polite. Although the possibility of losing his job causes him concern, he finds his worries about his breath to be intolerable. He has seen his doctor and dentist, both of whom tell him that he is healthy and does not have malodorous breath. What is the most appropriate diagnosis?

A. Social anxiety disorder (social phobia).
B. Obsessive-compulsive disorder.
C. Body dysmorphic disorder.
D. Other specified obsessive-compulsive and related disorder.
E. Illness anxiety disorder.

6.19   Which of the following substances, when abused, is most likely to cause symptoms mimicking obsessive-compulsive disorder?

A. Heroin.
B. Cocaine.
C. Alprazolam.
D. Marijuana.
E. Lysergic acid diethylamide (LSD).

CHAPTER 7

Trauma- and Stressor-Related Disorders

7.1 How does DSM-5 differ from DSM-IV in its classification of posttraumatic stress disorder (PTSD)?

A. In DSM-5, PTSD has been placed with the dissociative disorders.
B. In DSM-5, PTSD has been placed with the depressive disorders.
C. In DSM-5, PTSD has been placed in a newly created chapter.
D. In DSM-5, PTSD has been placed with "Other Conditions That May Be a Focus of Clinical Attention."
E. In DSM-5, PTSD has been placed with "Conditions for Further Study" in Section III.

7.2 Which of the following reactions to a traumatic event was required for the DSM-IV diagnosis of posttraumatic stress disorder (PTSD) but is not required for the DSM-5 diagnosis?

A. Intense fear, helplessness, or horror.
B. Insomnia or hypersomnia.
C. Avoidance.
D. A foreshortened sense of the future.
E. Flashbacks.

7.3 Which of the following statements about reactive attachment disorder (RAD) is *true*?

A. RAD occurs only in children who lack healthy attachments.
B. RAD occurs only in children who have secure attachments.
C. RAD occurs only in children who have impaired communication.
D. RAD occurs in children without a history of severe social neglect.
E. RAD is a common condition, with a prevalence of 25% of children seen in clinical settings.

7.4 A 4-year-old boy in day care often displays fear that does not seem to be related to any of his activities. Although frequently distressed, he does not seek contact with any of the staff and does not respond when a staff member tries to comfort him. What additional caregiver-obtained information about this child

would be important in deciding whether his symptoms represent reactive attachment disorder (RAD) or autism spectrum disorder (ASD)?

A. Age at first appearance of the behavior.
B. Family history about his siblings.
C. History of language delay.
D. Indications that he has experienced severe social neglect.
E. Presence of selective attachment behaviors.

7.5   For a child diagnosed with reactive attachment disorder, which of the follow-
        ing situations would qualify for a disorder specifier of "severe"?

A. The child has been in five foster homes.
B. The child never expresses positive emotions when interacting with caregiv-
   ers.
C. The disorder has been present for 18 months.
D. The child meets all symptoms of the disorder, with each symptom manifest-
   ing at relatively high levels.
E. There is a documented history of physical abuse of the child.

7.6   A 6-year-old girl has repeatedly approached strangers while in the park with
        her class. The teacher requests an evaluation of the behavior. The girl has a his-
        tory of being placed in several different foster homes over the past 3 years.
        Which diagnosis is suggested from this history?

A. Attention-deficit/hyperactivity disorder (ADHD).
B. Disinhibited social engagement disorder (DSED).
C. Autism spectrum disorder (ASD).
D. Bipolar I disorder.
E. Borderline personality disorder.

7.7   A 25-year-old woman, new to your practice, tells you that a little more than
        3 months ago she was accosted on her way home. The attacker told her he had
        a gun, was going to rape her, and would shoot her if she resisted. He walked
        her toward an alley. She was sure he would kill her afterward no matter what
        she did, and therefore she pushed away from him, aware that she might be
        shot. She was able to escape unharmed. She describes not being able to fall
        asleep for the first 2 nights after the attack and of avoiding that particular street
        in her neighborhood for 2 days following the event. She thinks that the attacker
        might have touched her breasts but cannot remember for sure. She has recently
        started feeling anxious all of the time and is tearful, and she has stopped going
        to work. She fears that something about her makes her "look like a victim."
        What is the most likely diagnosis?

A. Posttraumatic stress disorder.
B. Acute stress disorder.
C. Adjustment disorder.

D. Dissociative amnesia.

E. Personality disorder.

7.8 After a routine chest X ray, a 53-year-old man with a history of heavy cigarette use is told that he has a suspicious lesion in his lung. A bronchoscopy confirms the diagnosis of adenocarcinoma. The man delays scheduling a follow-up appointment with the oncologist for more than 2 weeks, describes feeling as if "all of this is not real," is having nightly dreams of seeing his own tombstone, and is experiencing intrusive flashbacks to the moment when he heard the physician saying, "The tests strongly suggest that you have cancer of the lung." He is tearful and is convinced he will die. He also feels intense guilt that his smoking caused the cancer and expresses the thought that he "deserves" to have cancer. What diagnosis best fits this clinical picture?

A. Acute stress disorder.

B. Posttraumatic stress disorder.

C. Adjustment disorder.

D. Major depressive disorder.

E. Generalized anxiety disorder.

7.9 Criterion B for acute stress disorder requires the presence of nine (or more) symptoms from any of five categories of response. Which of the following is *not* one of these five categories?

A. Intrusion.

B. Dissociation.

C. Confusion.

D. Avoidance.

E. Arousal.

7.10 Which of the following stressful situations would meet Criterion A for the diagnosis of acute stress disorder (ASD)?

A. Finding out that one's spouse has been fired.

B. Failing an important final examination.

C. Receiving a serious medical diagnosis.

D. Being in the cross fire of a police shootout but not being harmed.

E. Being in a subway train that gets stuck between stations.

7.11 Following discharge from the hospital, a 22-year-old man describes vivid and intrusive memories of his stay in the intensive care unit (ICU), where he received treatment for smoke inhalation. Now at home, he states that he has memories of people being tortured and hearing their screams. He dreams of this every night, waking from sleep in a terror. He talks about not feeling like himself after the experience, finding little pleasure in life after what happened to him, and being easily angered by his family; in addition, he avoids his physician out of fear that he will be told he needs to return to the ICU. What is the most likely explanation for this patient's symptoms?

A. He has acute stress disorder because his life was in danger during the ICU stay.
B. He has posttraumatic stress disorder because his life was in danger during the ICU stay.
C. He has a delirium persisting from the ICU stay.
D. He had a delirium in the ICU and now has an adjustment disorder.
E. He has a psychotic disorder.

7.12   Which of the following experiences would *not* qualify as exposure to a traumatic event (Criterion A) in the diagnosis of acute stress disorder or posttraumatic stress disorder?

A. Hearing that one's brother was killed in combat.
B. Hearing that one's close childhood friend survived a motor vehicle accident but is paralyzed.
C. Hearing that one's child has been kidnapped.
D. Hearing that one's company had suddenly closed.
E. Hearing that one's spouse has been shot.

7.13   A 31-year-old man narrowly escapes (without injury) from a house fire caused when he dropped the lighter while trying to light his crack pipe. Six weeks later, while smoking crack, he thinks he smells smoke and runs from the building in a panic, shouting, "It's on fire!" Which of the following symptoms or circumstances would rule out a diagnosis of posttraumatic stress disorder (PTSD) for this patient?

A. Having difficulty falling asleep.
B. Being uninterested in going back to work.
C. Inappropriately getting angry at family members.
D. Experiencing symptoms only when smoking crack cocaine.
E. Concluding that "the world is completely dangerous."

7.14   Criterion A4 of posttraumatic stress disorder requires "Experiencing repeated or extreme exposure to aversive details of the traumatic event." Which of the following would *not* qualify as an experiencing trauma under this criterion?

A. A police officer reviewing surveillance videotapes of homicides to identify perpetrators.
B. A social worker interviewing children who have been sexually abused and obtaining the details of the abuse.
C. A soldier sifting through the rubble of a collapsed building to retrieve remains of comrades.
D. A college student at a film festival watching a series of violent movies that contain graphic rape scenes.

E. A psychologist working with victims of torture who are seeking political asylum in the United States.

7.15 Which of the following statements about gender differences in the risk of developing posttraumatic stress disorder (PTSD) is *true?*

A. The risk is lower in females in preschool-age populations.
B. The risk is higher in females across the life span.
C. The risk is higher in males in elderly populations.
D. The risk is lower in middle-aged females than in middle-aged males.
E. The risk is higher in males across the life span.

7.16 A 5-year-old child was present when her babysitter was sexually assaulted. Which of the following symptoms would be most suggestive of posttraumatic stress disorder (PTSD) in this child?

A. Playing normally with toys.
B. Having dreams about princesses and castles.
C. Taking the clothing off her dolls while playing.
D. Expressing no fear when talking about the event.
E. Talking about the event with her parents.

7.17 Which of the following statements about risk factors for developing posttraumatic stress disorder (PTSD) is *true?*

A. Sustaining personal injury does not affect the risk of developing PTSD.
B. Severity of the trauma influences the risk of developing PTSD.
C. Dissociation has no impact on the risk of developing PTSD.
D. Perceived life threat is the only risk factor for developing PTSD.
E. Prior mental disorders have little influence on the risk of developing PTSD.

7.18 How does the 12-month prevalence of posttraumatic stress disorder (PTSD) in the United States compare with that in European and Latin American countries?

A. It is much lower than that in other countries.
B. It is much higher than that in other countries.
C. It is equal to that in other countries.
D. It is somewhat higher than that in other countries.
E. It is somewhat lower than that in other countries.

7.19 A woman complains of sad mood and feeling hopeless 3 months after her husband files for divorce. She finds it difficult to take care of her home or make meals for her family but has continued to fulfill her responsibilities. She denies suicidal ideation, feels she was a good wife who "has nothing to feel guilty about," and wishes she could "forget about the whole thing." She cannot stop thinking about her situation. Which diagnosis best fits this symptom picture?

A. Adjustment disorder, with depressed mood.

B. Adjustment disorder, with disturbance of conduct.

C. Adjustment disorder, with anxiety.

D. Adjustment disorder, with mixed disturbance of emotions and conduct.

E. Adjustment disorder, unspecified.

7.20　Six months after the death of her husband, a 70-year-old woman is seen for symptoms of overwhelming sadness, anger regarding her husband's unexpected death from a heart attack, intense yearning for him to come back, and repeated unsuccessful attempts to begin moving out of her large home (which she can no longer afford) due to inability to sort through and dispose of her husband's belongings. What is the most appropriate diagnosis?

A. Major depressive disorder.

B. Posttraumatic stress disorder.

C. Adjustment disorder, with depressed mood.

D. Other specified trauma- and stressor-related disorder (persistent complex bereavement disorder).

E. Normative stress reaction.

7.21　A 25-year-old woman with asthma becomes extremely anxious when she gets an upper respiratory infection. She presents to the emergency department with complaints of being unable to breathe. While there, she begins to hyperventilate and then reports feeling extremely dizzy. Her hyperventilation causes her to become fatigued, and when the medical evaluation indicates that she is retaining carbon dioxide (CO_2), it becomes necessary to admit her. The woman denies any other symptoms beyond anxiety. What is the most appropriate diagnosis?

A. Acute stress disorder.

B. Generalized anxiety disorder.

C. Adjustment disorder with anxiety.

D. Psychological factors affecting other medical conditions.

E. Factitious disorder.

7.22　How many Criterion B symptoms are required to be present for the diagnosis of acute stress disorder?

A. One.

B. Three.

C. Five.

D. Seven.

E. Nine.

7.23　How do the diagnostic criteria for posttraumatic stress disorder (PTSD) in preschool children differ from those for PTSD in individuals older than 6 years?

A. The preschool criteria incorporate simpler language that can be understood by children 6 years or younger.
B. The preschool criteria require one or more **intrusion** symptoms, one symptom representing *either* **avoidance** *or* **negative alterations in cognitions and mood,** and two or more **arousal/reactivity** symptoms, whereas the criteria for older individuals require symptoms in all four categories.
C. The criteria for individuals older than 6 years require one or more **intrusion** symptoms, one symptom representing *either* **avoidance** *or* **negative alterations in cognitions and mood,** and two or more **arousal/reactivity** symptoms, whereas the preschool criteria require symptoms in all four categories.
D. The preschool criteria require that the child directly experience the trauma, whereas the criteria for older individuals do not have this requirement.
E. The preschool criteria include only one type of traumatic exposure—witnessing of a traumatic event occurring to a parent or caregiving figure—as a qualifying traumatic event.

7.24 Criterion B in the DSM-5 diagnostic criteria for acute stress disorder (ASD) requires the presence of symptoms from **five** different categories: *Intrusion, Negative Mood, Dissociative, Avoidance,* and *Arousal.* Match each of the following symptoms to the appropriate category (each symptom may be placed into only one category).

a. Recurrent, involuntary, and intrusive distressing memories of the traumatic event(s).
b. Problems with concentration.
c. Persistent inability to experience positive emotions (e.g., inability to experience happiness, satisfaction, or loving feelings).
d. An altered sense of the reality of one's surroundings or oneself (e.g., seeing oneself from another's perspective, being in a daze, time slowing).
e. Efforts to avoid external reminders (people, places, conversations, activities, objects, situations) that arouse distressing memories, thoughts, or feelings about or closely associated with the traumatic event(s).
f. Irritable behavior and angry outbursts (with little or no provocation), typically expressed as verbal or physical aggression toward people or objects.
g. Inability to remember an important aspect of the traumatic event(s) (typically due to dissociative amnesia and not to other factors such as head injury, alcohol, or drugs).
h. Recurrent distressing dreams in which the content and/or affect of the dream is related to the event(s).
i. Hypervigilance.
j. Dissociative reactions (e.g., flashbacks) in which the individual feels or acts as if the traumatic event(s) were recurring.
k. Exaggerated startle response.

l. Efforts to avoid distressing memories, thoughts, or feelings about or closely associated with the traumatic event(s).

m. Sleep disturbance (e.g., difficulty falling or staying asleep, restless sleep).

n. Intense or prolonged psychological distress or marked physiological reactions in response to internal or external cues that symbolize or resemble an aspect of the traumatic event(s).

7.25 The DSM-5 diagnostic criteria for posttraumatic stress disorder (PTSD) require the presence of symptoms from **four** different categories: *Intrusion* (Criterion B), *Avoidance* (Criterion C), *Negative Alterations in Cognitions and Mood* (Criterion D), and *Arousal* (Criterion E). Match each of the following symptoms to the appropriate category (each symptom may be placed into only one category).

a. Irritable behavior and angry outbursts (with little or no provocation), typically expressed as verbal or physical aggression toward people or objects.

b. Avoidance of or efforts to avoid distressing memories, thoughts, or feelings about or closely associated with the traumatic event(s).

c. Recurrent, involuntary, and intrusive distressing memories of the traumatic event(s).

d. Inability to remember an important aspect of the traumatic event(s) (typically due to dissociative amnesia and not to other factors such as head injury, alcohol, or drugs).

e. Avoidance of or efforts to avoid external reminders (people, places, conversations, activities, objects, situations) that arouse distressing memories, thoughts, or feelings about or closely associated with the traumatic event(s).

f. Reckless or self-destructive behavior.

g. Recurrent distressing dreams in which the content and/or affect of the dream is related to the event(s).

h. Persistent and exaggerated negative beliefs or expectations about oneself, others, or the world (e.g., "I am bad," "No one can be trusted," "The world is completely dangerous," "My whole nervous system is permanently ruined").

i. Hypervigilance.

j. Dissociative reactions (e.g., flashbacks) in which the individual feels or acts as if the traumatic event(s) were recurring.

k. Persistent, distorted cognitions about the cause or consequences of the traumatic event(s) that lead the individual to blame himself/herself or others.

l. Exaggerated startle response.

m. Persistent negative emotional state (e.g., fear, horror, anger, guilt, or shame).

n. Problems with concentration.

o. Markedly diminished interest or participation in significant activities.

p. Intense or prolonged psychological distress at exposure to internal or external cues that symbolize or resemble an aspect of the traumatic event(s).

q. Sleep disturbance (e.g., difficulty falling or staying asleep, restless sleep).

r. Feelings of detachment or estrangement from others.

s. Marked physiological reactions to internal or external cues that symbolize or resemble an aspect of the traumatic event(s).

t. Persistent inability to experience positive emotions (e.g., inability to experience happiness, satisfaction, or loving feelings).

7.26 Eighteen months following the death of her son, a 49-year-old woman consults you for psychotherapy. She reports that her son died following a skiing accident on a trip that she gave him as a gift for his 17th birthday. She is preoccupied with the death and blames herself for providing the gift of the trip. Although she denies any overt suicidal plans, she describes longing for her son and an intense wish to be with him. She has not entered her son's room since his death, has difficulty relating to her husband and feels anger toward him for agreeing to allow their son to go on the ski trip, and reports arguments between them regarding her social isolation and her lack of interest in maintaining their home and preparing meals for their other children. She was treated with a selective serotonin reuptake inhibitor at full dose for 6 months after her son's death but reports that the medication had no impact on her symptoms. What is the most appropriate diagnosis?

A. Major depressive disorder.

B. Posttraumatic stress disorder.

C. Other specified trauma- and stressor-related disorder.

D. Normal grief.

E. Adjustment disorder.

CHAPTER 8

Dissociative Disorders

8.1   Which of the following is *not* a way in which DSM-5 classification of dissocia-
       tive disorders differs from DSM-IV?

    A. In DSM-IV, derealization occurring without depersonalization was classi-
       fied under dissociative disorder not otherwise specified (NOS), whereas in
       DSM-5 it is classified as depersonalization/derealization disorder.

    B. In DSM-IV, dissociative fugue was a separate diagnosis, whereas in DSM-5,
       it is a subtype of dissociative amnesia.

    C. In DSM-IV, experiences of possession could not be part of the diagnosis of
       dissociative identity disorder (DID); in DSM-5, they can be.

    D. In keeping with the empirical basis of DSM-5, DID can be diagnosed only
       if the clinician or a reliable family member witnesses the claimed disruption
       of identity; in DSM-IV, this restriction did not apply.

    E. The criteria for DID have been changed to indicate that gaps in the recall of
       events may occur for everyday events and not just traumatic events.

8.2   Dissociative disorders involve disruptions or discontinuities in the operation
       and integration of many areas of psychological functioning. Which of the fol-
       lowing is *not* a functional area affected in dissociative disorders?

    A. Memory.

    B. Consciousness.

    C. Perception.

    D. Delusional beliefs.

    E. Emotional responses.

8.3   Which of the following statements correctly describes the meanings of the ad-
       jectives *positive* and *negative* when applied to dissociative symptoms?

    A. When applied to dissociative disorder symptoms, the adjectives *positive*
       and *negative* have the same meanings as they do in schizophrenia.

    B. "Positive" dissociative symptoms refer to those accompanied by euphoric
       moods.

    C. "Negative" dissociative symptoms refer to inability to access mental con-
       tent or to control mental functions in a normal fashion.

    D. "Negative" dissociative symptoms refer to the belief that one has ceased to
       exist.

E. The adjectives *positive* and *negative* are not appropriately applied to dissociative symptoms because these symptoms are value neutral.

8.4   Which of the following statements about depersonalization/derealization disorder is *true?*

A. Although transient symptoms of depersonalization/derealization are common in the general population, symptomatology that meets full criteria for depersonalization/derealization disorder is markedly less common.
B. Women are 1.5 times more likely than men to develop depersonalization/derealization disorder.
C. Age at onset of the disorder is most commonly between 25 and 35 years.
D. During episodes of depersonalization/derealization, individuals may feel that they are "going crazy" and typically lose reality testing.
E. The most common childhood traumatic experience in persons with depersonalization/derealization disorder is sexual abuse.

8.5   Criterion A for the diagnosis of dissociative identity disorder (DID) requires the presence of two or more distinct personality states or an experience of possession. Which of the following symptom presentations would *not* qualify as a manifestation of an alternate identity?

A. An intrusive but nonhallucinatory voice that is not recognized as being part of one's own normal thought flow.
B. Suddenly emergent strong impulses or emotions.
C. Acute changes in personal preferences in areas such as food, clothing, or even political convictions.
D. An acute sense of being in a different body, such as an adult feeling like he or she is in a child's body.
E. A religious experience of being reborn into a new spiritual state that affects multiple domains of the individual's behavior.

8.6   Criterion B for the diagnosis of dissociative identity disorder (DID) requires recurrent gaps in the recall of everyday events, important personal information, and/or traumatic events that are inconsistent with ordinary forgetting. Which of the following statements about Criterion B–qualifying amnesia is *false?*

A. Gaps in recall of remote life events do not meet Criterion B definitions for amnesia.
B. It is common for individuals with DID to minimize their amnesia symptoms.
C. Individuals with DID may discover evidence of their past actions or experiences, such as finding clothing in the closet they do not recall buying, or seeing a photo of a trip they don't recall taking.

D. Forgetting of skills such as those involved in playing a musical instrument would count as amnesia for the purposes of Criterion B.

E. Dissociative fugues in which an individual finds him- or herself in a location with no memory of having traveled there are common in DID and represent a form of amnesia.

8.7 Dissociative amnesia most often involves which of the following types of amnesia?

A. Continuous amnesia.

B. Permanent, irreversible amnesia.

C. Localized or selective amnesia for specific events.

D. Generalized amnesia similar to that seen in neurological toxicity.

E. Systematized amnesia.

8.8 How does DSM-5 differ from DSM-IV in its classification of dissociative fugue?

A. Unlike DSM-IV, DSM-5 allows a fugue event to be diagnosed as dissociative identity disorder (DID) if it takes place in conjunction with the symptoms of DID.

B. Unlike DSM-IV, DSM-5 allows a fugue event secondary to temporal lobe epilepsy to be diagnosed as dissociative fugue.

C. Whereas dissociative fugue was a separate diagnosis in DSM-IV, it is a specifier of dissociative amnesia in DSM-5 (i.e., dissociative amnesia with dissociative fugue).

D. Unlike DSM-IV, DSM-5 recognizes that fugue states are more common in dissociative amnesia than in dissociative identity disorder.

E. Whereas DSM-IV treated dissociative fugue as an independent diagnostic entity, DSM-5 recognizes that fugue states most commonly present in the context of identity pathology.

CHAPTER 9

Somatic Symptom and Related Disorders

9.1 Somatoform Disorders in DSM-IV are referred to as Somatic Symptom and Related Disorders in DSM-5. Which of the following features characterizes the major diagnosis in this class, somatic symptom disorder?

A. Medically unexplained somatic symptoms.
B. Underlying psychic conflict.
C. Masochism.
D. Distressing somatic symptoms and abnormal thoughts, feelings, and behaviors in response to these symptoms.
E. Comorbidity with anxiety and depressive disorders.

9.2 In DSM-IV, a patient with a high level of anxiety about having a disease and many associated somatic symptoms would have been given the diagnosis of hypochondriasis. What DSM-5 diagnosis would apply to this patient?

A. Hypochondriasis.
B. Illness anxiety disorder.
C. Somatic symptom disorder.
D. Generalized anxiety disorder.
E. Unspecified somatic symptom and related disorder.

9.3 In DSM-III and DSM-IV, a large number of somatic symptoms were needed to qualify for the diagnosis of somatization disorder. How many somatic symptoms are needed to meet symptom criteria for the DSM-5 diagnosis of somatic symptom disorder?

A. Four: at least one pseudoneurological, one pain, one sexual, and one gastrointestinal symptom.
B. Fifteen, distributed across several organ systems.
C. One.
D. At least one that is medically unexplained.
E. None.

9.4 After an airplane flight, a 60-year-old woman with a history of chronic anxiety develops deep vein thrombophlebitis and a subsequent pulmonary embolism. Over the next year, she focuses relentlessly on sensations of pleuritic chest pain and repeatedly seeks medical attention for this symptom, which she worries is due to recurrent pulmonary emboli, despite negative test results. Review of systems reveals that she also has chronic back pain and that she has consulted many physicians for symptoms of culture-negative cystitis. What diagnosis best fits this clinical picture?

A. Post–pulmonary embolism syndrome.
B. Chest pain syndrome.
C. Hypochondriasis.
D. Pain disorder.
E. Somatic symptom disorder.

9.5 Which of the following is a descriptive specifier included in the diagnostic criteria for somatic symptom disorder?

A. With predominant pain.
B. With hypochondriasis.
C. With psychological comorbidity.
D. Psychotic type.
E. Undifferentiated.

9.6 A 60-year-old man has prostate cancer with bony metastases that cause persistent pain. He is treated with antiandrogen medications that result in hot flashes. He is unable to work because of his symptoms, but he is stoical, hopeful, and not anxious. What is the appropriate diagnosis?

A. Pain disorder.
B. Illness anxiety disorder.
C. Somatic symptom disorder.
D. Psychological factors affecting other medical conditions.
E. No diagnosis.

9.7 Illness anxiety disorder involves a preoccupation with having or acquiring a serious illness. How severe must the accompanying somatic symptoms be to meet criteria for the diagnosis of illness anxiety disorder?

A. Mild to moderate severity.
B. Moderate to high severity.
C. Any level of severity.
D. Mild severity at most, but there need not be any somatic symptoms.
E. None of the above; the presence of *any* somatic symptoms rules out the diagnosis of illness anxiety disorder.

9.8 Over a period of several years, a 50-year-old woman visits her dermatologist's office every few weeks to be evaluated for skin cancer, showing the dermatologist various freckles, nevi, and patches of dry skin about which she has become concerned. None of the skin findings have ever been abnormal, and the dermatologist has repeatedly reassured her. The woman does not have pain, itching, bleeding, or other somatic symptoms. She does have a history of occasional panic attacks. What is the most likely diagnosis?

A. Unspecified anxiety disorder.
B. Illness anxiety disorder.
C. Hypochondriasis.
D. Somatic symptom disorder.
E. Factitious disorder.

9.9 A 45-year-old man with a family history of early-onset coronary artery disease avoids climbing stairs, eschews exercise, and abstains from sexual activity for fear of provoking a heart attack. He frequently checks his pulse, reads extensively about preventive cardiology, and tries many health food supplements alleged to be good for the heart. When he experiences an occasional twinge of chest discomfort, he rests in bed for 24 hours; however, he does not go to doctors because he fears hearing bad news about his heart from them. What diagnosis best fits this clinical picture?

A. Persistent complex bereavement disorder.
B. Adjustment disorder.
C. Illness anxiety disorder.
D. Unspecified somatic symptom and related disorder.
E. Somatic symptom disorder.

9.10 A 25-year-old woman is hospitalized for evaluation of episodes in which she appears to lose consciousness, rocks her head from side to side, and moves her arms and legs in a nonsynchronous, bicycling pattern. The episodes occur a few times per day and last for 2–5 minutes. Electroencephalography during the episodes does not reveal any ictal activity. Immediately after a fit, her sensorium appears clear. What is the most likely diagnosis?

A. Epilepsy.
B. Malingering.
C. Somatic symptom disorder.
D. Conversion disorder (functional neurological symptom disorder), with attacks or seizures.
E. Factitious disorder.

9.11 Which of the following symptoms is incompatible with a diagnosis of conversion disorder (functional neurological symptom disorder)?

A. Light-headedness upon standing up.

B. Dystonic movements.

C. Tunnel vision.

D. Touch and temperature anesthesia with intact pinprick sensation over the left forearm.

E. Transient leg weakness in a patient with known multiple sclerosis.

9.12   Why is *la belle indifférence* (apparent lack of concern about the symptom) not included as a diagnostic criterion for conversion disorder (functional neurological symptom disorder)?

A. It has poor interrater reliability.

B. It has poor specificity.

C. It has poor sensitivity.

D. It pathologizes stoicism.

E. It has poor test-retest reliability.

9.13   A 20-year-old man presents with the complaint of acute onset of decreased visual acuity in his left eye. Physical, neurological, and laboratory examinations are entirely normal, including stereopsis testing, fogging test, and brain magnetic resonance imaging. The remainder of the history is negative except for the patient's report that since his midteens he has felt that his left cheekbone and eyebrow are too big. He spends a lot of time comparing the right and left sides of his face in the mirror. He is planning to have plastic surgery as soon as he graduates from college. Which of the following diagnoses are suggested?

A. Somatic symptom disorder and delusional disorder, somatic subtype.

B. Somatic symptom disorder and illness anxiety disorder.

C. Body dysmorphic disorder and conversion disorder (functional neurological symptom disorder).

D. Somatic symptom disorder, illness anxiety disorder, and body dysmorphic disorder.

E. Delusional disorder, somatic subtype.

9.14   A 50-year-old man with hard-to-control hypertension acknowledges to his physician that he regularly "takes breaks" from his medication regimen because he was brought up with the belief that pills are bad and natural remedies are better. He is well aware that his blood pressure becomes dangerously high when he does not follow the regimen. Which diagnosis best fits this case?

A. Nonadherence to medical treatment.

B. Unspecified anxiety disorder.

C. Denial of medical illness.

D. Adjustment disorder.

E. Psychological factors affecting other medical conditions.

9.15   A 60-year-old man has prostate cancer with bony metastases that cause persistent pain. He is being treated with antiandrogen medications that result in hot flashes. Although (by his own assessment) his pain is well controlled with analgesics, he states that he is unable to work because of his symptoms. Despite reassurance that his medications are controlling his metastatic disease, every instance of pain leads him to worry that he has new bony lesions and is about to die, and he continually expresses fears about his impending death to his wife and children. Which diagnosis best fits this patient's presentation?

   A. Panic disorder.
   B. Illness anxiety disorder.
   C. Somatic symptom disorder.
   D. Psychological factors affecting other medical conditions.
   E. Adjustment disorder with anxious mood.

9.16   A 60-year-old man with a history of coronary disease and emphysema continues to smoke one pack of cigarettes daily despite his doctor's clear advice that abstinence is important for his survival. He says he's tried to quit a dozen times but has always relapsed due to withdrawal symptoms or feelings of tension relieved by smoking. What is the most likely diagnosis?

   A. Psychological factors affecting other medical conditions.
   B. Tobacco use disorder.
   C. Denial of illness.
   D. Nonadherence to medical treatment.
   E. Adjustment disorder.

9.17   What is the essential diagnostic feature of factitious disorder?

   A. Somatic symptoms.
   B. Conscious misrepresentation and deception.
   C. External gain associated with illness.
   D. Absence of another medical disorder that may cause the symptoms.
   E. Normal physical examination and laboratory tests.

9.18   A 19-year-old man is brought to the emergency department by his family with acute onset of hemoptysis. Although he denies any role in the genesis of the symptom, he is observed in the waiting area to be surreptitiously inhaling a solution that provokes violent coughing. On confrontation he eventually acknowledges his action but explains that he heard an angel's voice instructing him to purify himself for a divine mission for which he will receive a heavenly reward. He was therefore trying to expunge all "evil vapors" from his lungs but felt obliged to keep this a secret. Why would this patient *not* be considered to have factitious disorder?

A. Consequences of religious or culturally normative practices are exempt from consideration as fabricated illnesses.
B. Factitious disorder occurs almost exclusively in women.
C. Repeated instances of illness fabrication are necessary for a diagnosis of factitious disorder.
D. The patient expects to receive an external reward and therefore should be considered to be malingering.
E. The presence of a psychotic illness that better accounts for the symptoms precludes the diagnosis of factitious disorder.

9.19 When a mother knowingly and deceptively reports signs and symptoms of illness in her preschool-aged child, resulting in the child's hospitalization and subjection to numerous tests and procedures, what diagnosis would be recorded for the child?

A. Munchausen syndrome by proxy.
B. Factitious disorder by proxy.
C. No diagnosis.
D. Munchausen syndrome imposed on another.
E. Factitious disorder imposed on another.

9.20 A 25-year-old woman with a history of intravenous heroin abuse is admitted to the hospital with infective endocarditis. Blood cultures are positive for several fungal species. Search of the patient's belongings discloses hidden syringes and needles and a small bag of dirt, which, when cultured, yields the same fungal species. Which of the following diagnoses are likely to apply?

A. Infective endocarditis, opioid use disorder, malingering, factitious disorder, and antisocial personality disorder.
B. Opioid use disorder and malingering.
C. Infective endocarditis, opioid use disorder, and factitious disorder.
D. Malingering and antisocial personality disorder.
E. Malingering and factitious disorder.

9.21 After finding a breast lump, a 50-year-old woman with a family history of breast cancer is overwhelmed by feelings of anxiety. Consultation with a breast surgeon, mammogram, and biopsy show the lump to be benign. The surgeon tells her that she requires no treatment; however, she continues to ruminate about the possibility of cancer and surgery that will result in disfigurement. Her sleep is restless, and she is having trouble concentrating at work. After 6 weeks of these symptoms, her primary physician refers her for psychiatric consultation. Her medical and psychiatric history is otherwise negative. Which diagnosis best fits this presentation?

A. Somatic symptom disorder.
B. Illness anxiety disorder.

C. Unspecified somatic symptom and related disorder.

D. Other specified somatic symptom and related disorder.

E. Adjustment disorder with anxious mood.

9.22 After finding a breast lump, a 53-year-old woman with a family history of breast cancer is overwhelmed by feelings of anxiety. Consultation with a breast surgeon, mammogram, and biopsy show the lump to be benign. The surgeon indicates that she requires no treatment; however, she continues to ruminate about the possibility of cancer and surgery that will result in disfigurement. Her sleep is restless and she is having trouble concentrating at work. After 6 weeks in this state, her primary physician requests that she consult a psychiatrist. On initial evaluation the patient weeps throughout the interview, and is so distraught that the evaluator is unable to elicit details of her medical and psychiatric history beyond reviewing the current "crisis." Which diagnosis best fits this presentation?

A. Somatic symptom disorder.

B. Illness anxiety disorder.

C. Unspecified somatic symptom and related disorder.

D. Other specified somatic symptom and related disorder.

E. Adjustment disorder with anxious mood.

CHAPTER 10

Feeding and Eating Disorders

10.1   Which DSM-5 diagnosis replaced the DSM-IV diagnosis of feeding disorder of infancy or early childhood?

A. Anorexia nervosa.
B. Unspecified feeding or eating disorder.
C. Anorexia nervosa of early childhood.
D. Avoidant/restrictive food intake disorder.
E. Pica.

10.2   Which of the following statements about DSM-5 changes in the diagnostic criteria for anorexia nervosa is *true?*

A. The requirement for menorrhagia has been eliminated.
B. The requirement for amenorrhea has been eliminated.
C. The requirements for amenorrhea and menorrhagia have been eliminated.
D. Low body weight is no longer required.
E. Developmental stage is no longer a significant issue.

10.3   Which of the following statements about DSM-5 changes in the diagnostic criteria for bulimia nervosa is *true?*

A. There is an increase in the required numbers of binge-eating episodes and inappropriate compensatory behaviors per week, from twice to three times weekly.
B. There is an increase in the numbers of episodes of using ipecac or vomiting per week, from three to four.
C. There is a reduction in the required minimum frequency of binge eating and inappropriate compensatory behavior frequency, from twice to once weekly.
D. There is a requirement for an episode of pica, at least once in the last year.
E. There is a requirement for electrolyte imbalances to be demonstrated at least twice in the past 2 years.

10.4   What is the minimum average frequency of binge eating required for a diagnosis of DSM-5 binge-eating disorder?

A. Once weekly for the last 3 months.
B. Once weekly for the last 4 months.
C. Every other week for the last 3 months.
D. Every other week for the last 4 months.
E. Once a month for the last 3 months.

10.5   In avoidant/restrictive food intake disorder, the eating or feeding disturbance is manifested by persistent failure to meet appropriate nutritional and/or energy needs associated with one or more of four specified features. Which of the following options correctly lists these four features?

A. Manic or hypomanic symptoms; ruminative behaviors; compulsive thoughts; marked interference with psychosocial functioning.
B. Significant weight loss; significant nutritional deficiency; dependence on enteral feeding or oral nutritional supplements; marked interference with psychosocial functioning.
C. Significant weight loss; ruminative behaviors; delusions or hallucinations; manic or hypomanic symptoms.
D. Significant nutritional deficiency; increased use of alcohol or other substances; manic or hypomanic symptoms; delusions or hallucinations.
E. Dependence on enteral feeding or oral nutritional supplements; ruminative behaviors; delusions or hallucinations; manic or hypomanic symptoms.

10.6   Which of the following statements about onset and prevalence of avoidant/restrictive food intake disorder is *true*?

A. The disorder occurs mostly in females, with onset typically in older adolescence.
B. The disorder occurs mostly in males, with onset typically in early childhood.
C. The disorder is more common in childhood and more common in females than in males.
D. The disorder is more common in childhood and equally common in males and females.
E. The disorder is extremely common in elderly adults, who often manifest an age-related reduction in intake.

10.7   A 45-year-old woman had a choking episode 3 years ago after eating salad. Since that time she has been afraid to eat a wide range of foods, fearing that she will choke. This fear has affected her functionality and her ability to eat out with friends and has contributed to weight loss. Which diagnosis best fits this clinical picture?

A. Bulimia nervosa.
B. Schizophrenia.

C. Avoidant/restrictive food intake disorder.
D. Binge-eating disorder.
E. Adjustment disorder.

10.8 What are the two subtypes of anorexia nervosa?

A. Restricting type and binge-eating/purging type.
B. Energy-sparing type and binge-eating/purging type.
C. Low-calorie/low-carbohydrate type and restricting type.
D. Low-carbohydrate/low-fat type and restricting type.
E. Restricting type and low-weight type.

10.9 What are the three essential diagnostic features of anorexia nervosa?

A. Persistently low self-confidence, intense fear of becoming fat, and disturbance in motivation.
B. Low self-esteem, disturbance in self-perceived weight or shape, and persistent energy restriction.
C. Restricted affect, disturbance in motivation, and low calorie intake.
D. Persistent restriction of energy intake, intense fear of becoming fat, and disturbance in self-perceived weight or shape.
E. Persistent lack of weight gain, disturbance in motivation, and restricted affect.

10.10 What laboratory abnormalities are commonly found in individuals with anorexia nervosa?

A. Elevated blood urea nitrogen (BUN); low triiodothyronine (T_3); hyperadrenocorticism; low serum estrogen (females) or testosterone (males); bradycardia; low bone mineral density.
B. Low BUN; hypercholesterolemia; high thyroxine (T_4); hypoadrenocorticism; short QTc; low bone mineral density.
C. Blast cells; thrombocytosis; hyperphosphatemia; hypoamylasemia; high serum estrogen (females) or testosterone (males).
D. Hyperzincemia; hypermagnesemia; hyperchloremia; hyperkalemia.
E. C and D.

10.11 A 27-year-old graduate student has a 10-year history of anorexia nervosa. Her boyfriend is quite concerned because she has extreme fears related to cleanliness. She washes her hands more than 12 times a day and is excessively worried about contamination. What would be the best decision by the mental health professional at this point regarding these symptoms?

A. Assume that the patient's obsessive-compulsive symptoms are related to her anorexia nervosa.

B. Further evaluate the obsessive-compulsive features, because if they are not related to anorexia nervosa, a new diagnosis of obsessive-compulsive disorder might be warranted.

C. Ask the patient to wait 1 year and see how this evolves.

D. Make a diagnosis of body dysmorphic disorder.

E. Refer the patient for a colonoscopy.

10.12 What are the three essential diagnostic features of bulimia nervosa?

A. Recurrent episodes of binge eating; recurrent inappropriate compensatory behaviors to prevent weight gain; self-evaluation that is unduly influenced by body shape and weight.

B. Recurrent restriction of food; self-evaluation that is unduly influenced by body shape and weight; mood instability.

C. Delusions regarding body habitus; obsessional focus on food; recurrent purging.

D. Hypomanic symptoms for 1 month; mood instability; self-evaluation that is unduly influenced by body shape and weight.

E. Self-evaluation that is unduly influenced by body shape and weight; history of anorexia nervosa; recurrent inappropriate compensatory behaviors to gain weight.

10.13 What are the subtypes of bulimia nervosa?

A. Restrictive.

B. Purging.

C. Restrictive and purging.

D. None.

E. With normal weight/abnormal weight.

10.14 What minimum average frequency of binge eating is required to qualify for a diagnosis of binge-eating disorder?

A. At least once a week for 3 months.

B. At least twice a week for 3 months.

C. At least once a week for 6 months.

D. At least twice a week for 6 months.

E. None of the above.

CHAPTER 11

Elimination Disorders

11.1 A 7-year-old boy with mild to moderate developmental delay presents with a chronic history of wetting his clothes during the day about once weekly, even during school. He is now refusing to go to school for fear of wetting his pants and being ridiculed by his classmates. Which of the following statements accurately describes the diagnostic options regarding enuresis in this case?

A. He should not be diagnosed with enuresis because the frequency is less than twice per week.
B. He should be diagnosed with enuresis because the incontinence is resulting in impairment of age-appropriate role functioning.
C. He should not be diagnosed with enuresis because his mental age is likely less than 5 years old.
D. He should be diagnosed with enuresis, diurnal only subtype.
E. He should not be diagnosed with enuresis because the events are restricted to the daytime.

11.2 Which of the following statements about enuresis is *true?*

A. Over 60% of children diagnosed with enuresis have a comorbid DSM-5 disorder.
B. Developmental delays are no more common in children with enuresis than in other children.
C. Urinary tract infections are more common in children with enuresis.
D. While embarrassing, enuresis has no effect on children's self-esteem.
E. Prevalence rates for enuresis at age 10 are similar to those at age 5.

11.3 Which of the following statements about the diurnal-only subtype of enuresis is *true?*

A. This subtype is more common in males.
B. This subtype is more common after age 9 years.
C. This subtype is sometimes referred to as *monosymptomatic enuresis.*
D. This subtype is more common than the nocturnal-only subtype.
E. This subtype includes a subgroup of individuals with "voiding postponement," in which micturition is consciously deferred because of a social reluctance to use the bathroom or to interrupt a play activity.

11.4 Which of the following statements correctly identifies a distinction between primary enuresis and secondary enuresis?

   A. Secondary enuresis is due to an identified medical condition; primary enuresis has no known etiology.
   B. Children with secondary enuresis have higher rates of psychiatric comorbidity than do children with primary enuresis.
   C. Primary enuresis has a typical onset at age 10, much later than the onset of secondary enuresis.
   D. Primary enuresis is never preceded by a period of continence, whereas secondary enuresis is always preceded by a period of continence.
   E. Unlike primary enuresis, secondary enuresis tends to persist into late adolescence.

11.5 Which of the following statements correctly describes factors related to the etiology and/or onset of enuresis?

   A. Enuresis has been shown to be heritable, with a child being twice as likely to have the diagnosis if either parent has had it.
   B. Mode of toilet training or its neglect can affect rates of enuresis, as shown by high rates seen in orphanages.
   C. In girls with enuresis, nocturnal enuresis is the more common form.
   D. Rates of enuresis are much higher in European countries than in developing countries.
   E. The development of modern diapers is believed to speed toilet training and reduce enuresis.

11.6 A 6-year-old boy with mild to moderate developmental delay presents with a history of passing feces into his underwear during the day about once every 2 weeks, even during school. He is now refusing to go to school for fear of soiling his pants and being ridiculed by his classmates. Which of the following statements accurately describes the diagnostic options regarding encopresis in this case?

   A. He should not be diagnosed with encopresis because the frequency is less than twice per week.
   B. He should be diagnosed with encopresis because the incontinence is resulting in impairment of age-appropriate role functioning.
   C. He should not be diagnosed with encopresis because his mental age is likely less than 4 years old.
   D. He should be diagnosed with encopresis.
   E. He should not be diagnosed with encopresis because the events are restricted to the daytime.

11.7 Which of the following statements about encopresis is *true?*

A. When oppositional defiant disorder or conduct disorder is present, one cannot diagnose encopresis.
B. When constipation is present, one cannot diagnose encopresis.
C. Urinary tract infections can be comorbid with encopresis and are more common in girls.
D. Although it is embarrassing, encopresis has no effect on children's self-esteem.
E. Prevalence rates for encopresis at age 5 are estimated to be 5%.

11.8 Which of the following statements correctly describes clinical aspects of the diagnosis of encopresis?

A. Encopresis with constipation and overflow incontinence is often involuntary.
B. Encopresis with constipation and overflow incontinence always involves well-formed stool.
C. Encopresis with constipation and overflow incontinence cannot be diagnosed if the behavior results from avoidance of defecation that develops for psychological reasons.
D. In encopresis with constipation and overflow incontinence, leakage usually occurs during sleep.
E. Encopresis with constipation and overflow incontinence rarely resolves after treatment of the constipation.

CHAPTER 12

Sleep-Wake Disorders

12.1 Which of the following is a core feature of insomnia disorder?

A. Depressed mood.
B. Dissatisfaction with sleep quantity or quality.
C. Cognitive impairment.
D. Abnormal behaviors during sleep.
E. Daytime fatigue.

12.2 Which of the following is necessary to make a diagnosis of insomnia disorder?

A. Difficulty being fully awake after awakening.
B. Difficulty with sleep initiation or sleep maintenance, or early-morning awakening with inability to return to sleep.
C. Absence of a coexisting mental disorder.
D. Documented insufficient opportunity for sleep.
E. Persistence of sleep difficulties despite use of sedative-hypnotic agents.

12.3 An 80-year-old man has a history of myocardial infarction and had coronary artery bypass graft surgery 8 years ago. He plays tennis three times a week, takes care of his grandchildren 2 afternoons each week, generally enjoys life, and manages all of his activities of daily living independently; however, he complains of excessively early morning awakening. He goes to sleep at 9:00 P.M. and sleeps well, with nocturia once nightly, but wakes at 3:30 A.M. although he would like to rise at 5:00 A.M. He does not endorse daytime sleepiness as a problem. His physical examination, mental status, and cognitive function are normal. What is the most likely sleep-wake disorder diagnosis?

A. Insomnia disorder.
B. Rapid eye movement (REM) sleep behavior disorder.
C. Restless legs syndrome.
D. Obstructive sleep apnea hypopnea.
E. The man is a short sleeper, which is not a DSM-5 diagnosis.

12.4 Which of the following symptoms is most likely to indicate the presence of hypersomnolence disorder?

A. Sleep inertia.
B. Nonrefreshing sleep in main sleep episode.

C. Automatic behavior.
D. Frequent napping.
E. Headache.

12.5   An obese 52-year-old man complains of daytime sleepiness, and his partner
        confirms that he snores, snorts, and gasps during nighttime sleep. What poly-
        somnographic finding is needed to confirm the diagnosis of obstructive sleep
        apnea hypopnea?

        A. No polysomnography is necessary.
        B. Polysomnographic evidence of at least 5 apnea or hypopnea episodes per
           hour of sleep.
        C. Polysomnographic evidence of at least 10 apnea or hypopnea episodes per
           hour of sleep.
        D. Polysomnographic evidence of at least 15 apnea or hypopnea episodes per
           hour of sleep.
        E. Polysomnographic evidence of resolution of apneas/hypopneas with ap-
           plication of continuous positive airway pressure.

12.6   In addition to requiring recurrent sleep attacks, the diagnostic criteria for nar-
        colepsy require the presence of cataplexy, hypocretin deficiency, *or* characteris-
        tic abnormalities on sleep polysomnography or multiple sleep latency testing.
        Which of the following is a defining characteristic of cataplexy?

        A. It is sudden.
        B. It is induced by suggestion.
        C. It occurs unilaterally.
        D. It persists for hours.
        E. It is accompanied by hypertonia.

12.7   In DSM-IV, the diagnosis of breathing-related sleep disorder would be given to
        an individual complaining of excessive daytime sleepiness, with nocturnal
        polysomnography demonstrating episodic loss of ventilatory effort and result-
        ing apneic episodes occurring 10–20 times per hour, whose symptoms cannot
        be attributed to another mental disorder, a medication or substance, or another
        medical condition. What is the appropriate DSM-5 diagnosis for the same in-
        dividual?

        A. Insomnia disorder.
        B. Narcolepsy.
        C. Obstructive sleep apnea hypopnea.
        D. Central sleep apnea.
        E. Other specified hypersomnolence disorder.

12.8 Which of the following metabolic changes is the cardinal feature of sleep-related hypoventilation?

A. Insulin resistance.
B. Hypoxia.
C. Hypercapnia.
D. Low arterial hemoglobin oxygen saturation.
E. Elevated vasopressin.

12.9 A 51-year-old man presents with symptoms of chronic fatigue and excessive worrying about current life stressors. He has a strong family history of depression and a past history of a major depressive episode, with some improvement while maintained on antidepressants. On weekday nights, it takes him several hours to fall asleep, and he then has difficulty getting up to go to work in the morning, experiencing sleepiness for the first few hours of awake time. On weekends, he awakens later in the morning and feels less fatigue and sleepiness. Which of the following diagnoses apply?

A. Major depressive disorder, in partial remission.
B. Generalized anxiety disorder.
C. Insomnia disorder.
D. Major depressive disorder in partial remission and circadian rhythm sleep-wake disorder, delayed sleep phase type.
E. Major depressive disorder in partial remission; generalized anxiety disorder; circadian rhythm sleep-wake disorder, delayed sleep phase type; and insomnia disorder.

12.10 A 67-year-old woman complains of insomnia. She does not have trouble falling asleep between 10 and 11 P.M., but after 1–2 hours she awakens for several hours in the middle of the night, sleeps again for 2–4 hours in the early morning, and then naps three or four times during the day for 1–3 hours at a time. She has a family history of dementia. On exam she appears fatigued and has deficits in short-term memory, calculation, and abstraction. What is the most likely diagnosis?

A. Major neurocognitive disorder (NCD).
B. Circadian rhythm sleep-wake disorder, irregular sleep-wake type, and unspecified NCD.
C. Narcolepsy.
D. Insomnia disorder.
E. Major depressive disorder.

12.11 Following a traumatic brain injury resulting in blindness, a 50-year-old man develops waxing and waning daytime sleepiness interfering with daytime activity. Serial actigraphy (a method of measuring human activity/rest cycles) demonstrates that the time of onset of the major sleep period occurs progressively later day after day, with a normal duration of the major sleep period. What is the most likely diagnosis?

A. Circadian rhythm sleep-wake disorder, unspecified type.
B. Circadian rhythm sleep-wake disorder, delayed sleep phase type.
C. Circadian rhythm sleep-wake disorder, non-24-hour sleep-wake type.
D. Pineal gland injury.
E. Malingering.

12.12 A 50-year-old emergency department nurse complains of sleepiness at work interfering with her ability to function. She recently switched from the 7 A.M.– 4 P.M. day shift to the 11 P.M.–8 A.M. night shift in order to have her afternoons free. Even with this schedule change, she finds it difficult to sleep in the mornings at home, has little energy for recreational activities or household chores in the afternoon, and feels exhausted by the middle of her overnight shift. What is the most likely diagnosis?

A. Normal variation in sleep secondary to shift work.
B. Circadian rhythm sleep-wake disorder, shift work type.
C. Bipolar disorder.
D. Insomnia disorder.
E. Hypersomnolence disorder.

12.13 A 14-year-old girl frequently wakes in the morning with clear recollection of very frightening dreams. Once she awakens, she is normally alert and oriented, but the dreams are a persistent source of distress. Her mother reports that the girl sometimes murmurs or groans but does not talk or move during the period before waking. Her history is otherwise notable for having been homeless and living with her mother in a series of temporary shelter accommodations for 1 year when she was 10 years old. What is the most likely diagnosis?

A. Unspecified anxiety disorder.
B. Rapid eye movement (REM) sleep behavior disorder.
C. Non–rapid eye movement sleep arousal disorders.
D. Posttraumatic stress disorder.
E. Nightmare disorder.

12.14 Which of the following is a type of non–rapid eye movement (REM) sleep arousal disorder in DSM-5?

A. REM sleep behavior disorder.
B. Sleep terrors.
C. Nightmare disorder.
D. Fugue.
E. Obstructive sleep apnea hypopnea.

12.15 Which of the following is a specific subtype of non–rapid eye movement sleep arousal disorder, sleepwalking type?

  A. Rapid eye movement (REM) sleep behavior disorder.
  B. Sleep-related seizure disorder.
  C. Sleep-related sexual behavior (sexsomnia).
  D. Complex motor behavior during alcoholic blackout.
  E. Nocturnal panic attack.

12.16 What is the difference between sleep terrors and nightmare disorder?

  A. In nightmare disorder, arousal or awakening from the nightmare is incomplete, whereas sleep terrors result in complete awakening.
  B. In sleep terrors, episodes are concentrated in the final hours of the sleep period, whereas nightmares occur mostly early in the sleep period.
  C. Sleep terrors are characterized by clear recall of vivid dreams with frightening content, whereas nightmares are not recalled.
  D. Sleep terrors occur during rapid eye movement (REM) sleep, whereas nightmares occur in non-REM sleep.
  E. Sleep terrors are precipitous but incomplete awakenings from sleep beginning with a panicky scream or cry, with little recall, whereas nightmares are characterized by full arousal and vivid recall.

12.17 What is the key abnormality in sleep physiology in rapid eye movement (REM) sleep behavior disorder?

  A. REM starts earlier than normal in the sleep cycle.
  B. There is more REM sleep than normal.
  C. Delta wave activity is increased.
  D. Skeletal muscle tone is preserved during REM sleep.
  E. Total sleep time is greater than normal.

12.18 Which of the following conditions is commonly associated with rapid eye movement (REM) sleep behavior disorder?

  A. Attention-deficit/hyperactivity disorder.
  B. Synucleinopathies.
  C. Tourette's syndrome.
  D. Sleep terrors.
  E. Epilepsy.

12.19 Which of the following classes of psychotropic drugs may result in rapid eye movement (REM) sleep without atonia and REM sleep behavior disorder?

  A. Selective serotonin reuptake inhibitors.
  B. Benzodiazepines.

C. Phenothiazines.

D. Second-generation antipsychotics.

E. Monoamine oxidase inhibitors.

12.20 A 10-year-old boy is referred by his teacher for evaluation of his difficulty sitting still in school, which is interfering with his academic performance. The boy complains of an unpleasant "creepy-crawly" sensation in his legs and an urge to move them when sitting still that is relieved by movement. This symptom bothers him most of the day, but less when playing sports after school or watching television in the evening, and it generally does not bother him in bed at night. What aspect of his clinical presentation rules out a diagnosis of restless legs syndrome (RLS)?

A. He is too young for a diagnosis of RLS.

B. He does not have a sleep complaint.

C. He does not complain of daytime fatigue or sleepiness.

D. His symptoms occur in the daytime as much as or more than in the evening or at night.

E. He does not have impaired social functioning.

12.21 A 28-year-old woman who is in her thirty-fourth week of pregnancy reports that for the past few weeks she has experienced restlessness and difficulty falling asleep at the onset of the sleep period, as well as daytime fatigue. She works during the day and has not changed her schedule. She states that as she becomes increasingly tired, she feels more irritable and depressed. What sleep disorder is suggested by the onset of these symptoms in the third trimester of pregnancy?

A. Circadian rhythm sleep-wake disorder, delayed sleep phase type.

B. Insomnia disorder.

C. Rapid eye movement (REM) sleep behavior disorder.

D. Restless legs syndrome.

E. Hypersomnolence disorder.

12.22 Which of the following sleep disturbances or disorders occurs during rapid eye movement (REM) sleep?

A. Nightmare disorder.

B. Confusional arousals.

C. Sleep terrors.

D. Obstructive sleep apnea hypopnea.

E. Central sleep apnea.

12.23 Which of the following sleep disturbances is associated with chronic opiate use?

A. Excessive daytime sleepiness.
B. Insomnia.
C. Periodic limb movements in sleep.
D. Obstructive sleep apnea hypopnea.
E. Parasomnias.

12.24 Which of the following substances is associated with parasomnias?

A. Cannabis.
B. Zolpidem.
C. Methadone.
D. Cocaine.
E. Mescaline.

12.25 A psychiatric consultation is requested for evaluation and help with management of severe insomnia in a 65-year-old man, beginning the day after elective hip replacement surgery and continuing for 2 days. On evaluation the patient acknowledges heavy drinking until the day before surgery, and he appears to be in alcohol withdrawal, with autonomic instability, confusion, and tremor. Why would a diagnosis of substance/medication-induced sleep disorder be inappropriate in this situation?

A. The insomnia is an understandable emotional reaction to the anxiety provoked by having surgery.
B. The insomnia is not causing functional impairment.
C. The insomnia has not been documented with polysomnography or actigraphy.
D. The insomnia is occurring during acute alcohol withdrawal.
E. The insomnia might be related to postoperative pain.

12.26 A 56-year-old college professor complains of having difficulty sleeping for more than 5 hours per night over the past few weeks, leaving her feeling tired in the daytime. She awakens an hour or two before her intended waking time in the morning, experiencing restless sleep with frequent awakenings until it is time to get up. She does not have initial insomnia and is not depressed. The patient attributes the sleep trouble to intrusive thoughts that arise, after she initially awakens momentarily, about the need to complete an overdue academic project. What is the most appropriate diagnosis?

A. Adjustment disorder with anxious mood.
B. Obsessive-compulsive personality disorder.
C. Insomnia disorder.
D. Other specified insomnia disorder (brief insomnia disorder).
E. Unspecified insomnia disorder.

12.27 A 74-year-old woman has a history of daytime sleepiness interfering with her ability to carry out her daily routine. She reports that it has become progressively worse over the past year. Polysomnography reveals sleep apnea without evidence of airway obstruction with two or three apneic episodes per hour. What is the most appropriate diagnosis?

A. Central sleep apnea.
B. Other specified sleep-wake disorder (atypical central sleep apnea).
C. Unspecified sleep-wake disorder.
D. Rapid eye movement (REM) sleep behavior disorder.
E. Circadian rhythm sleep-wake disorder.

CHAPTER 13

Sexual Dysfunctions

13.1 According to "Highlights of Changes From DSM-IV to DSM-5" in the DSM-5 Appendix, which of the following DSM-IV sexual dysfunction diagnoses is still included in DSM-5?

A. Sexual aversion disorder.
B. Female orgasmic disorder.
C. Dyspareunia.
D. Vaginismus.
E. None of the above.

13.2 Female sexual interest/arousal disorder requires a lack of, or significantly reduced, sexual interest/arousal, as manifested by at least three of six possible indicators. Which of the following is *not* one of these six indicators?

A. No/reduced initiation of sexual activity, and typically unreceptive to a partner's attempts to initiate.
B. Absent/reduced sexual excitement/pleasure during sexual activity with the opposite sex.
C. Absent/reduced genital or nongenital sensations during sexual activity in almost all or all sexual encounters.
D. Absent/reduced interest in sexual activity.
E. Absent/reduced sexual/erotic thoughts or fantasies.

13.3 Several of the sexual dysfunctions have criteria that contain the phrase "almost all or all"; for example, "Absent/reduced sexual excitement/pleasure during sexual activity in almost all or all sexual encounters." How is "almost all or all" defined?

A. At least 75%.
B. At least 90%.
C. Approximately 75%–100%.
D. Approximately 90%–100%.
E. In the clinician's best estimate.

13.4 Which of the following is a subtype of sexual dysfunction in DSM-5?

A. Lifelong.
B. Secondary to a medical condition.
C. Due to relationship factors.

D. Due to psychological factors.

E. None of the above.

13.5 In all of the sexual dysfunctions except substance/medication-induced sexual dysfunction, symptoms must be present for what minimum duration to qualify for the diagnosis?

A. Approximately 1 month.

B. Approximately 3 months.

C. Approximately 6 months.

D. Approximately 1 year.

E. Approximately 2 years.

13.6 A 65-year-old man who presented with difficulty in obtaining an erection due to diabetes and severe vascular disease had received a DSM-IV diagnosis of Sexual Dysfunction Due to…[Indicate the General Medical Condition] (coded as *607.84 male erectile disorder due to diabetes mellitus*). What DSM-5 diagnosis would be given to a person with this presentation?

A. Sexual dysfunction due to a general medical condition.

B. Erectile disorder.

C. Somatic symptom disorder.

D. A dual diagnosis of erectile disorder and somatic symptom disorder.

E. No diagnosis.

13.7 A 35-year-old man with new-onset diabetes presents with a 6-month history of inability to maintain an erection. His erectile dysfunction had a sudden onset: he was fired from his job a month before the symptoms began. His serum glucose is well controlled with oral hypoglycemic medication. What is the appropriate DSM-5 diagnosis?

A. Sexual dysfunction due to a general medical condition.

B. Erectile disorder.

C. Adjustment disorder.

D. Unspecified sexual dysfunction.

E. No diagnosis.

13.8 Which of the following factors should be considered during assessment and diagnosis of a sexual dysfunction?

A. Partner factors.

B. Relationship factors.

C. Cultural or religious factors.

D. Individual vulnerability factors, psychiatric comorbidity, or stressors.

E. All of the above.

13.9 A 30-year-old woman comes to your office and reports that she is there only because her mother pleaded with her to see you. She tells you that although she has a good social network with friends of both sexes, she has never had any feelings of sexual arousal in response to men or women, does not have any erotic fantasies, and has little interest in sexual activity. She has found other like-minded individuals, and she and her friends accept themselves as asexual. What is the appropriate diagnosis, if any?

A. Female sexual interest/arousal disorder, lifelong, mild.
B. Female sexual interest/arousal disorder, lifelong, severe.
C. Hypoactive sexual desire disorder.
D. No diagnosis, because she does not have the minimum number of symptoms required (Criterion A) for female sexual interest/arousal disorder.
E. No diagnosis, because she does not have clinically significant distress or impairment.

13.10 Which of the following symptoms or conditions would rule out a diagnosis of erectile disorder?

A. Presence of diabetes mellitus.
B. Marked decrease in erectile rigidity.
C. Age over 60 years.
D. Presence of alcohol use disorder.
E. Presence of symptom for less than 3 months.

13.11 Which of the following statements about the diagnoses of premature (early) ejaculation and delayed ejaculation is *true?*

A. Criterion A for both diagnoses includes a specific time period following penetration during which ejaculation must or must not have occurred.
B. Criterion A for both diagnoses specifies "partnered sexual activity."
C. Early ejaculation, but not delayed ejaculation, may be diagnosed even when there is no clinically significant distress.
D. Estimated and measured intravaginal ejaculatory latencies are poorly correlated.
E. For both diagnoses, the severity is based on the level of distress experienced by the individual.

13.12 Which of the following statements about sexual dysfunction occurring in the context of substance or medication use is *true?*

A. It is more frequently caused by buprenorphine than by methadone.
B. It occurs more commonly in 3,4-methylenedioxymethamphetamine (MDMA) abusers than in heroin abusers.
C. It occurs in approximately 50% of patients taking antipsychotics.

D. Less than 10% of individuals with orgasm delay from antidepressants will experience spontaneous remission of the dysfunction within 6 months.
E. The overall incidence and prevalence of medication-induced sexual dysfunction are well delineated, based on extensive research.

13.13 Which of the following conditions would be appropriately diagnosed as "other specified sexual dysfunction"?

A. Substance/medication-induced sexual dysfunction.
B. Sexual aversion.
C. Erectile dysfunction.
D. Female sexual interest/arousal disorder.
E. Delayed ejaculation.

CHAPTER 14

Gender Dysphoria

14.1   In order for a child to meet criteria for a diagnosis of gender dysphoria, which of the following *must* be present?

   A. A co-occurring disorder of sex development.
   B. A strong desire to be of the other gender or an insistence that one *is* the other gender.
   C. A strong dislike of one's sexual anatomy.
   D. A stated wish to change gender.
   E. A strong desire for the primary and/or secondary sex characteristics that match one's experienced gender.

14.2   Which of the following statements about the diagnosis of gender dysphoria in adolescents and adults is *true*?

   A. The "posttransition" specifier is used to indicate that the individual has undergone or is pursuing treatment procedures to support the new gender assignment.
   B. To qualify for the diagnosis, the individual must be pursuing some kind of sex reassignment treatment.
   C. To qualify for the diagnosis, the individual must have a strong desire to be the other gender or must insist that he or she *is* the other gender.
   D. To qualify for the diagnosis, the individual must have an associated disorder of sex development.
   E. To qualify for the diagnosis, the individual must engage in cross-dressing behavior.

14.3   Match each of the following terms (A–E) to its correct definition (i–v).

   A. Transgender.
   B. Gender.
   C. Sex.
   D. Transsexual.
   E. Gender dysphoria.

   i. The biological indicators of male or female seen in an individual.
   ii. The distress that may accompany the incongruence between one's experienced or expressed gender and one's assigned gender.
   iii. An individual's lived role in society as boy or girl, man or woman.

iv. An individual who transiently or persistently identifies with a gender different from his or her natal gender.

v. An individual who seeks, or has undergone, a social transition from male to female or female to male.

14.4 Which of the following statements about gender is *true*?

A. An individual's gender cannot always be predicted from his or her biological indicators.
B. An individual's gender is determined by cultural factors.
C. An individual's gender is determined by assignment at birth (natal gender).
D. An individual's gender is determined by psychological factors.
E. An individual's gender cannot be determined when there is a concurrent disorder of sexual development.

14.5 What new DSM-5 diagnosis has re placed the former DSM-IV diagnosis of gender identity disorder?

A. Gender aversion disorder.
B. Gender dysmorphic disorder.
C. Gender dysphoria.
D. Cross-gender identity disorder.
E. Gender incongruence.

CHAPTER 15

Disruptive, Impulse-Control, and Conduct Disorders

15.1 An 11-year-old boy has shown extreme stubbornness and defiance since early childhood. This behavior is seen primarily at home and does not typically involve significant mood instability or anger, although he occasionally can be spiteful and vindictive. These symptoms have affected his sibling relationships in an extremely negative fashion, and more recently this behavior has been seen with peers and has begun to affect his friendships. His parents demonstrate a somewhat hostile parenting style. Which of the following statements correctly summarizes the appropriateness of a diagnosis of oppositional defiant disorder (ODD) for this patient?

A. The boy does not qualify for a diagnosis of ODD because his symptoms lack a significant mood component and seem to be confined primarily to the home setting.

B. Although the boy does not have a persistently negative mood, he may nevertheless qualify for a diagnosis of ODD if he meets the other symptom criteria.

C. If as a preschooler the boy had demonstrated temper outbursts that occurred on a weekly basis on most days during a 6-week period, he might have received a diagnosis of ODD at that point, as long as he had four or more of the required symptoms for 6 months.

D. The boy does not qualify for a diagnosis of ODD; the hostile parenting style is probably the cause of his oppositional behavior.

E. If the boy meets criteria for ODD, then he probably has begun to acknowledge his own role in overreacting to reasonable demands.

15.2 A 3-year-old boy has rather severe temper tantrums that have occurred at least weekly for a 6-week period. Although the tantrums can sometimes be associated with defiant behavior, they often result from a change in routine, fatigue, or hunger, and he only rarely does anything destructive. He is generally well behaved in nursery school and during periods between his tantrums. Which of the following conclusions best fits this child's presentation?

A. The boy does not meet criteria for oppositional defiant disorder (ODD).

B. The boy meets criteria for ODD because of the presence of tantrums and defiant behavior.

C. The boy could be diagnosed with ODD as long as it does not appear that his home environment is harsh, neglectful, or inconsistent.

D. The boy's symptoms more likely represent intermittent explosive disorder than ODD.

E. The boy's symptoms more likely represent disruptive mood dysregulation disorder than ODD.

15.3 The diagnostic criteria for oppositional defiant disorder (ODD) include specifiers for indicating severity of the disorder as manifested by pervasiveness of symptoms across settings and relationships. Which of the following specifiers would be appropriate for an 11-year-old boy who meets Criterion A symptoms in two settings?

A. Mild.

B. Moderate.

C. Severe.

D. Extreme.

E. There is not enough information to code the specifier.

15.4 A previously well-behaved 13-year-old girl begins to display extremely defiant and oppositional behavior, with vindictiveness. She is angry, argumentative, and refuses to accept responsibility for her behavior, which is affecting both her home life and school life in a significant way. What is the *least likely* diagnosis?

A. Major depressive disorder.

B. Bipolar disorder.

C. Oppositional defiant disorder.

D. Adjustment disorder.

E. Substance use disorder.

15.5 Which of the following statements about prevalence/course of and risk factors for oppositional defiant disorder (ODD) is *false?*

A. ODD is more prevalent in boys than in girls by a ratio of 1.4:1.

B. Harsh, inconsistent, or neglectful child-rearing practices are common in the families of individuals with ODD.

C. ODD tends to be moderately stable across childhood and adolescence.

D. Individuals with ODD as children or adolescents are at higher risk as adults for difficulties with antisocial behavior, impulse-control problems, anxiety, substance abuse, and depression.

E. Biological factors such as lower heart rate and skin conductance reactivity, reduced basal cortisol reactivity, and abnormalities in the prefrontal cortex and the amygdala have been associated with ODD and can be used diagnostically.

15.6　A 16-year-old boy with a long history of defiant behavior toward authority figures also has a history of aggression toward peers (gets into fights at school), toward his parents, and toward objects (punching holes in walls, breaking doors). He frequently lies, and he has recently begun to steal merchandise from stores and money and jewelry from his parents. He does not seem pervasively irritable or depressed, and he has no sleep disturbance or psychotic symptoms. What is the most likely diagnosis?

A. Oppositional defiant disorder (ODD).
B. Conduct disorder.
C. Attention-deficit/hyperactivity disorder (ADHD).
D. Major depressive disorder.
E. Disruptive mood dysregulation disorder.

15.7　A 15-year-old boy has a history of episodic violent behavior that is out of proportion to the precipitant. During a typical episode, which will escalate rapidly, he will become extremely angry, punching holes in walls or destroying furniture in the home. There seems to be no specific purpose or gain associated with the outbursts, and within 30 minutes he is calm and "back to himself," a state that is not associated with any predominant mood disturbance. What diagnosis best fits this clinical picture?

A. Bipolar disorder.
B. Disruptive mood dysregulation disorder (DMDD).
C. Intermittent explosive disorder (IED).
D. Conduct disorder.
E. Attention-deficit/hyperactivity disorder (ADHD).

15.8　Which of the following statements about the risk and prognostic factors in intermittent explosive disorder (IED) is *true?*

A. First-degree relatives of individuals with IED show no increased risk of having IED themselves.
B. The etiology for the disorder is thought to be predominantly environmentally determined, and twin studies have not demonstrated a significant genetic influence for the impulsive aggression.
C. Individuals with antisocial personality disorder or borderline personality disorder and those who have a history of disorders with disruptive behaviors (e.g., attention-deficit/hyperactivity disorder [ADHD], conduct disorder, oppositional defiant disorder) are at greater risk of comorbid IED.
D. The course of IED is usually not chronic and persistent.
E. The prevalence in males versus females across cultures and studies is consistently about 4:1.

15.9   Which of the following biological markers is associated with intermittent explosive disorder (IED)?

A. Serotonergic abnormalities globally and in the limbic system and orbitofrontal cortex.
B. Reduced amygdala responses to anger stimuli during functional magnetic resonance imaging (fMRI) scanning.
C. Atrophy of the cerebral cortex.
D. Abnormalities in adrenal function.
E. Increased urinary catecholamines.

15.10   Which of the following statements about the differential diagnosis of intermittent explosive disorder (IED) is *false?*

A. The diagnosis of IED can be made even if the impulsive aggressive outbursts occur in the context of an adjustment disorder.
B. In contrast to IED, disruptive mood dysregulation disorder is characterized by a persistently negative mood state (i.e., irritability, anger) most of the day, nearly every day, between impulsive aggressive outbursts.
C. The level of impulsive aggression in individuals with antisocial personality disorder or borderline personality disorder is lower than that in individuals with IED.
D. A diagnosis of IED should not be made when aggressive outbursts are judged to result from the physiological effects of another diagnosable medical condition.
E. Aggression in oppositional defiant disorder is typically characterized by temper tantrums and verbal arguments with authority figures, whereas impulsive aggressive outbursts in IED are in response to a broader array of provocation and include physical assault.

15.11   A 17-year-old boy with a history of bullying and initiating fights using bats and knives has also stolen from others, set fires, destroyed property, broken into homes, and "conned" others. This pattern of disturbed conduct covers all of the Criterion A behavior categories *except*

A. Aggression to people and animals.
B. Destruction of property.
C. Deceitfulness or theft.
D. Serious violations of rules.
E. Malevolent intent.

15.12   A 15-year-old girl with a history of cruelty to animals, stealing, school truancy, and running away from home shows no remorse when caught, or when she is confronted with how her behavior is affecting the rest of her family. She disregards the feelings of others and seems to not care that her conduct is compromising her school performance. The behavior has been present for over a year and in multiple relationships and settings. Which of the following components of the "With limited prosocial emotions" specifier is absent in this clinical picture?

A. Lack of remorse or guilt.
B. Callous—lack of empathy.
C. Lack of concern about performance.
D. Shallow or deficient affect.
E. The required time duration.

15.13 Which of the following does *not* qualify as aggressive behavior under Criterion A definitions for the diagnosis of conduct disorder?

A. Cyberbullying.
B. Forcing someone into sexual activity.
C. Stealing while confronting a victim.
D. Being physically cruel to people.
E. Aggression in the context of a mood disorder.

15.14 In order to be considered a symptom of conduct disorder, running away must have occurred with what frequency?

A. At least three times.
B. At least five times.
C. Only once if the individual did not return for a lengthy period.
D. Twice, in response to physical or sexual abuse.
E. Six times over a 3-month period.

15.15 Which of the following statements about childhood versus adolescent onset of conduct disorder (CD) is *true*?

A. Compared with individuals with adolescent-onset CD, those with child-hood-onset CD are more often female and tend to get along better with peers.
B. Compared with individuals with adolescent-onset CD, those with child-hood-onset CD are less aggressive and less likely to have oppositional defiant disorder (ODD) or attention-deficit/hyperactivity disorder (ADHD).
C. Compared with individuals with childhood-onset CD, those with adolescent-onset CD are more likely to have CD that persists into adulthood.
D. Compared with individuals with childhood-onset CD, those with adolescent-onset CD are more likely to display aggressive behaviors and to have disturbed peer relationships.
E. Compared with individuals with childhood-onset CD, those with adolescent-onset CD are less likely to have CD that persists into adulthood.

15.16 Which of the following statements about individuals who qualify for the "With limited prosocial emotions" specifier for conduct disorder is *true*?

A. These individuals generally display personality features such as risk avoidance, fearfulness, and extreme sensitivity to punishment.
B. These individuals are less likely than other individuals with conduct disorder to engage in aggression that is planned for instrumental gain.
C. These individuals generally exert more effort in their activities compared with other individuals with conduct disorder, and consequently are more successful.
D. These individuals are more likely to have a severity specifier rating of mild.
E. These individuals are more likely to have the childhood-onset type of conduct disorder.

15.17 Which of the following statements about the prevalence of conduct disorder is *true*?

A. One-year prevalence rates range from 5% to 15%, with a median of 7%.
B. The prevalence varies widely across countries that differ in race and ethnicity.
C. Prevalence rates are higher among males than among females.
D. Callous unemotional traits are present in more than half of individuals with conduct disorder.
E. Prevalence rates remain fairly constant from childhood to adolescence.

15.18 Which of the following statements about the onset and developmental course of conduct disorder is *true*?

A. Onset may occur as early as the preschool years and is rare after age 16 years.
B. Onset typically occurs in adolescence.
C. Age at onset has no bearing on the developmental course of the disorder.
D. Oppositional defiant disorder is generally not a precursor to the childhood-onset type of conduct disorder.
E. Those with the adolescent-onset type of conduct disorder are less likely to adjust successfully as adults.

15.19 Which of the following statements about risk factors in conduct disorder is *false*?

A. A difficult undercontrolled infant temperament and lower-than-average verbal IQ are risk factors for conduct disorder.
B. Family-based risk factors include parental rejection and neglect, inconsistent child-rearing practices, harsh discipline, physical or sexual abuse, lack of supervision, early institutional living, frequent changes of caregivers, large family size, and substance-related disorders.

C. Community-level risk factors include association with a delinquent peer group and neighborhood exposure to violence.

D. The risk of conduct disorder is increased in children who have a biological or adoptive parent or sibling with conduct disorder.

E. Parental history of attention-deficit/hyperactivity disorder (ADHD) does not constitute a risk factor for conduct disorder in offspring.

15.20 Which of the following statements about risk and prognostic factors in conduct disorder (CD) is *false?*

A. Individuals with CD are at risk of later depressive and bipolar disorders, anxiety disorders, posttraumatic stress disorder, impulse control disorders, somatic symptom disorders, and substance-related disorders as adults.

B. Temperamental risk factors for CD include a difficult undercontrolled infant temperament and lower-than-average intelligence, particularly in regard to verbal IQ.

C. Structural and functional differences in brain areas associated with affect regulation and affect processing have been consistently noted in individuals with CD.

D. The risk that CD will persist into adulthood is increased by co-occurring attention-deficit/hyperactivity disorder and by substance abuse.

E. Increased autonomic fear conditioning, particularly high skin conductance, is well documented and diagnostic of CD.

15.21 Which of the following statements about the differential diagnosis of conduct disorder (CD) and oppositional defiant disorder (ODD) is *true?*

A. In both diagnoses, individuals tend to have conflict with authority figures.

B. In both diagnoses, individuals display significant emotional dysregulation.

C. In both diagnoses, individuals display aggression toward people or animals.

D. In both diagnoses, individuals destroy property, steal, or lie.

E. If criteria for CD are met, then an individual cannot also receive a diagnosis of ODD.

15.22 Which of the following comorbid disorders is associated with pyromania?

A. Antisocial personality disorder.

B. Substance use disorders.

C. Mood disorders.

D. Gambling disorder.

E. All of the above.

15.23 A 15-year-old male student in private school, without known psychiatric history, has been caught stealing other students' laptops and cell phones, even though he comes from a wealthy family and his parents continue to purchase the newest electronics for him in an effort to deter him from stealing. Which of the following would raise your clinical suspicion that he may have kleptomania?

A. He demonstrates recurrent failure to resist impulses to steal objects that are not needed for personal use or for their monetary value.
B. He demonstrates recurrent failure to resist impulses to steal objects during periods of detachment or boredom.
C. He experiences increased tension before committing the theft but does not experience relief, pleasure, or gratification while committing the theft.
D. He has a strong family history for antisocial personality disorder and conduct disorder.
E. He has a strong family history for bipolar disorder.

15.24 Which of the following statements about kleptomania is *false?*

A. The prevalence of kleptomania in the general population is generally very low, and the disorder more frequent among females.
B. First-degree relatives of individuals with kleptomania may have higher rates of obsessive-compulsive disorder and/or substance use disorders than the general population.
C. Kleptomania is similar to ordinary theft in that the act of shoplifting, whether planned or impulsive, is deliberate and often motivated by the usefulness of the object.
D. The age at onset is variable, but the disorder often begins in adolescence.
E. Individuals with kleptomania generally do not preplan their thefts.

C H A P T E R   1 6

Substance-Related and Addictive Disorders

16.1 The diagnostic criteria for substance abuse, substance dependence, substance intoxication, and substance withdrawal were not equally applicable to all substances in DSM-IV. In DSM-5, this remains true, although *substance use disorder* now replaces the diagnoses of *substance abuse* and *substance dependence*. For which of the following substance classes is there adequate evidence to support diagnostic criteria in DSM-5 for the three major categories of *use disorder, intoxication,* and *withdrawal?*

A. Caffeine.
B. Cannabis.
C. Tobacco.
D. Hallucinogen.
E. Inhalant.

16.2 Almost all of the possible physical and behavioral symptom criteria included in the DSM-IV definitions of *substance abuse* and *substance dependence* are included in the DSM-5 definition of *substance use disorder*. Which of the following possible criteria included in DSM-IV were intentionally *omitted* in DSM-5?

A. There is a persistent desire or unsuccessful efforts to cut down or control substance use.
B. The substance is often taken in larger amounts or over a longer period than was intended.
C. The recurrent substance use results in a failure to fulfill major role obligations at work, school, or home.
D. There is continued substance use despite having persistent or recurrent social or interpersonal problems caused or exacerbated by the effects of the substance.
E. There are recurrent substance-related legal problems.

16.3 Whereas in DSM-IV, there were 11 recognized substance classes, DSM-5 has only 10, because certain related substances have been combined into a single class. Which of the following pairs of drugs falls into a single class in DSM-5?

A. Cocaine and phencyclidine (PCP).
B. Cocaine and methamphetamine.

C. 3,4-Methylenedioxymethamphetamine (MDMA [Ecstasy]) and methamphetamine.

D. Lorazepam and alcohol.

E. Lorazepam and oxycodone.

16.4 Tolerance and withdrawal were each considered valid criteria for the diagnosis of substance dependence in DSM-IV, although neither was required. Which of the following statements about tolerance and withdrawal in the DSM-5 diagnosis of substance use disorder is *true*?

A. Tolerance and withdrawal are no longer considered to be valid diagnostic symptoms of substance use disorder.

B. The definitions of tolerance and withdrawal have been updated because the previous definitions had poor interrater reliability.

C. The presence of either tolerance or withdrawal is now required to make a diagnosis of substance use disorder.

D. The presence of either tolerance or withdrawal is now required to make a substance use disorder diagnosis for some but not all classes of substances.

E. Both tolerance and withdrawal are still listed as possible criteria, but if they occur during appropriate medically supervised treatment, they may not be counted toward the diagnosis of a substance use disorder.

16.5 Which of the following is *not* a recognized alcohol-related disorder in DSM-5?

A. Alcohol dependence.

B. Alcohol use disorder.

C. Alcohol intoxication.

D. Alcohol withdrawal.

E. Alcohol-induced sexual dysfunction.

16.6 Which of the following statements about caffeine-related disorders is *true*?

A. Culturally appropriate levels of caffeine intake should be considered when making the diagnosis of caffeine intoxication.

B. In order to diagnose caffeine intoxication, at least one symptom must begin during caffeine use.

C. The diagnosis of caffeine withdrawal requires the preceding use of caffeine on a daily basis.

D. Caffeine withdrawal may be diagnosed even in the absence of clinically significant distress or impairment in social, occupational, or other important areas of functioning.

E. Extensive data are available regarding the prevalence of caffeine use disorder.

16.7 Which of the following symptoms is a recognized consequence of the abrupt termination of daily or near-daily cannabis use?

A. Hallucinations.
B. Delusions.
C. Hunger.
D. Irritability.
E. Apathy.

16.8 The Criterion A symptoms listed for *other hallucinogen use disorder* are the same as those listed for use disorders of most other substance classes, with one exception. Which of the following is *not* a recognized symptom associated with hallucinogen use?

A. Withdrawal.
B. Tolerance.
C. A persistent desire or unsuccessful efforts to cut down or control use of the substance.
D. Recurrent use of the substance in situations in which it is physically hazardous.
E. Craving, or a strong desire or urge to use the substance.

16.9 To meet proposed criteria for the Section III condition *neurobehavioral disorder associated with prenatal alcohol exposure,* an individual's prenatal alcohol exposure must have been "more than minimal." How is "more than minimal" exposure defined, in terms of how much alcohol was used by the mother during gestation?

A. Fewer than 7 drinks per month, and no more than 1 drink per drinking occasion.
B. Fewer than 7 drinks per month, and no more than 2 drinks per drinking occasion.
C. Fewer than 7 drinks per month, and no more than 3 drinks per drinking occasion.
D. Fewer than 14 drinks per month, and no more than 1 drink per drinking occasion.
E. Fewer than 14 drinks per month, and no more than 2 drinks per drinking occasion.

16.10 Which of the following is the only non-substance-related disorder to be included in the DSM-5 chapter "Substance-Related and Addictive Disorders"?

A. Gambling disorder.
B. Internet gaming disorder.
C. Electronic communication addiction disorder.

D. Compulsive computer use disorder.

E. Compulsive shopping.

16.11 In most substance/medication-induced mental disorders (with the exception of substance/medication-induced major or mild neurocognitive disorder and hallucinogen persisting perception disorder), if the person abstains from substance use, the disorder will eventually disappear or no longer be clinically relevant even without formal treatment. In what time frame is this likely to happen?

A. One hour.

B. One month.

C. Three months.

D. One year.

E. "Relatively quickly" but no specific period of time.

16.12 Because opioid withdrawal and sedative, hypnotic, or anxiolytic withdrawal can involve very similar symptoms, distinguishing between the two can be difficult. Which of the following presenting symptoms would aid in making the correct diagnosis?

A. Nausea or vomiting.

B. Anxiety.

C. Yawning.

D. Restlessness or agitation.

E. Insomnia.

16.13 In DSM-5, the sedative, hypnotic, or anxiolytic class contains all prescription sleeping medications and almost all prescription antianxiety medications. What is the reason that nonbenzodiazepine antianxiety agents (e.g., buspirone, gepirone) are *not* included in this class?

A. They are not generally available in nonparenteral (intravenous or intramuscular) formulations.

B. They do not appear to be associated with significant misuse.

C. They are not associated with illicit manufacturing or diversion (e.g., Schedule I–V drugs in the United States, or included in the list of psychotropic substances recognized by the International Narcotics Control Board and the United Nations).

D. They are not respiratory depressants.

E. They do not appear to be associated with cravings or tolerance.

16.14 Which of the following criteria for substance use disorder in DSM-5 was *not* one of the criteria for either substance abuse or substance dependence in DSM-IV?

A. Important social, occupational, or recreational activities are given up or reduced because of substance use.
B. The substance is often taken in larger amounts or over a longer period than was intended.
C. Craving, or a strong desire or urge to use the substance, is present.
D. Recurrent substance use results in a failure to fulfill major role obligations at work, school, or home.
E. A great deal of time is spent in activities necessary to obtain the substance, use the substance, or recover from its effects.

16.15 A 27-year-old woman presents for psychiatric evaluation after almost hitting someone with her car while driving under the influence of marijuana. She reports that she was prompted to seek treatment by her husband, with whom she has had several conflicts over the past year about her ongoing marijuana use. She has continued to smoke two joints daily and drive while under the influence of marijuana since this event. What is the appropriate diagnosis?

A. Cannabis abuse.
B. Cannabis dependence.
C. Cannabis intoxication.
D. Cannabis use disorder.
E. Unspecified cannabis-related disorder.

16.16 A 45-year-old man with a long-standing history of heavy alcohol use is referred for psychiatric evaluation after his recent admission to the hospital for acute hepatitis. The patient reports that he drank almost daily in college. Over the past 10 years, he has gradually increased his nightly alcohol intake from a single 6-pack to two 12-packs of beer, and this nightly drinking habit has resulted in his frequently oversleeping and missing work. He has tried to moderate his alcohol use on numerous occasions with little success, particularly after developing complications associated with alcoholic cirrhosis. The patient admits that he becomes anxious and gets hand tremors when he doesn't drink. This patient meets the criteria for which of the following diagnoses?

A. Alcohol abuse.
B. Alcohol dependence.
C. Alcohol use disorder, mild.
D. Alcohol use disorder, moderate.
E. Alcohol use disorder, severe.

16.17 Which of the following statements about alcohol withdrawal is *true?*

A. Fewer than 10% of individuals undergoing alcohol withdrawal experience dramatic symptoms such as severe autonomic hyperactivity, tremors, or alcohol withdrawal delirium.
B. Delirium occurs in the majority of individuals who meet criteria for alcohol withdrawal.

C. Approximately 80% of all patients with alcohol use disorder will experience alcohol withdrawal.

D. Tonic-clonic seizures occur in about 15% of individuals who meet criteria for alcohol withdrawal.

E. Alcohol withdrawal symptoms typically begin between 24 and 48 hours after alcohol use has been stopped or reduced.

16.18 How many remission specifiers are included in the DSM-5 diagnostic criteria for substance use disorders?

A. One.
B. Two.
C. Three.
D. Four.
E. Five.

16.19 A 25-year-old woman is brought to the emergency department by her friends after a party. They report that the woman had been seen ingesting some unknown pills earlier in the evening. She became increasingly confused throughout the course of the night. She eventually had a witnessed seizure on the street, prompting activation of emergency medical services. Vital signs indicate that the patient is tachycardic and hypertensive. On evaluation, the patient is observed to be thin with dilated pupils. She is smiling to herself, is fidgety, and is oriented to self, place, and date. When queried about auditory hallucinations, the patient admits that she is hearing voices but is unconcerned, stating, "I only hear them while I'm partying, Doc." Which diagnosis best fits this clinical presentation?

A. Stimulant-induced manic episode.
B. Stimulant-induced psychotic disorder.
C. Stimulant intoxication, with perceptual disturbances.
D. Other hallucinogen-induced psychotic disorder.
E. Other hallucinogen intoxication.

16.20 Which of the following substances is most likely to be associated with poly-drug use?

A. Cannabis.
B. Tobacco.
C. 3,4-Methylenedioxymethamphetamine (MDMA [Ecstasy]).
D. Methamphetamine.
E. Alcohol.

16.21 Alcohol intoxication, inhalant intoxication, and sedative, hypnotic, or anxiolytic intoxication have which of the following Criterion C signs/symptoms in
common?

A. Depressed reflexes.
B. Generalized muscle weakness.
C. Blurred vision.
D. Impairment in attention or memory.
E. Nystagmus.

16.22 In DSM-IV, caffeine withdrawal was included in Appendix B as a criteria set
provided for further study. Which of the following statements correctly describes how caffeine withdrawal is classified in DSM-5?

A. Caffeine withdrawal is no longer considered a valid psychiatric diagnosis.
B. Caffeine withdrawal remains a proposed diagnosis in DSM-5 and is in-
cluded in "Conditions for Further Study" in Section III.
C. Caffeine withdrawal is classified under *other (or unknown) substance with-
drawal* in DSM-5.
D. Caffeine withdrawal is classified under *stimulant withdrawal* in DSM-5.
E. Caffeine withdrawal was moved to the main body of DSM-5 and is now in-
cluded in the "Substance-Related and Addictive Disorders" chapter.

16.23 A 25-year-old medical student presents to the student health service at 7 A.M.
complaining of having a "panic attack." He reports that he stayed up all night
studying for his final gross anatomy exam, which starts in an hour, but he feels
too anxious to go. He reports vomiting twice. The patient is restless and appears flushed, with visible muscle twitching. He is urinating excessively, has
tachycardia, and his electrocardiogram shows premature ventricular complexes. His thoughts and speech appear to be rambling in nature. His urine toxicology screen is negative. What is the most likely diagnosis?

A. Panic disorder.
B. Amphetamine intoxication, amphetamine-like substance.
C. Caffeine intoxication.
D. Cocaine intoxication.
E. Alcohol withdrawal.

16.24 Which substance use disorder of an illicit substance is the most prevalent in the
United States?

A. Alcohol use disorder.
B. Caffeine use disorder.
C. Cannabis use disorder.
D. Opioid use disorder.
E. Stimulant use disorder.

16.25 Which of the following laboratory tests can be used in combination with gamma-glutamyltransferase (GGT) to monitor abstinence from alcohol?

A. Alanine aminotransferase (ALT).
B. Alkaline phosphatase.
C. Carbohydrate-deficient transferrin (CDT).
D. Mean corpuscular volume (MCV).
E. Triglycerides.

16.26 Which substance or class of substances in the Substance-Related and Addictive Disorders chapter of DSM-5 is *not* associated with a substance use disorder?

A. Caffeine.
B. Hallucinogens.
C. Inhalants.
D. Stimulants.
E. Tobacco.

16.27 What is the hallmark feature of caffeine withdrawal?

A. Vomiting.
B. Drowsiness.
C. Flu-like symptoms.
D. Headache.
E. Dysphoria.

16.28 Which mental disorder or disorder class has the highest prevalence among individuals with cannabis use disorder?

A. Major depressive disorder.
B. Bipolar I disorder.
C. Anxiety disorders.
D. Schizophrenia spectrum and other psychotic disorders.
E. Conduct disorder.

16.29 Which personality disorder has the highest prevalence among individuals with cannabis use disorder?

A. Obsessive-compulsive personality disorder.
B. Paranoid personality disorder.
C. Schizotypal personality disorder.
D. Borderline personality disorder.
E. Antisocial personality disorder.

16.30 What are the three main chemical classes of hallucinogens?

A. Ethnobotanical compounds, ergolines, and phenylalkylamines.
B. Ethnobotanical compounds, ergolines, and indoleamines.
C. Indoleamines, ergolines, and phenylalkylamines.
D. Tryptoamines, indoleamines, and ergolines.
E. Tryptoamines, phenylalkylamines, and hydrocarbons.

16.31 Which of the following statements about 3,4-methylenedioxymethamphet-amine (MDMA [Ecstasy]) is *false?*

A. Relative to use of other hallucinogenic drugs, use of MDMA increases the risk of developing a hallucinogen use disorder.
B. MDMA has both hallucinogenic and stimulant properties.
C. MDMA is more likely than other drugs in this class to be associated with withdrawal symptoms.
D. MDMA has a shorter half-life relative to other hallucinogens.
E. MDMA can be administered via inhalation and injection whereas most other hallucinogens are ingested orally and occasionally smoked.

16.32 Which of the following substance use disorders is more common among adolescent males than among adolescent females?

A. Other hallucinogen use disorder.
B. Inhalant use disorder.
C. Sedative, hypnotic, or anxiolytic use disorder.
D. Stimulant use disorder, cocaine subtype.
E. Stimulant use disorder, amphetamine-type substance subtype.

16.33 Which two groups of inhalant agents are *not* among the recognized substances qualifying for the DSM-5 inhalant use disorder diagnosis?

A. Butane lighters and toluene.
B. Xylene and butane.
C. Trichloroethane and hexane.
D. Nitrous oxide and nitrite gases.
E. Gasoline and cleaning compounds.

16.34 Match each of the following substances (A–E) with the population subgroup (i–v) most associated with its use, according to epidemiological data included in DSM-5.

A. Amphetamines.
B. *Salvia divinorum.*
C. Air fresheners and hair sprays.

D. Gasoline.

E. Cannabis.

   i. 18- to 29-year-olds.

   ii. 18- to 25-year-olds with risk-taking behaviors.

  iii. Adolescent boys.

  iv. Adolescent girls.

   v. Adult males.

16.35 A 22-year-old university student presents to his primary care physician complaining of progressive worsening of numbness, tingling, and weakness in both of his legs over the past several weeks. His gait is unsteady, and he has difficulty grasping objects in his hands. He did not use any substances on the day of presentation but admits that over the past 3 months he has been consistently using one particular substance on a daily basis. Which substance use disorder most likely accounts for this patient's symptoms?

A. Cannabis use disorder.

B. Other hallucinogen use disorder.

C. Inhalant use disorder.

D. Opioid use disorder.

E. Other (or unknown) substance use disorder.

16.36 Which organ system or anatomical function is most commonly affected by chronic use of 3,4-methylenedioxymethamphetamine (MDMA [Ecstasy])?

A. Neurological.

B. Respiratory.

C. Cardiopulmonary.

D. Oral cavity.

E. Immunological/infectious.

16.37 What percentage of individuals who undergo untreated sedative, hypnotic, or anxiolytic withdrawal experience a grand mal seizure?

A. 5%–10%.

B. 10%–20%.

C. 20%–30%.

D. 30%–40%.

E. 40%–50%.

16.38 Which route of stimulant use is most prevalent among individuals who are in treatment for a stimulant use disorder?

A. Oral.

B. Intranasal.

C. Smoking.
D. Intravenous.
E. Mixed routes.

16.39 What is the most common co-occurring psychiatric diagnosis among individuals with a history of significant prenatal alcohol exposure?

A. Major depressive disorder.
B. Generalized anxiety disorder.
C. Attention-deficit/hyperactivity disorder.
D. Oppositional defiant disorder.
E. Substance use disorder.

CHAPTER 17

Neurocognitive Disorders

17.1 The essential feature of the DSM-5 diagnosis of delirium is a disturbance in attention/awareness and in cognition that develops over a short period of time, represents a change from baseline, and tends to fluctuate in severity during the course of a day. Which of the following additional conditions must apply?

A. There must be laboratory evidence of an evolving dementia.
B. The disturbance must be associated with a disruption of the sleep-wake cycle.
C. The disturbance must not occur in the context of a severely reduced level of arousal, such as coma.
D. The disturbance must be a direct physiological consequence of a substance use disorder.
E. The disturbance must not be superimposed on a preexisting neurocognitive disorder.

17.2 Both major and mild neurocognitive disorders can increase the risk of delirium and complicate its course. Traditionally, delirium is distinguished from dementia on the basis of the key features of acute onset, impairment in attention, and which of the following?

A. Fluctuating course.
B. Steady course.
C. Presence of mania.
D. Presence of depression.
E. Cogwheeling movements.

17.3 A 79-year-old woman with a history of depression is being evaluated at a nursing home for a suspected urinary tract infection. She is easily distracted, perseverates on answers to questions, asks the same question repeatedly, is unable to focus, and cannot answer questions regarding orientation. The mental status changes evolved over a single day. Her family reports that they thought she "wasn't herself" when they saw her the previous evening, but the nursing report this morning indicates that the patient was cordial and appropriate. What is the most likely diagnosis?

A. Major depressive disorder, recurrent episode.
B. Depressive disorder due to another medical condition.
C. Delirium.

D. Major depressive disorder, with anxious distress.

E. Obsessive-compulsive disorder.

17.4 The diagnostic criteria for major or mild neurocognitive disorder with Lewy bodies (NCDLB) include fulfillment of criteria for major or mild neurocognitive disorder and presence of "a combination of core diagnostic features and suggested diagnostic features for either probable or possible neurocognitive disorder with Lewy bodies." Another feature necessary for the diagnosis is that "the disturbance is not better explained by cerebrovascular disease, another neurodegenerative disease, the effects of a substance, or another mental, neurological, or systemic disorder." Which of the following completes the list of features necessary for the diagnosis?

A. An acute onset and rapid progression.

B. An insidious onset and gradual progression.

C. An insidious onset and rapid progression.

D. A waxing and waning presentation.

E. A characteristic finding on ultrasound of the neck.

17.5 Which of the following is *not* a diagnostic criterion, feature, or marker of major or mild neurocognitive disorder with Lewy bodies (NCDLB)?

A. Concurrent symptoms of rapid eye movement (REM) sleep behavior disorder.

B. High striatal dopamine transporter uptake in basal ganglia demonstrated by single-photon emission computed tomography (SPECT) or positron emission tomography (PET) imaging.

C. Low striatal dopamine transporter uptake in basal ganglia demonstrated by SPECT or PET imaging.

D. Severe neuroleptic sensitivity.

E. Insidious onset and gradual progression.

17.6 A 72-year-old man with no history of alcohol or other substance use disorders and no psychiatric history is brought to the emergency department (ED) because of transient episodes of unexplained loss of consciousness. His wife reports that he has experienced repeated falls and syncope over the past year, as well as auditory and visual hallucinations. A thorough workup for cardiac disease has found no evidence of structural heart disease or arrhythmias. In the ED, he is found to have severe autonomic dysfunction, including orthostatic hypotension and urinary incontinence. What is the best provisional diagnosis for this patient?

A. New-onset schizophrenia.

B. New-onset schizoaffective disorder.

C. Possible major or mild neurocognitive disorder with Lewy bodies.

D. Possible major or mild neurocognitive disorder due to Alzheimer's disease.

E. New-onset seizure disorder.

17.7　The diagnostic criteria for neurocognitive disorder (NCD) due to HIV infection include fulfillment of criteria for major or mild NCD and documented infection with human immunodeficiency virus (as confirmed by established laboratory methods). Which of the following is a prominent feature of NCD due to HIV infection?

A. Impairment in executive functioning.
B. Conspicuous aphasia.
C. Significant delusions and hallucinations at onset of the disorder.
D. Marked difficulty with recall of learned information.
E. Rapid progression to profound neurocognitive impairment.

17.8　In addition to documented infection with HIV and fulfillment of criteria for major or mild neurocognitive disorder (NCD), what other requirement must be met to qualify for a diagnosis of major or mild NCD due to HIV infection?

A. Presence of HIV in the cerebrospinal fluid.
B. A pattern of cognitive impairment characterized by early predominance of aphasia and impaired memory for previously learned information.
C. Presence of progressive multifocal leukoencephalopathy.
D. Inability to attribute the NCD to non-HIV conditions (including secondary brain diseases), another medical condition, or a mental disorder.
E. Presence of Kayser-Fleisher rings.

17.9　Which of the following features characterizes alcohol-induced major or mild neurocognitive disorder, amnestic-confabulatory type?

A. Amnesia for new information and confabulation.
B. Seizures.
C. Amnesia for previously learned information and downward gaze paralysis.
D. Aphasia.
E. Anosognosia and apraxia.

17.10　Which of the following statements about the diagnosis of neurocognitive disorder due to Huntington's disease (NCDHD) is *true?*

A. NCDHD is a laboratory-based diagnosis/disorder.
B. NCDHD is a disorder that requires positive neuroimaging for diagnosis.
C. NCDHD is a clinical diagnosis based on abnormal physical findings and family history/genetic findings.
D. NCDHD is a diagnosis that is best defined as patients who have a pill-rolling tremor.
E. NCDHD is a diagnosis mostly based on radiological examination.

17.11 Depression, irritability, anxiety, obsessive-compulsive symptoms, and apathy are frequently associated with Huntington's disease and often precede the onset of motor symptoms. Psychosis more rarely precedes the onset of motor symptoms. Which of the following is a core feature of major or mild neurocognitive disorder due to Huntington's disease?

A. Progressive cognitive impairment with early changes in executive function.
B. Prominent early memory impairment, mostly affecting short-term memory.
C. Psychosis in the early stages, with marked olfactory hallucinations.
D. Voluntary jerking movements.
E. Diminished hearing and smell.

17.12 Genetic testing is the primary laboratory test for the determination of Huntington's disease. Which of the following best characterizes the genetic nature of Huntington's disease?

A. X-linked recessive inheritance with incomplete penetrance.
B. Autosomal recessive inheritance with complete penetrance.
C. Autosomal dominant inheritance with complete penetrance.
D. Random mutation.
E. X-linked dominant inheritance.

17.13 Major or mild neurocognitive disorder (NCD) due to prion disease encompasses NCDs associated with a group of subacute spongiform encephalopathies caused by transmissible agents known as *prions*. What is the most common prion disease?

A. Creutzfeldt-Jakob disease.
B. Wernicke-Korsakoff syndrome.
C. Bovine spongiform encephalopathy.
D. Huntington's disease.
E. Neurosyphilis.

17.14 Prion disease has been reported to occur in individuals of all ages, from the teenage years to late life. Which of the following best characterizes the time frame of disease progression?

A. Over a few months.
B. Over several days.
C. Over several weeks.
D. Over 5 years.
E. Over 10 years.

17.15 Major and mild neurocognitive disorders (NCDs) exist on a spectrum of cognitive and functional impairment. Which of the following constitutes an important threshold differentiating the two diagnoses?

A. Whether or not the individual is concerned about the decline in cognitive function.
B. Whether or not there is impairment in cognitive performance as measured by standardized testing or clinical assessment.
C. Whether or not the cognitive impairment is sufficient to interfere with independent completion of activities of daily living.
D. Whether or not the cognitive deficits occur exclusively in the context of a delirium.
E. Whether or not the cognitive deficits are better explained by another mental disorder.

17.16 Expressed as a percentile, what is the typical performance on neuropsychological testing of individuals with major neurocognitive disorder (NCD)?

A. Sixtieth percentile or below.
B. Fiftieth percentile or below.
C. Twenty-fifth percentile or below.
D. Sixteenth percentile or below.
E. Third percentile or below.

17.17 A 68-year-old semiretired cardiologist with responsibility for electrocardiogram (ECG) interpretation at his community hospital is referred by the hospital's Employee Assistance Program for clinical evaluation because of concerns expressed by other clinicians that he has been making many mistakes in his ECG interpretations over the past few months. The patient discloses symptoms of persistent sadness since the death of his wife 6 months prior to the evaluation, with frequent thoughts of death, trouble sleeping, and escalating usage of sedative-hypnotics and alcohol. He has some trouble concentrating, but he has been able to maintain his household, pay his bills, shop, and prepare meals by himself without difficulty. He scores 28/30 on the Mini-Mental State Examination (MMSE). Which of the following would be the primary consideration in the differential diagnosis?

A. Major neurocognitive disorder (NCD).
B. Mild NCD.
C. Adjustment disorder.
D. Major depressive disorder.
E. No diagnosis.

17.18 A 69-year-old semiretired radiologist with responsibility for chest x-ray interpretation at his academic medical center has been referred by the hospital's Employee Assistance Program for clinical evaluation because of concerns expressed by other clinicians that he has been making many mistakes in his x-ray interpretations over the past few months. Evaluation discloses a remote history of alcohol dependence with sobriety for the past 20 years, and a depressive episode following the death of his wife 9 years before the current problem, treated with cognitive-behavioral therapy with full resolution of symptoms after 6 months and no recurrence. He acknowledges some trouble concentrating but no other symptoms, and he minimizes the alleged x-ray interpretation problems. He cannot state the correct date or day of the week and cannot recall the previous day's news events, but he can describe highlights of his long career in medicine in great detail. Collateral history from his children reveals that on several occasions in the past year neighbors in his apartment building had complained that he forgot to turn off his stove while cooking, resulting in a smoke-filled apartment. He scores 21/30 on the Mini-Mental State Examination. What diagnosis best fits this clinical picture?

A. Major neurocognitive disorder (NCD).
B. Mild NCD.
C. Adjustment disorder.
D. Major depressive disorder.
E. No diagnosis.

17.19 In a patient with *mild* neurocognitive disorder (NCD), which of the following would distinguish *probable* from *possible* Alzheimer's disease?

A. Evidence of a causative Alzheimer's disease genetic mutation from either genetic testing or family history.
B. Clear evidence of decline in memory and learning.
C. Steadily progressive, gradual decline in cognition, without extended plateaus.
D. No evidence of mixed etiology.
E. Onset after age 80.

17.20 In major or mild frontotemporal neurocognitive disorder, which of the following is a diagnostic feature of the language variant?

A. Severe semantic memory impairment.
B. Severe deficits in perceptual-motor function.
C. Receptive aphasia.
D. Grammar, word-finding, or word-generation difficulty.
E. Hyperorality.

17.21 Which of the following neurocognitive disorders (NCDs) is especially characterized by deficits in domains such as speech production, word finding, object naming, or word comprehension, whereas episodic memory, perceptual-motor abilities, and executive function are relatively preserved?

A. Major or mild NCD due to Alzheimer's disease.
B. Major or mild NCD with Lewy bodies.

C. Major or mild vascular NCD.

D. Behavioral-variant major or mild frontotemporal NCD.

E. Language-variant major or mild frontotemporal NCD.

17.22 Which of the following is a core feature of major or mild neurocognitive disorder with Lewy bodies?

A. Fluctuating cognition with pronounced variations in attention and alertness.

B. Recurrent auditory hallucinations.

C. Spontaneous features of parkinsonism, with onset at least 1 year prior to development of cognitive decline.

D. Fulfillment of criteria for rapid eye movement (REM) sleep behavior disorder.

E. Evidence of low striatal dopamine transporter uptake in basal ganglia as demonstrated by single photon emission computed tomography (SPECT) or positron emission tomography (PET) imaging.

17.23 A previously healthy 67-year-old man, who is experiencing an acute change in mental status, is brought to the emergency department by his family. There is no evidence in the initial history, physical examination, and laboratory studies to indicate substance intoxication or withdrawal, or to suggest another medical problem as the cause of his altered mental state. Over the course of 1 hour of observation, his level of alertness varies from alert but distractible, with apparent auditory and visual hallucinations, to somnolent; he has difficulty sustaining attention to an examiner, and he cannot perform simple tasks such as serial subtractions or spelling words backwards. What is the most appropriate diagnosis?

A. Delirium.

B. Delirium due to another medical condition.

C. Delirium due to substance intoxication.

D. Delirium due to multiple etiologies.

E. Unspecified delirium.

17.24 A 35-year-old man brings his 60-year-old father for evaluation of cognitive and functional decline, stating that he thinks his father has dementia; the son is also worried about the possibility of a hereditary illness. The physician notes to herself that the patient has substantial cognitive impairment and features suggestive of the diagnosis of major neurocognitive disorder due to Huntington's disease, but she is not sure about the cause of the neurocognitive disorder. She also notes that the patient's son appears extremely anxious. She has a tight schedule and cannot provide a counseling session for the patient's son until the next day. What is the most appropriate diagnosis to record on the insurance claim form that the patient's son will submit on his father's behalf?

A. Unspecified central nervous system (CNS) disorder.
B. Unspecified neurocognitive disorder.
C. Unspecified mild neurocognitive disorder.
D. Huntington's disease.
E. Problem related to living alone (V code category reflecting other problems related to the social environment).

CHAPTER 18

Personality Disorders

18.1   Which of the following DSM-IV personality disorder diagnoses is no longer present in DSM-5?

A. Antisocial personality disorder.
B. Avoidant personality disorder.
C. Borderline personality disorder.
D. Personality disorder not otherwise specified (NOS).
E. Schizotypal personality disorder.

18.2   While collaborating on a presentation to their customers, the members of a sales team become increasingly frustrated with their team leader. The leader insists that the members of the team adhere to his strict rules for developing the project. This involves approaching the task in sequential manner such that no new task can be begun until the prior one is perfected. When other members suggest alternative approaches, the leader becomes frustrated and insists that the team stick to his approach. Although the results are inarguably of high quality, the team is convinced that they will not finish in time for the scheduled presentation. When voicing these concerns to the leader, he suggests that the real problem is that the other members of the team simply don't share his high standards. Which of the following disorders would best explain the behavior of this team leader?

A. Narcissistic personality disorder.
B. Obsessive-compulsive disorder (OCD).
C. Avoidant personality disorder.
D. Obsessive-compulsive personality disorder (OCPD).
E. Unspecified personality disorder.

18.3   Individuals with obsessive-compulsive personality disorder are primarily motivated by a need for which of the following?

A. Efficiency.
B. Admiration.
C. Control.
D. Intimacy.
E. Autonomy.

18.4   Which of the following findings would rule out the diagnosis of obsessive-compulsive personality disorder (OCPD)?

    A. A concurrent diagnosis of obsessive-compulsive disorder.
    B. A concurrent diagnosis of antisocial personality disorder.
    C. Evidence of psychotic symptoms.
    D. Evidence that the behavioral patterns reflect culturally sanctioned interpersonal styles.
    E. A concurrent diagnosis of cocaine use disorder.

18.5   A 36-year-old woman is approached by her new boss, who has noticed that despite working for her employer for many years, she has not advanced beyond an entry level position. The boss hears that she is a good employee who works long hours. The woman explains that she has not asked for a promotion because she knows she's not as good as other employees and doesn't think she deserves it. She explains her long hours by saying that she is not very smart and has to check over all her work, because she's afraid that people will laugh at her if she makes any mistakes. On reviewing her past evaluations, her boss notes that there are only minor critiques and her overall evaluations have been very positive. Which of the following personality disorders would best explain this woman's lack of job advancement?

    A. Narcissistic personality disorder.
    B. Avoidant personality disorder.
    C. Obsessive-compulsive personality disorder.
    D. Schizoid personality disorder.
    E. Borderline personality disorder.

18.6   A cardiologist requests a psychiatric consultation for her patient, a 46-year-old man, because even though he is adherent to treatment, she is concerned that he "seems crazy." On evaluation, the patient makes poor eye contact, tends to ramble, and makes unusual word choices. He is modestly disheveled and wears clothes with mismatched colors. He expresses odd beliefs about supernatural phenomena, but these beliefs do not seem to be of delusional intensity. Collateral information from his sister elicits the observation that "He's always been like this—weird. He keeps to himself, and likes it that way." Which of the following conditions best explains this man's odd behaviors and beliefs?

    A. Schizoid personality disorder.
    B. Schizotypal personality disorder.
    C. Paranoid personality disorder.
    D. Delusional disorder.
    E. Schizophrenia.

18.7 Which of the following statements about the development, course, and prognosis of borderline personality disorder (BPD) is *true?*

A. The risk of suicide in individuals with BPD increases with age.
B. A childhood history of neglect, rather than abuse, is unusual in individuals with BPD.
C. Follow-up studies of individuals with BPD identified in outpatient clinics have shown that 10 years later, as many as half of these individuals no longer meet full criteria for the disorder.
D. Individuals with BPD have relatively low rates of improvement in social or occupational functioning.
E. There is little variability in the course of BPD.

18.8 Which of the following is *not* a characteristic of narcissistic personality disorder (NPD)?

A. Excessive reference to others for self-definition and self-esteem regulation.
B. Impaired ability to recognize or identify with the feelings and needs of others.
C. Excessive attempts to attract and be the focus of the attention of others.
D. Persistence at tasks long after the behavior has ceased to be functional or effective.
E. Preoccupation with fantasies of unlimited success or power.

18.9 Which of the following cognitive or perceptual disturbances are associated with borderline personality disorder?

A. Odd thinking and speech.
B. Ideas of reference.
C. Odd beliefs.
D. Transient, stress-related paranoid ideation.
E. Superstitiousness.

18.10 A 43-year-old warehouse security guard comes to your office complaining of vague feelings of depression for the last few months. He denies any particular sense of fear or anxiety. As he gets older, he wonders if he should try harder to form relationships with other people. He feels little desire for this but notes that his coworkers seem happier than he, and they have many relationships. He has never felt comfortable with other people, not even with his own family. He has lived alone since early adulthood and has been self-sufficient. He almost always works night shifts to avoid interactions with others. He tries to remain low-key and undistinguished to discourage others from striking up conversations with him, as he does not understand what they want when they talk to him. Which personality disorder would best fit with this presentation?

A. Paranoid.
B. Schizoid.

C. Schizotypal.
D. Avoidant.
E. Dependent.

18.11 Which of the following behaviors or states would be highly unusual in an individual with schizoid personality disorder?

A. An angry outburst at a colleague who criticizes his work.
B. Turning down an invitation to a party.
C. Lacking desire for sexual experiences.
D. Drifting with regard to life goals.
E. Difficulty working in a collaborative work environment.

18.12 What is the relationship between a history of conduct disorder before age 15 and the diagnosis of antisocial personality after age 18?

A. A history of some conduct disorder symptoms before age 15 is one of the required criteria for a diagnosis of antisocial personality disorder in adulthood.
B. All children with conduct disorder will go on to receive a diagnosis of antisocial personality disorder in adulthood.
C. Antisocial personality disorder diagnosis is independent of conduct disorder.
D. Conduct disorder is the same as antisocial personality disorder, except that financial irresponsibility is also a required feature of antisocial personality disorder.
E. Conduct disorder is the same as antisocial personality disorder except that remorse is present in conduct disorder.

18.13 A 25-year-old man has a childhood history of repeated instances of torturing animals, setting fires, stealing, running away from home, and school truancy, beginning at the age of 9 years. As an adult he has a history of repeatedly lying to others; engaging in petty thefts, con games, and frequent fights (including episodes in which he used objects at hand—pipe wrenches, chairs, steak knives—to injure others); and using aliases to avoid paying child support. There is no history of manic, depressive, or psychotic symptoms. He is dressed in expensive clothing and displays an expensive wristwatch for which he demands admiration; he expresses feelings of specialness and entitlement; the belief that he deserves exemption from ordinary rules; feelings of anger that his special talents have not been adequately recognized by others; devaluation, contempt, and lack of empathy for others; and lack of remorse for his behavior. There is no sign of psychosis. What is the appropriate diagnosis?

A. Antisocial personality disorder.
B. Malignant narcissism.
C. Narcissistic personality disorder.

D. Antisocial personality disorder and narcissistic personality disorder.

E. Other specified personality disorder (mixed personality features).

18.14 Which of the following is one of the general criteria for a personality disorder in DSM-5?

A. An enduring pattern of inner experience that deviates markedly from the expectations of the individual's culture.

B. The pattern is flexible and confined to a single personal or social situation.

C. The pattern is fluctuating and of short duration.

D. The pattern leads to occasional mild distress.

E. The pattern's onset can be traced to a specific traumatic event in the individual's recent history.

18.15 Which of the following presentations is characteristic of histrionic personality disorder?

A. A pattern of acute discomfort in close relationships, cognitive or perceptual distortions, and eccentricities of behavior.

B. A pattern of submissive and clinging behavior related to an excessive need to be taken care of.

C. A pattern of instability in interpersonal relationships, self-image, and affects, and marked impulsivity.

D. A pattern of grandiosity, need for admiration, and lack of empathy.

E. A pattern of excessive emotionality and attention seeking.

18.16 Which of the following presentations is characteristic of borderline personality disorder?

A. A pattern of acute discomfort in close relationships, cognitive or perceptual distortions, and eccentricities of behavior.

B. A pattern of submissive and clinging behavior related to an excessive need to be taken care of.

C. A pattern of instability in interpersonal relationships, self-image, and affects, and marked impulsivity.

D. A pattern of grandiosity, need for admiration, and lack of empathy.

E. A pattern of excessive emotionality and attention seeking.

18.17 Which of the following presentations is characteristic of dependent personality disorder?

A. A pattern of acute discomfort in close relationships, cognitive or perceptual distortions, and eccentricities of behavior.

B. A pattern of submissive and clinging behavior related to an excessive need to be taken care of.

C. A pattern of instability in interpersonal relationships, self-image, and affects, and marked impulsivity.

D. A pattern of grandiosity, need for admiration, and lack of empathy.

E. A pattern of social inhibition, feelings of inadequacy, and hypersensitivity to negative evaluation.

18.18 Which of the following presentations is characteristic of avoidant personality disorder?

A. A pattern of social inhibition, feelings of inadequacy, and hypersensitivity to negative evaluation.

B. A pattern of acute discomfort in close relationships, cognitive or perceptual distortions, and eccentricities of behavior.

C. A pattern of submissive and clinging behavior related to an excessive need to be taken care of.

D. A pattern of instability in interpersonal relationships, self-image, and affects, and marked impulsivity.

E. A pattern of grandiosity, need for admiration, and lack of empathy.

18.19 Which of the following presentations is characteristic of schizotypal personality disorder?

A. A pattern of social inhibition, feelings of inadequacy, and hypersensitivity to negative evaluation.

B. A pattern of acute discomfort in close relationships, cognitive or perceptual distortions, and eccentricities of behavior.

C. A pattern of submissive and clinging behavior related to an excessive need to be taken care of.

D. A pattern of instability in interpersonal relationships, self-image, and affects, and marked impulsivity.

E. A pattern of grandiosity, need for admiration, and lack of empathy.

18.20 Which of the following presentations is characteristic of paranoid personality disorder?

A. A pattern of social inhibition, feelings of inadequacy, and hypersensitivity to negative evaluation.

B. A pattern of distrust and suspiciousness such that others' motives are interpreted as malevolent.

C. A pattern of submissive and clinging behavior related to an excessive need to be taken care of.

D. A pattern of instability in interpersonal relationships, self-image, and affects, and marked impulsivity.

E. A pattern of grandiosity, need for admiration, and lack of empathy.

18.21 Which of the following presentations is characteristic of narcissistic personality disorder?

A. A pattern of social inhibition, feelings of inadequacy, and hypersensitivity to negative evaluation.
B. A pattern of acute discomfort in close relationships, cognitive or perceptual distortions, and eccentricities of behavior.
C. A pattern of submissive and clinging behavior related to an excessive need to be taken care of.
D. A pattern of instability in interpersonal relationships, self-image, and affects, and marked impulsivity.
E. A pattern of grandiosity, need for admiration, and lack of empathy.

18.22 Which of the following presentations is characteristic of schizoid personality disorder?

A. A pattern of social inhibition, feelings of inadequacy, and hypersensitivity to negative evaluation.
B. A pattern of acute discomfort in close relationships, cognitive or perceptual distortions, and eccentricities of behavior.
C. A pattern of detachment from social relationships and a restricted range of emotional expression.
D. A pattern of instability in interpersonal relationships, self-image, and affects, and marked impulsivity.
E. A pattern of grandiosity, need for admiration, and lack of empathy.

18.23 Which of the following presentations is characteristic of antisocial personality disorder?

A. A pattern of preoccupation with orderliness, perfectionism, and control.
B. A pattern of detachment from social relationships and a restricted range of emotional expression.
C. A pattern of distrust and suspiciousness such that others' motives are interpreted as malevolent.
D. A pattern of disregard for, and violation of, the rights of others.
E. A pattern of social inhibition, feelings of inadequacy, and hypersensitivity to negative evaluation.

18.24 Which of the following presentations is characteristic of obsessive-compulsive personality disorder?

A. A pattern of social inhibition, feelings of inadequacy, and hypersensitivity to negative evaluation.
B. A pattern of acute discomfort in close relationships, cognitive or perceptual distortions, and eccentricities of behavior.

C. A pattern of preoccupation with orderliness, perfectionism, and control.
D. A pattern of detachment from social relationships and a restricted range of emotional expression.
E. A pattern of grandiosity, need for admiration, and lack of empathy.

CHAPTER 19

Paraphilic Disorders

19.1   What changes were made to the diagnosis of paraphilias and paraphilic disorders in DSM-5?

    A. A distinction has been made between paraphilias and paraphilic disorders.
    B. Three specifiers have been added to paraphilic disorders: "in a controlled environment," 'in remission," and "benign."
    C. Transvestic disorder has been eliminated.
    D. To be diagnosed as a paraphilic disorder, a paraphilia must go beyond fantasy or urge to include behavior.
    E. Paraphilic disorders are grouped in a chapter with sexual disorders.

19.2   Which of the following statements about paraphilias is *false?*

    A. The presence of a paraphilia does not always justify clinical intervention.
    B. Most paraphilias can be divided into those that involve an unusual activity and those that involve an unusual target.
    C. Paraphilias may coexist with normophilic sexual interests.
    D. It is rare for an individual to manifest more than one paraphilia.
    E. The propensity to act on a paraphilia is difficult to assess "in a controlled environment."

19.3   Which of the following is *not* a paraphilic disorder?

    A. Sexual masochism disorder.
    B. Transvestic disorder.
    C. Transsexual disorder.
    D. Voyeuristic disorder.
    E. Fetishistic disorder.

19.4   Which of the following statements about pedophilic disorder is *true?*

    A. Pedophilic disorder is found in 10%–12% of the male population.
    B. There is no evidence that neurodevelopmental perturbation in utero increases the probability of development of a pedophilic orientation.
    C. Adult males with pedophilia often report that they were sexually abused as children.

D. To meet criteria for the diagnosis, the individual must experience sexually arousing fantasies, sexual urges, or behaviors involving sexual activity with children age 8 years or younger.

E. To meet criteria for the diagnosis, the individual must be at least 8 years older than the victim(s).

19.5   Which of the following statements about pedophilic disorder is *true?*

A. The extensive use of pornography depicting prepubescent or early pubescent children is not a useful diagnostic indicator of pedophilic disorder.

B. Pedophilic disorder is stable over the course of a lifetime.

C. There is an association between pedophilic disorder and antisocial personality disorder.

D. Although normophilic sexual interest declines with age, pedophilic sexual interest remains constant.

E. Vaginal plethysmography is a more reliable diagnostic instrument for pedophilia in women than is penile plethysmography for pedophilia in men.

19.6   A 35-year-old woman tells her therapist that she has recently become intensely aroused while watching movies in which people are tortured and that she regularly fantasizes about torturing people while masturbating. She is not distressed by these thoughts and denies ever having acted on these new fantasies, though she fantasizes about these activities several times a day. Which of the following best summarizes the diagnostic implications of this patient's presentation?

A. She meets all of the criteria for sexual sadism disorder.

B. She does not meet the criteria for sexual sadism disorder because the fantasies are not sexual in nature.

C. She does not meet the criteria for sexual sadism disorder because she has never acted on the fantasies.

D. She does not meet the criteria for sexual sadism disorder because the interest and arousal began after age 35.

E. She does not meet the criteria for sexual sadism disorder as the diagnosis is only made in men.

19.7   While intoxicated at a Mardi Gras celebration, a 19-year-old woman lifts her blouse and bra as a float goes by to get beads. The event appears on a cable news program watched by friends of her parents, who inform her parents. They insist that she get a psychiatric evaluation. She denies any other similar events in her life but admits that the experience was "sort of sexy." She is currently extremely anxious and distressed—to the point of being unable to focus on her work at college—about her parents' anger at her and their refusal to allow her to attend parties or go away on vacation. What is the most appropriate diagnosis?

A. Exhibitionistic disorder.
B. Frotteuristic disorder.
C. Voyeuristic disorder.
D. Adjustment disorder.
E. Antisocial personality disorder.

CHAPTER 20

Assessment Measures (DSM-5 Section III)

20.1 Although the DSM classification represents a categorical approach to the diagnosis of mental disorders, such approaches have a number of shortcomings. Which of the following is *not* a limitation of categorical approaches as described in DSM-5?

A. Failure to find "zones of rarity" between diagnoses.
B. Need to create intermediate categories.
C. Low rates of comorbidity.
D. Frequent use of "not otherwise specified (NOS)" diagnoses.
E. Lack of treatment specificity for various diagnostic categories.

20.2 Which of the following statements about the World Health Organization Disability Assessment Schedule, Version 2.0 (WHODAS 2.0), is *true?*

A. It is a clinician-administered scale.
B. It focuses only on disabilities due to psychiatric illness.
C. It assesses a patient's ability to perform activities in six functional areas.
D. It is available in both an adult self-rated version and a parent/guardian-rated version.
E. It primarily measures physical disability.

20.3 Which of the following statements about the DSM-5 Level 1 Cross-Cutting Symptom Measure is *true?*

A. It is intended to help clinicians assess a patient's ability to perform activities in six areas of daily life functioning.
B. It asks about the presence and frequency of symptoms in 13 psychiatric domains.
C. It focuses only on symptoms present *at the time of the interview.*
D. It lacks validity data in clinical settings and is primarily intended as a research tool.
E. Because it is self-rated, it cannot be used with patients who have communication or cognitive disorders.

20.4　In clinician review of item scores on the DSM-5 Level 1 Cross-Cutting Symptom Measure for an adult patient, a rating of "slight" would call for further inquiry if found for any item in which of the following domains?

A. Depression.
B. Mania.
C. Anger.
D. Psychosis.
E. Personality functioning.

20.5　If a parent answers "I don't know" to the question "In the past TWO (2) WEEKS, has your child had an alcoholic beverage (beer, wine, liquor, etc.)?" in the parent/guardian-rated version of the DSM-5 Level 1 Cross-Cutting Symptom Measure, what is the appropriate clinician response?

A. Advise that the child be hospitalized before further workup proceeds.
B. Ask the child questions from the substance use domain of the child-rated Level 2 Cross-Cutting Symptom Measure.
C. Rely on other questions from the substance use domain and do not incorporate this answer into the final score.
D. Ask the parent to ask the child, and schedule a follow-up visit to readminister the questionnaire.
E. Consider reporting the parent to child protective services.

20.6　If a patient selects "mild/several days" in response to the question "During the past TWO (2) WEEKS, how much (or how often) have you been bothered by...Little interest or pleasure in doing things?" in the DSM-5 Self-Rated Level 1 Cross-Cutting Symptom Measure—Adult, what is the appropriate clinician response?

A. Continue asking additional questions from that domain and rely on the total score when assessing for depression.
B. Suggest that the patient begin treatment for depression and describe treatment options.
C. Follow up with a Level 2 assessment focusing on depressive symptoms.
D. Note the score and continue with the rest of the examination.
E. Immediately begin an assessment for suicidal ideation.

20.7　When reviewing a patient's responses to items on the World Health Organization Disability Assessment Schedule 2.0 (WHODAS 2.0), the clinician asks the patient, "How much time did you spend on your health condition or its consequences?" The patient answers, "Hardly any." The clinician, who has treated the patient for several years, is surprised to hear this because she is quite certain that the patient spends most of the day dealing with health concerns. What is the appropriate action for this clinician?

A. Confront the patient about the clinician's concerns and ask the patient to re-consider.
B. Record the patient's response as is and score accordingly.
C. Indicate on the form that the clinician is making a correction and revise the score.
D. Attempt to obtain additional information from family members in order to clarify the discrepancy.
E. Take the average of the patient's and clinician's differing scores and use that for the final score.

20.8 The cross-cutting symptom measures in DSM-5 are modeled on which of the following?

A. The International Classification of Functioning, Disability, and Health.
B. The general medical review of systems.
C. The Brief Psychiatric Rating Scale.
D. The Clinical Global Impression Scale.
E. The DSM-IV Global Assessment of Functioning scale.

20.9 Which of the following statements about severity measures in DSM-5 is *true*?

A. They are not related to specific disorders.
B. They are administered once in the course of diagnosis and treatment.
C. They are completed only by the clinician.
D. They have only a loose correspondence to diagnostic criteria.
E. They may be administered to patients who have a clinically significant syndrome that falls short of meeting full diagnostic criteria.

CHAPTER 21

Cultural Formulation (DSM-5 Section III) and Glossary of Cultural Concepts of Distress (DSM-5 Appendix)

21.1   The DSM-5 Outline of Cultural Formulation is an update of the framework introduced in DSM-IV for assessing cultural features of a person's mental health presentation. Which of the following is *not* a category in the updated framework?

A. Cultural identity of the individual.
B. Cultural conceptualizations of distress.
C. Cultural stressors and cultural features of vulnerability and resilience.
D. Cultural preferences in leisure and entertainment choices.
E. Cultural features of the relationship between the individual and the clinician.

21.2   *Cultural identity of the individual* is one of several categories in the DSM-5 Outline for Cultural Formulation. Which of the following is *not* a feature of cultural identity of the individual?

A. Self-defined racial or ethnic reference group.
B. For immigrants or minorities, the degree of involvement with both culture of origin and host culture.
C. Language abilities and preferences.
D. Political party affiliation.
E. Sexual orientation.

21.3   Which of the following statements about the Cultural Formulation Interview (CFI) is *true?*

A. The CFI tests how well the patient is versed in the cultural heritage from which he or she originates.

B. By determining the patient's culture of origin, the CFI helps the clinician predict the patient's attitudes toward the illness concept and the acceptability of treatments.

C. The CFI is a carefully formulated, structured interview and should be followed closely to maintain the validity and accuracy of elicited responses.

D. The CFI takes a person-centered approach to culture, focusing on an individual's beliefs and attitudes as well as those of others in the patient's social networks.

E. Basic demographic information is elicited by the CFI, eliminating the need to obtain it separately.

21.4 In which of the following clinical situations would the Cultural Formulation Interview (CFI) *not* be directly useful?

A. The clinician and the patient come from very different cultural backgrounds.

B. The clinician and patient have a shared belief system regarding the nature of the problem and the appropriate therapeutic approach.

C. The patient presents with a symptom complex that is distressing but does not fit any DSM-5 diagnosis.

D. The clinician is finding it difficult to get a sense of the severity of the patient's presenting problems.

E. The clinician and patient are having trouble agreeing on an approach to treatment.

21.5 The DSM-5 Cultural Formulation Interview (CFI) is intended not only as an adjunct to diagnosis but also as a holistic clinical approach to the patient. Which of the following clinician communications would be consistent with the spirit of the CFI?

A. "I want you to understand the medical approach to depression, so we can clarify any misunderstandings you may have."

B. "You need not worry, I have worked with many Latino patients who have been depressed, and I know how Latinos think about this."

C. "There is no need to feel ashamed—depression is an illness, like asthma, and it affects everybody in a similar way."

D. "How does your family view your illness?"

E. "The most important thing is to take medication regularly, and the depression will go away, just as an infection would disappear with antibiotics."

21.6 In DSM-5 the term *cultural concepts of distress* encompasses three main types of concepts. Which of the following options correctly lists these three subtypes?

A. Cultural syndromes, cultural idioms of distress, cultural explanations or perceived causes.

B. Cultural identity, culture-bound syndromes, cultural bias.

C. Cultural boundaries, cultural identity, cultural arts.

D. Culturally based sexuality, culture-based faith, cultural causes.

E. Culturally recognized etiologies, cultural grievances, cultural healers.

21.7   Information on cultural concepts to improve the comprehensiveness of clinical assessment is contained in various locations in DSM-5. Which of the following is *not* one of those locations?

A. The Cultural Formulation Interview (CFI) section of the "Cultural Formulation" chapter in Section III.

B. The "Glossary of Cultural Concepts of Distress" in the Appendix.

C. Culturally relevant information embedded in the DSM-5 criteria and text for specific disorders.

D. The Z and V codes in the "Other Conditions That May Be a Focus of Clinical Attention" chapter at the end of Section II.

E. The DSM-5 multiaxial diagnostic system.

21.8   Which of the following statements about *ataque de nervios* is *false?*

A. *Ataque* is a cultural syndrome as well as a cultural idiom of distress.

B. *Ataque* is related to panic disorder, other specified or unspecified dissociative disorder, conversion disorder (functional neurological symptom disorder), and other specified or unspecified trauma- and stressor-related disorder.

C. *Ataque* is most often associated with withdrawn and reserved behaviors and limited interaction.

D. *Ataque* often involves a sense of being out of control.

E. Community studies have found *ataque* to be associated with suicidal ideation, disability, and outpatient psychiatric service utilization.

21.9   Which of the following statements about *dhat syndrome* is *false?*

A. It is a cultural syndrome found in South Asia.

B. It is related to widespread ideas regarding the harmful effects of loss of semen on sexual as well as general health.

C. The central feature of *dhat syndrome* is distress about loss of semen, to which is attributed diverse symptoms, including fatigue, weakness, and depressive mood.

D. The syndrome is most common among young men of lower socioeconomic status.

E. The estimated rate of *dhat syndrome* in men attending general medical clinics in Pakistan is 30%.

21.10 A 22-year-old man from Zimbabwe presents to a clinic with a complaint of anxiety and pain in his chest. He tells the clinician that the cause of his symptoms is *kufungisisa*, or "thinking too much." Which of the following statements about *kufungisisa* is *true?*

A. In cultures in which *kufungisisa* is a shared concept, thinking a lot about troubling issues is considered to be a helpful way of dealing with them.
B. The term *kufungisisa* is used as both a cultural explanation and a cultural idiom of distress.
C. *Kufungisisa* involves concerns about bodily deformity.
D. *Kufungisisa* is related to schizophrenia.
E. B and C.

21.11 A young Haitian man from a prominent family becomes severely depressed after his first semester of university studies. The family brings the young man to a clinician and states that *maladi moun* has caused his problem. Which of the following statements about *maladi moun* is *false?*

A. It is similar to Mediterranean concepts of the "evil eye," in which a person's good fortune is envied by others who in turn cause misfortune to the individual.
B. It can present with a wide variety of symptoms, from anxiety to psychosis.
C. It is based on a shared social assumption that "rising tides lift all boats."
D. It is a Haitian cultural explanation for a diverse set of medical and emotional presentations.
E. It is also referred to as "sent sickness."

21.12 A 19-year-old man presents to the clinic complaining of headaches, irritability, emotional lability, and difficulty concentrating. He is accompanied by his mother, who tells you that her son has had *nervios* since childhood. Which of the following statements about *nervios* is *false?*

A. Unlike *ataque de nervios,* which is a syndrome, *nervios* is a cultural idiom of distress implying a state of vulnerability to stressful experiences.
B. The term *nervios* is used only when the individual has serious loss of functionality or intense symptoms.
C. *Nervios* can manifest with emotional symptoms, somatic disturbances, and an inability to function.
D. *Nervios* can be related to both trait characteristics of an individual and episodic psychiatric symptoms such as depression and dissociative episodes.
E. *Nervios* is a common term used by Latinos in the United States and Latin America.

21.13   Which of the following statements about *shenjing shuairuo* is *false?*

    A. In the *Chinese Classification of Mental Disorders,* it is defined by a presentation of three out of five symptom clusters.

    B. One of the psychosocial precipitants is an acute sense of failure.

    C. It is related to traditional Chinese medicine concepts of depletion of *qi* (vital energy) and dysregulation of *jing* (bodily channels that convey vital forces).

    D. Prominent psychotic symptoms must be present.

    E. It is believed to be related in some cases to the inability to change a chronically frustrating and distressing situation.

CHAPTER 22

Alternative DSM-5 Model for Personality Disorders (DSM-5 Section III)

22.1   Which of the following terms best describes the diagnostic approach proposed in the Alternative DSM-5 Model for Personality Disorders?

A. Categorical.
B. Dimensional.
C. Hybrid.
D. Polythetic.
E. Socratic.

22.2   In addition to an assessment of pathological personality traits, a personality disorder diagnosis in the alternative DSM-5 model requires an assessment of which of the following?

A. Level of impairment in personality functioning.
B. Comorbidity with Axis I disorders.
C. Degree of introversion versus extroversion.
D. Stability of the personality traits over time.
E. Familial inheritance of specific traits.

22.3   Which of the following is a domain of the Alternative DSM-5 Model for Personality Disorders?

A. Neuroticism.
B. Extraversion.
C. Disinhibition.
D. Agreeableness.
E. Conscientiousness.

22.4   In addition to negative affectivity, which of the following maladaptive trait domains is most associated with avoidant personality disorder?

A. Detachment.
B. Antagonism.
C. Disinhibition.

D. Compulsivity.

E. Psychoticism.

22.5 The diagnosis of personality disorder—trait specified in the Alternative DSM-5 Model of Personality Disorders differs from the DSM-IV diagnosis of personality disorder not otherwise specified in that the DSM-5 diagnosis includes personality trait domains based on which of the following?

A. The level of impairment.

B. Their resemblance to Axis I disorders.

C. The five-factor model of personality.

D. Cognitive theories of behavior.

E. Neurobiological correlates of behavior.

22.6 In the Alternative DSM-5 Model for Personality Disorders, personality functioning includes both **self functioning** (involving *identity* and *self-direction*) and **interpersonal functioning** (involving *empathy* and *intimacy*). Which of the following is a characteristic of healthy self functioning?

A. Comprehension and appreciation of others' experiences and motivations.

B. Variability of self-esteem.

C. Tolerance of differing perspectives.

D. Fluctuating boundaries between self and others.

E. Experience of oneself as unique.

22.7 Which of the following is *not* a personality disorder criterion in the Alternative DSM-5 Model for Personality Disorders?

A. The impairments in personality functioning and the individual's personality trait expression are relatively inflexible and pervasive across a broad range of personal and social situations.

B. The impairments in personality functioning and the individual's personality trait expression are relatively stable across time, with onsets that can be traced back to at least adolescence or early adulthood.

C. The impairments in personality functioning and the individual's personality trait expression are not solely attributable to the physiological effects of a substance or another medical condition (e.g., severe head trauma).

D. The impairments in personality functioning are not comorbid with another mental disorder.

E. The impairments in personality functioning and the individual's personality trait expression are not better understood as normal for an individual's developmental stage or sociocultural environment.

22.8　In order to meet the proposed diagnostic criteria for antisocial personality disorder (ASPD) in the Alternative DSM-5 Model for Personality Disorders, an individual must have maladaptive personality traits in which of the following domains?

A. Negative affectivity.
B. Detachment.
C. Antagonism.
D. Suicidality.
E. Psychoticism.

22.9　In the Alternative DSM-5 Model for Personality Disorders, which of the following is *not* an element used to assess level of impairment in personality functioning?

A. Identity.
B. Self-direction.
C. Empathy.
D. Work performance.
E. Intimacy.

22.10　Which of the following statements about the relationship between severity of personality dysfunction—as rated on the Level of Personality Functioning Scale (LPFS)—and presence of a personality disorder is *false?*

A. A patient must have "some impairment" as rated on the LPFS in order to be diagnosed with a personality disorder.
B. "Moderate impairment" on the LPFS predicts the presence of a personality disorder.
C. "Severe impairment" on the LPFS predicts the presence of more than one personality disorder.
D. "Severe impairment" on the LPFS predicts the presence of one of the more severe personality disorders.
E. The LPFS does not take into account the level of impairment, merely the presence or absence of functional impairment.

22.11　Which of the following statements about the Level of Personality Functioning Scale (LPFS) is *false?*

A. An assessment indicating "moderate impairment" as described by the LPFS is necessary for diagnosis of a personality disorder.
B. An assessment indicating "moderate impairment" as described by the LPFS is sufficient for diagnosis of a personality disorder.
C. The LPFS can be used without specification of a personality disorder diagnosis.

D. The LPFS can be used to describe individuals with personality characteristics that do not reach the threshold for a personality disorder diagnosis.

E. The LPFS can be used to describe a person's level of impairment at any given time.

CHAPTER 23

Glossary of Technical Terms (DSM-5 Appendix)

23.1   Match each term with the appropriate description.

   A. Affect.
   B. Alogia.
   C. Anhedonia.
   D. Autogynephilia
   E. Catalepsy.
   F. Cataplexy.
   G. Compulsion.
   H. Conversion symptom.
   I. Depressivity.
   J. Dissociation.
   K. Dysphoria.
   L. Euphoria.
   M. Flashback.
   N. Flight of ideas.
   O. Gender dysphoria.
   P. Hypervigilance.
   Q. Ideas of reference.
   R. Language pragmatics.
   S. Magical thinking.
   T. Mood.
   U. Panic attacks.
   V. Perseveration.
   W. Personality disorder—trait specified (PD-TS).
   X. Separation insecurity.
   Y. Subsyndromal.
   Z. Traumatic stressor.

   i. A condition in which a person experiences intense feelings of depression, discontent, and in some cases indifference to the world around them.
   ii. A pattern of observable behaviors that is the expression of a subjectively experienced feeling state (emotion). Examples include sadness, elation, and anger.

iii. Distress that accompanies the incongruence between one's experienced and expressed gender and one's assigned or natal gender.

iv. Below a specified level or threshold required to qualify for a particular condition. These conditions *(formes frustes)* are medical conditions that do not meet full criteria for a diagnosis—for example, because the symptoms are fewer or less severe than a defined syndrome—but that nevertheless can be identified and related to the "full-blown" syndrome.

v. In Section III "Alternative DSM-5 Model for Personality Disorders," a proposed diagnostic category for use when a personality disorder is considered present but the criteria for a specific disorder are not met.

vi. The splitting off of clusters of mental contents from conscious awareness. This mechanism is central to dissociative disorders. The term is also used to describe the separation of an idea from its emotional significance and affect, as seen in the inappropriate affect in schizophrenia.

vii. Sexual arousal of a natal male associated with the idea or image of being a woman.

viii. The feeling that casual incidents and external events have a particular and unusual meaning that is specific to the person.

ix. A mental and emotional condition in which a person experiences intense feelings of well-being, elation, happiness, excitement, and joy.

x. Passive induction of a posture held against gravity.

xi. Lack of enjoyment from, engagement in, or energy for life's experiences; deficits in the capacity to feel pleasure and take interest in things.

xii. Persistence at tasks or in particular way of doing things long after the behavior has ceased to be functional or effective; continuance of the same behavior despite repeated failures or clear reasons for stopping.

xiii. The erroneous belief that one's thoughts, words, or actions will cause or prevent a specific outcome in some way that defies commonly understood laws of cause and effect.

xiv. Repetitive behaviors (e.g., hand washing, ordering, checking) or mental acts (e.g., praying, counting, repeating words silently) that the individual feels driven to perform in response to an obsession, or according to rules that must be applied rigidly.

xv. A nearly continuous flow of accelerated speech with abrupt changes from topic to topic that are usually based on understandable associations, distracting stimuli, or plays on words. When the condition is severe, speech may be disorganized and incoherent.

xvi. Any event (or events) that may cause or threaten death, serious injury, or sexual violence to an individual, a close family member, or a close friend.

xvii. Fears of being alone due to rejection by and/or separation from significant others, based in a lack of confidence in one's ability to care for oneself, both physically and emotionally.

xviii. The understanding and use of language in a given context. For example, the warning "Watch your hands" when issued to a child who is dirty is intended not only to prompt the child to look at his or her hands but also to communicate the admonition "Don't get anything dirty."

xix. An enhanced state of sensory sensitivity accompanied by an exaggerated intensity of behaviors whose purpose is to detect threats. Other symptoms include abnormally increased arousal, a high responsiveness to stimuli, and a continual scanning of the environment for threats.

xx. A dissociative state during which aspects of a traumatic event are reexperienced as though they were occurring at that moment.

xxi. A loss of, or alteration in, voluntary motor or sensory functioning, with or without apparent impairment of consciousness. The symptom is not fully explained by a neurological or another medical condition or the direct effects of a substance and is not intentionally produced or feigned.

xxii. Episodes of sudden bilateral loss of muscle tone resulting in the individual collapsing, often occurring in association with intense emotions such as laughter, anger, fear, or surprise.

xxiii. A pervasive and sustained emotion that colors the perception of the world. Common examples include depression, elation, anger, and anxiety.

xxiv. An impoverishment in thinking that is inferred from observing speech and language behavior. There may be brief and concrete replies to questions and restriction in the amount of spontaneous speech (termed *poverty of speech*). Sometimes the speech is adequate in amount but conveys little information because it is overconcrete, overabstract, repetitive, or stereotyped (termed *poverty of content*).

xxv. Discrete periods of sudden onset of intense fear or terror, often associated with feelings of impending doom. During these events there are symptoms such as shortness of breath or smothering sensations; palpitations, pounding heart, or accelerated heart rate; chest pain or discomfort; choking; and fear of going crazy or losing control.

xxvi. Feelings of being intensely sad, miserable, and/or hopeless. Some patients describe an absence of feelings and/or dysphoria; difficulty recovering from such moods; pessimism about the future; pervasive shame and/or guilt; feelings of inferior self-worth; and thoughts of suicide and suicidal behavior.

PART II

Answer Guide

DSM-5 Introduction

I.1   DSM-IV employed a multiaxial diagnostic system. Which of the following statements best describes the multiaxial system in DSM-5?

    A. There is a different multiaxial system in DSM-5.
    B. The multiaxial system in DSM-IV has been retained in DSM-5.
    C. DSM-5 has moved to a nonaxial documentation of diagnosis.
    D. Axis I (Clinical Disorders) and Axis II (Personality Disorders) have been retained in DSM-5.
    E. Axis IV (Psychosocial and Environmental Problems) and Axis V (Global Assessment of Functioning) have been retained in DSM-5.

Correct Answer: C. DSM-5 has moved to a nonaxial documentation of diagnosis.

Explanation: Despite widespread use and its adoption by certain insurance and governmental agencies, the multiaxial system in DSM-IV was not required to make a mental disorder diagnosis. DSM-5 has moved to a nonaxial documentation of diagnosis (formerly Axes I, II, and III), with separate notations for important psychosocial and contextual factors (formerly Axis IV) and disability (formerly Axis V). The approach of separately noting diagnosis from psychosocial and contextual factors is consistent with established World Health Organization (WHO) and *International Classification of Diseases* (ICD) guidance to consider the individual's functional status separately from his or her diagnoses or symptom status. In DSM-5, Axis III has been combined with Axes I and II. Clinicians should continue to list medical conditions that are important to the understanding or management of an individual's mental disorder(s).

I.1—The Multiaxial System (p. 16)

I.2   True or False: The Global Assessment of Functioning (GAF) Scale (DSM-IV Axis V) remains a separate category that should be coded in DSM-5.

    A. True.
    B. False.

Correct Answer: B. False.

Explanation: DSM-IV Axis V consisted of the GAF Scale, representing the clinician's judgment of the individual's overall level of "functioning on a hypothetical continuum of mental health–illness." It was recommended that the GAF be dropped from DSM-5 for several reasons, including its conceptual lack of clarity (i.e., including symptoms, suicide risk, and disabilities in its descriptors) and questionable psychometrics in routine practice.

I.2—The Multiaxial System (p. 16)

I.3   To enhance diagnostic specificity, DSM-5 replaced the previous "not otherwise specified" (NOS) designation with two options for clinical use: Other Specified [disorder] and Unspecified [disorder]. Which of the following statements about use of the Unspecified designation is *true?*

A. The Unspecified designation is used when the clinician chooses not to specify the reason that criteria for a specific disorder were not met.
B. The Unspecified designation is used when there is no recognized Other Specified disorder (e.g., recurrent brief depression, sexual aversion).
C. The Unspecified designation is used when the individual has fewer than three symptoms of any of the recognized disorders within the diagnostic class.
D. The Unspecified designation is used when the individual presents with symptomatology of disorders in two or more diagnostic classes.
E. The Unspecified designation is used when the clinician believes the condition is of a temporary nature.

Correct Answer: A. The Unspecified designation is used when the clinician chooses not to specify the reason that criteria for a specific disorder were not met.

Explanation: To enhance diagnostic specificity, DSM-5 replaced the previous NOS designation with two options for clinical use: Other Specified disorder and Unspecified disorder. The Other Specified category is provided to allow the clinician to communicate the specific reason that the presentation does not meet the criteria for any specific category within a diagnostic class. This is done by recording the name of the category, followed by the specific reason. For example, for an individual with clinically significant depressive symptoms lasting 4 weeks but whose symptomatology falls short of the diagnostic threshold for a major depressive episode, the clinician would record "other specified depressive disorder, depressive episode with insufficient symptoms." If the clinician chooses not to specify the reason that the criteria are not met for a particular disorder, then "unspecified depressive disorder" would be diagnosed. Note that the differentiation between Other Specified and Unspecified disorders is based on the clinician's decision, providing maximum flexibility for diagnosis. Clinicians do not have to differentiate between Other Specified and Unspecified disorders based on some feature of the presentation itself. When the clinician determines that there is evidence to specify the nature of the clinical presentation, the Other Specified diagnosis can be given. When the clinician is not able to further specify and describe the clinical presentation, the Unspecified diagnosis can be given. This is left entirely up to clinical judgment.

I.3—Use of Other Specified and Unspecified Disorders (pp. 15–16)

CHAPTER 1

Neurodevelopmental Disorders

1.1   Which of the following is *not* required for a DSM-5 diagnosis of intellectual disability (intellectual developmental disorder)?

A. Full-scale IQ below 70.
B. Deficits in intellectual functions confirmed by clinical assessment.
C. Deficits in adaptive functioning that result in failure to meet developmental and sociocultural standards for personal independence and social responsibility.
D. Symptom onset during the developmental period.
E. Deficits in intellectual functions confirmed by individualized, standardized intelligence testing.

Correct Answer: A. Full-scale IQ below 70.

Explanation: The essential features of intellectual disability (intellectual developmental disorder) relate to both intellectual impairment and deficits in adaptive function. In contrast to DSM-IV, which specified "an IQ of approximately 70 or below" for the former diagnosis of "mental retardation," DSM-5 has no specific requirement for IQ in the renamed diagnosis of intellectual disability.

1.1—Intellectual Disability (Intellectual Developmental Disorder) diagnostic criteria (p. 33); Diagnostic Features (p. 37)

1.2   A 7-year-old boy in second grade displays significant delays in his ability to reason, solve problems, and learn from his experiences. He has been slow to develop reading, writing, and mathematics skills in school. All through development, these skills lagged behind peers, although he is making slow progress. These deficits significantly impair his ability to play in an age-appropriate manner with peers and to begin to acquire independent skills at home. He requires ongoing assistance with basic skills (dressing, feeding, and bathing himself; doing any type of schoolwork) on a daily basis. Which of the following diagnoses best fits this presentation?

A. Childhood-onset major neurocognitive disorder.
B. Specific learning disorder.
C. Intellectual disability (intellectual developmental disorder).

D. Communication disorder.

E. Autism spectrum disorder.

Correct Answer: C. Intellectual disability (intellectual developmental disorder).

Explanation: Intellectual disability is characterized by deficits in general mental abilities, which result in impairments of intellectual and adaptive functioning. In specific learning disorder and communication disorders, there is no general intellectual impairment. Autism spectrum disorder must include history suggesting "persistent deficits in social communication and social interaction across multiple contexts" (Criterion A) or "restricted, repetitive patterns of behavior, interests, or activities" (Criterion B). Intellectual disability is categorized as a neurodevelopmental disorder and is distinct from the neurocognitive disorders, which are characterized by a *loss* of cognitive functioning. There is no evidence for a neurocognitive disorder in this case, although major neurocognitive disorder may co-occur with intellectual disability (e.g., an individual with Down syndrome who develops Alzheimer's disease, or an individual with intellectual disability who loses further cognitive capacity following a head injury). In such cases, the diagnoses of intellectual disability and neurocognitive disorder may both be given.

1.2—Intellectual Disability (Intellectual Developmental Disorder) / Differential Diagnosis (pp. 39–40)

1.3   A 7-year-old boy in second grade displays significant delays in his ability to reason, solve problems, and learn from his experiences. He has been slow to develop reading, writing, and mathematics skills in school. All through development, these skills lagged behind peers, although he is making slow progress. These deficits significantly impair his ability to play in an age-appropriate manner with peers and to begin to acquire independent skills at home. He requires ongoing assistance with basic skills (dressing, feeding, and bathing himself; doing any type of schoolwork) on a daily basis. What is the appropriate severity rating for this patient's current presentation?

A. Mild.

B. Moderate.

C. Severe.

D. Profound.

E. Cannot be determined without an IQ score.

Correct Answer: B. Moderate.

Explanation: With respect to severity, the "moderate" qualifier reflects this patient's skills (which have chronically lagged behind those of peers) and his need for assistance in most activities of daily living; however, it also takes into account the fact that he is slowly developing these skills (which would peak at roughly the elementary school level, according to DSM-5).

Although IQ testing would be informative in diagnosing intellectual disability (in previous DSM classifications, subtypes of mild, moderate, severe, and profound were categories based on IQ scores), DSM-5 specifies that *the various levels of severity are defined on the basis of adaptive functioning, and not IQ scores, because it is adaptive functioning that determines the level of supports required*" (p. 33). Deficits in adaptive functioning refer to how well a person meets community standards of personal independence and social responsibility, in comparison to others of similar age and sociocultural background. Adaptive functioning is assessed using both clinical evaluation and individualized, culturally appropriate, psychometrically sound measures.

Adaptive functioning involves adaptive reasoning in three domains: conceptual, social, and practical. The *conceptual (academic) domain* involves competence in memory, language, reading, writing, math reasoning, acquisition of practical knowledge, problem solving, and judgment in novel situations, among others. The *social domain* involves awareness of others' thoughts, feelings, and experiences; empathy; interpersonal communication skills; friendship abilities; and social judgment, among others. The *practical domain* involves learning and self-management across life settings, including personal care, job responsibilities, money management, recreation, self-management of behavior, and school and work task organization, among others. Intellectual capacity, education, motivation, socialization, personality features, vocational opportunity, cultural experience, and coexisting general medical conditions or mental disorders influence adaptive functioning.

1.3—Intellectual Disability (Intellectual Developmental Disorder) / Diagnostic Features (p. 37)

1.4 Which of the following statements about intellectual disability (intellectual developmental disorder) is *false?*

A. Individuals with intellectual disability have deficits in general mental abilities and impairment in everyday adaptive functioning compared with age- and gender-matched peers from the same linguistic and sociocultural group.
B. For individuals with intellectual disability, the full-scale IQ score is a valid assessment of overall mental abilities and adaptive functioning, even if subtest scores are highly discrepant.
C. Individuals with intellectual disability may have difficulty in managing their behavior, emotions, and interpersonal relationships and in maintaining motivation in the learning process.
D. Intellectual disability is generally associated with an IQ that is 2 standard deviations from the population mean, which equates to an IQ score of about 70 or below (±5 points).

E. Assessment procedures for intellectual disability must take into account factors that may limit performance, such as sociocultural background, native language, associated communication/language disorder, and motor or sensory handicap.

Correct Answer: B. For individuals with intellectual disability, the full-scale IQ score is a valid assessment of overall mental abilities and adaptive functioning, even if subtest scores are highly discrepant.

Explanation: The single IQ score is an approximation of conceptual functioning, but insufficient alone for assessing mastery of practical tasks and reasoning in real-life situations. Highly discrepant individual subtest scores may make an overall IQ score invalid. Thus, the profile of weaknesses on subtest scores is generally a more accurate reflection of an individual's overall mental abilities than the full-scale IQ.

> 1.4—Intellectual Disability (Intellectual Developmental Disorder) / Diagnostic Features (p. 37)

1.5   Which of the following statements about the diagnosis of intellectual disability (intellectual developmental disorder) is *false?*

A. An individual with an IQ of less than 70 would receive the diagnosis if there were no significant deficits in adaptive functioning.
B. An individual with an IQ above 75 would not meet diagnostic criteria even if there were impairments in adaptive functioning.
C. In forensic assessment, severe deficits in adaptive functioning might allow for a diagnosis with an IQ above 75.
D. Adaptive functioning must take into account the three domains of conceptual, social, and practical functioning.
E. The specifiers mild, moderate, severe, and profound are based on IQ scores.

Correct Answer: E. The specifiers mild, moderate, severe, and profound are based on IQ scores.

Explanation: Severity specifiers are included in the diagnostic criteria for intellectual disability (intellectual developmental disorder). The various levels of severity are defined on the basis of adaptive functioning, and not IQ scores, because it is adaptive functioning that determines the level of supports required. Moreover, IQ measures are less valid in the lower end of the IQ range. This represents a change from DSM-IV, in which mental retardation severity levels were based on IQ scores.

> 1.5—Intellectual Disability (Intellectual Developmental Disorder) / Specifiers (p. 33)

1.6 Which of the following is *not* a diagnostic feature of intellectual disability (intellectual developmental disorder)?

A. A full-scale IQ of less than 70.
B. Inability to perform complex daily living tasks (e.g., money management, medical decision making) without support.
C. Gullibility, with naiveté in social situations and a tendency to be easily led by others.
D. Lack of age-appropriate communication skills for social and interpersonal functioning.
E. All of the above are diagnostic features of intellectual disability.

Correct Answer: A. A full-scale IQ of less than 70.

Explanation: The DSM-5 diagnosis does not require a full-scale IQ less than 70, because impairment in adaptive functioning is also required. In general, individuals with intellectual disability may have difficulty with social judgment. Lack of communication skills may also predispose them to disruptive and aggressive behaviors. Communication, conversation, and language are more concrete or immature than expected for any given age. Furthermore, gullibility is an important feature of intellectual developmental disorder. It is especially important in forensic situations and may affect judgment.

1.6—Intellectual Disability (Intellectual Developmental Disorder) / Diagnostic Features (p. 37)

1.7 Which of the following statements about adaptive functioning in the diagnosis of intellectual disability (intellectual developmental disorder) is *true?*

A. Adaptive functioning is based on an individual's IQ score.
B. "Deficits in adaptive functioning" refers to problems with motor coordination.
C. At least two domains of adaptive functioning must be impaired to meet Criterion B for the diagnosis of intellectual disability.
D. Adaptive functioning in intellectual disability tends to improve over time, although the threshold of cognitive capacities and associated developmental disorders can limit it.
E. Individuals diagnosed with intellectual disability in childhood will typically continue to meet criteria in adulthood even if their adaptive functioning improves.

Correct Answer: D. Adaptive functioning tends to improve over time, although the threshold of cognitive capacities and associated developmental disorders can limit it.

Explanation: In the DSM-5 diagnosis of intellectual disability (intellectual developmental disorder), unlike the DSM-IV diagnosis of mental retardation, the various levels of severity are defined on the basis of adaptive functioning rather than IQ scores alone, because it is adaptive functioning that determines the level of support required. Moreover, IQ measures are less valid in the lower end of the IQ range. Severity levels are meant to refer only to functioning at the time of the assessment, and they can change over time in a positive direction if the individual receives support and can develop compensatory strategies. Improvement in adaptive functioning can occur to a degree such that the individual no longer meets criteria for the diagnosis in adulthood.

> **1.7—Intellectual Disability (Intellectual Developmental Disorder) / Specifiers (pp. 33–36); Diagnostic Features (pp. 37–38); Development and Course (pp. 38–39)**

1.8   Which of the following statements about development of and risk factors for intellectual disability (intellectual developmental disorder) is *true?*

    A. Intellectual developmental disorder should not be diagnosed in the presence of a known genetic syndrome, such as Lesch-Nyhan or Prader-Willi syndrome.
    B. Etiologies are confined to perinatal and postnatal factors and exclude prenatal events.
    C. In severe acquired forms of intellectual developmental disorder, onset may be abrupt following an illness (e.g., meningitis) or head trauma occurring during the developmental period.
    D. When intellectual disability results from a loss of previously acquired cognitive skills, as in severe traumatic brain injury (TBI), only the TBI diagnosis is assigned.
    E. Prenatal, perinatal, and postnatal etiologies of intellectual developmental disorder are demonstrable in approximately 33% of cases.

Correct Answer: C. In severe acquired forms of intellectual developmental disorder, onset may be abrupt following an illness (e.g., meningitis) or head trauma occurring during the developmental period.

Explanation: The presence of a known genetic syndrome is *not* exclusionary if the criteria for intellectual developmental disorder are met. Prenatal, perinatal, and postnatal etiologies are demonstrable in approximately 70% of cases. If the diagnosis results from TBI, both diagnoses are given.

> **1.8—Intellectual Disability (Intellectual Developmental Disorder) / Development and Course (pp. 38–39); Risk and Prognostic Factors (p. 39)**

1.9   Which of the following statements about the developmental course of intellectual disability (intellectual developmental disorder) is *true?*

A. Delayed motor, language, and social milestones are not identifiable until after the first 2 years of life.
B. Intellectual disability caused by an illness (e.g., encephalitis) or by head trauma occurring during the developmental period would be diagnosed as a neurocognitive disorder, not as intellectual disability (intellectual developmental disorder).
C. Intellectual disability is always nonprogressive.
D. Major neurocognitive disorder may co-occur with intellectual developmental disorder.
E. Even if early and ongoing interventions throughout childhood and adulthood lead to improved adaptive and intellectual functioning, the diagnosis of intellectual disability would continue to apply.

Correct Answer: D. Major neurocognitive disorder may co-occur with intellectual developmental disorder.

Explanation: Intellectual disability is categorized as a neurodevelopmental disorder and is distinct from the neurocognitive disorders, which are characterized by a loss of cognitive functioning. Major neurocognitive disorder may co-occur with intellectual disability (e.g., an individual with Down syndrome who develops Alzheimer's disease, or an individual with intellectual disability who loses further cognitive capacity following a head injury). In such cases, the diagnoses of intellectual disability and neurocognitive disorder may both be given.

Delayed motor, language, and social milestones may be identifiable within the first 2 years of life among those with more severe intellectual disability. Head trauma with subsequent cognitive deficits would represent an acquired form of intellectual developmental disorders. Although intellectual disability is generally nonprogressive, in certain genetic disorders (e.g., Rett syndrome) there are periods of worsening, followed by stabilization, and in others (e.g., San Phillippo syndrome) progressive worsening of intellectual function. After early childhood, the disorder is generally lifelong, although severity levels may change over time. If early and ongoing interventions improve adaptive functioning and significant improvement of intellectual functioning occurs, the diagnosis of intellectual disability may no longer be appropriate.

1.9—Intellectual Disability (Intellectual Developmental Disorder) / Development and Course (pp. 38–39); Differential Diagnosis (pp. 39–40); Comorbidity (p. 40)

1.10 The DSM-5 diagnosis of intellectual developmental disorder includes severity specifiers—Mild, Moderate, Severe, and Profound—with which to indicate the level of supports required in various domains of adaptive functioning. Which of the following features would *not* be characteristic of an individual with a "Severe" level of impairment?

A. The individual generally has little understanding of written language or of concepts involving numbers, quantity, time, and money.

B. The individual's spoken language is quite limited in terms of vocabulary and grammar.

C. The individual requires support for all activities of daily living, including meals, dressing, bathing, and toileting.

D. In adulthood, the individual may be able to sustain competitive employment in a job that does not emphasize conceptual skills.

E. The individual cannot make responsible decisions regarding the well-being of self or others.

Correct Answer: D. In adulthood, the individual may be able to sustain competitive employment in a job that does not emphasize conceptual skills.

Explanation: Competitive employment may be attainable by individuals with a "Mild" level of impairment but would not be characteristic of those with a "Severe" level of impairment. Intellectual disability (intellectual developmental disorder) is a disorder with onset during the developmental period that includes both intellectual and adaptive functioning deficits in conceptual, social, and practical domains (DSM-5 Table 1, pp. 34–36). The *conceptual (academic) domain* involves competence in memory, language, reading, writing, math reasoning, acquisition of practical knowledge, problem solving, and judgment in novel situations, among others. The *social domain* involves awareness of others' thoughts, feelings, and experiences; empathy; interpersonal communication skills; friendship abilities; and social judgment, among others. The *practical domain* involves learning and self-management across life settings, including personal care, job responsibilities, money management, recreation, self-management of behavior, and school and work task organization, among others.

> 1.10—Intellectual Disability (Intellectual Developmental Disorder) / diagnostic criteria (p. 33) / Table 1 [Severity levels for intellectual disability (intellectual developmental disorder)] (pp. 33–36); Diagnostic Features (p. 37)

1.11 A 10-year-old boy with a history of dyslexia, who is otherwise developmentally normal, is in a skateboarding accident in which he experiences severe traumatic brain injury. This results in significant global intellectual impairment (with a persistent reading deficit that is more pronounced than his other newly acquired but stable deficits, along with a full-scale IQ of 75). There is mild impairment in his adaptive functioning such that he requires support in some areas of functioning. He is also displaying anxious and depressive symptoms in response to his accident and hospitalization. What is the *least likely* diagnosis?

A. Intellectual disability (intellectual developmental disorder).

B. Traumatic brain injury.

C. Specific learning disorder.

D. Major neurocognitive disorder due to traumatic brain injury.

E. Adjustment disorder.

Correct Answer: D. Major neurocognitive disorder due to traumatic brain injury.

Explanation: There are no exclusion criteria for a diagnosis of intellectual developmental disorder in DSM-5, which notes that both specific learning disorder and communication disorders can co-occur if the criteria are met. Although his full-scale IQ is 75, the statistical model associated with his intellect would allow for his actual IQ to be ±5 points. His adaptive functioning would be the key factor in his receiving the diagnosis of intellectual developmental disorder, with a mild level of severity due to needing to receive only some support in most of his areas of functioning. With his reading skills remaining disproportionately impaired in comparison with the rest of his cognitive profile, and because onset of these impairments was during the developmental period, he would continue to receive a diagnosis of specific learning disorder (dyslexia). His emotional symptoms in response to the accident would yield a potential diagnosis of an adjustment disorder. The boy's deficits are not severe enough to qualify for a diagnosis of major neurocognitive disorder.

1.11—Intellectual Disability (Intellectual Developmental Disorder) / Differential Diagnosis (p. 40)

1.12 In which of the following situations would a diagnosis of global developmental delay be *inappropriate?*

A. The patient is a child who is too young to fully manifest specific symptoms or to complete requisite assessments.

B. The patient, a 7-year-old boy, has a full-scale IQ of 65 and severe impairment in adaptive functioning.

C. The patient's scores on psychometric tests suggest intellectual disability (intellectual developmental disorder), but there is insufficient information about the patient's adaptive functional skills.

D. The patient's impaired adaptive functioning suggests intellectual developmental disorder, but there is insufficient information about the level of cognitive impairment measured by standardized instruments.

E. The patient's cognitive and adaptive impairments suggest intellectual developmental disorder, but there is insufficient information about age at onset of the condition.

Correct Answer: B. The patient, a 7-year-old boy, has a full-scale IQ of 65 and severe impairment in adaptive functioning.

Explanation: Enough information is present to diagnose intellectual disability (intellectual developmental disorder) in this boy. The diagnosis of global developmental delay is used when there is insufficient information to make the diagnosis of intellectual developmental disorder.

1.12—Global Developmental Delay (p. 41)

1.13   Which of the following statements about global developmental delay is *true*?

A. The diagnosis is typically made in children younger than 5 years of age.
B. The etiology can usually be determined.
C. The prevalence is estimated to be between 0.5% and 2%.
D. The condition is progressive.
E. The condition does not generally occur with other neurodevelopmental disorders.

Correct Answer: A. The diagnosis is typically made in children younger than 5 years of age.

Explanation: The diagnosis of global developmental delay is reserved for individuals under the age of 5 years who fail to meet expected developmental milestones in several areas of intellectual functioning, when the clinical severity level cannot be reliably assessed during early childhood. The diagnosis is used for individuals who are unable to undergo systematic assessments of intellectual functioning, including children who are too young to participate in standardized testing.

1.13—Global Developmental Delay (p. 41)

1.14   A 3½-year-old girl with a history of lead exposure and a seizure disorder demonstrates substantial delays across multiple domains of functioning, including communication, learning, attention, and motor development, which limit her ability to interact with same-age peers and require substantial support in all activities of daily living at home. Unfortunately, her mother is an extremely poor historian, and the child has received no formal psychological or learning evaluation to date. She is about to be evaluated for readiness to attend preschool. What is the most appropriate diagnosis?

A. Major neurocognitive disorder.
B. Developmental coordination disorder.
C. Autism spectrum disorder.
D. Global developmental delay.
E. Specific learning disorder.

Correct Answer: D. Global developmental delay.

Explanation: Although this girl's deficits may be suggestive of intellectual disability (intellectual developmental disorder), that diagnosis cannot be made in this case because information is lacking (e.g., about age at onset of her symptoms), and she is too young to participate in standardized testing. At this point, there is no information to suggest that this child has dementia (major neurocognitive disorder), an autism spectrum disorder (no evidence of symptoms in the core autism spectrum disorder categories), a specific disorder relating to coordination, or a specific area of learning weakness (which generally would not be able to be diagnosed until the elementary years).

1.14—Global Developmental Delay (p. 41)

1.15   A 5-year-old boy has difficulty making friends and problems with initiating and sustaining back-and-forth conversation; reading social cues; and sharing his feelings with others. He makes good eye contact, has normal speech intonation, displays facial gestures, and has a range of affect that generally seems appropriate to the situation. He demonstrates an interest in trains that seems abnormal in intensity and focus, and he engages in little imaginative or symbolic play. Which of the following diagnostic requirements for autism spectrum disorder are *not* met in this case?

A. Deficits in social-emotional reciprocity.
B. Deficits in nonverbal communicative behaviors used for social interaction.
C. Deficits in developing and maintaining relationships.
D. Restricted, repetitive patterns of behavior, interests, or activities as manifested by symptoms in two of the specified four categories.
E. Symptoms with onset in early childhood that cause clinically significant impairment.

Correct Answer: B. Deficits in nonverbal communicative behaviors used for social interaction.

Explanation: DSM-5 Criterion A for autism spectrum disorder specifies that all three symptom clusters (summarized in options A, B, and C above) must be met. This boy's nonverbal communication is reported to be unimpaired (although this should be confirmed with a standard instrument such as the Autism Diagnostic Observation Schedule). Based on the current history, he could not be diagnosed with autism spectrum disorder in DSM-5. In order to meet Criterion B, at least two symptom clusters must be met. Although the boy has "highly restricted, fixated interests that are abnormal in intensity or focus," he would need to have at least one other symptom from categories in Criterion B (which includes stereotyped or repetitive motor movements, use of objects, or speech; insistence on sameness, inflexible adherence to routines, or ritualized patterns of verbal or nonverbal behavior; or hyper- or hyporeactivity to sensory input or unusual interest in sensory aspects of the environment).

1.15—Autism Spectrum Disorder / diagnostic criteria (p. 50)

1.16   Which of the following statements about the development and course of autism spectrum disorder (ASD) is *false?*

A. Symptoms of ASD are typically recognized during the second year of life (12–24 months of age).
B. Symptoms of ASD are usually not noticeable until 5–6 years of age or later.
C. First symptoms frequently involve delayed language development, often accompanied by lack of social interest or unusual social interactions.
D. ASD is not a degenerative disorder, and it is typical for learning and compensation to continue throughout life.
E. Because many normally developing young children have strong preferences and enjoy repetition, distinguishing restricted and repetitive behaviors that are diagnostic of ASD can be difficult in preschoolers.

Correct Answer: B. Symptoms are not typically noticeable until 5–6 years of age or later.

Explanation: Details about the age and pattern of onset are important and should be noted in the history. Symptoms of ASD are typically recognized during the second year of life (12–24 months of age) but may be seen earlier than 12 months if developmental delays are severe, or noted later than 24 months if symptoms are more subtle. The pattern of onset description might include information about early developmental delays or any losses of social or language skills. In cases where skills have been lost, parents or caregivers may give a history of a gradual or relatively rapid deterioration in social behaviors or language skills. Typically, this would occur between 12 and 24 months of age and is distinguished from the rare instances of developmental regression occurring after at least 2 years of normal development (previously described as childhood disintegrative disorder).

1.16—Autism Spectrum Disorder / Development and Course (pp. 55–56)

1.17   Which of the following was a criterion symptom for autistic disorder in DSM-IV that was eliminated from the diagnostic criteria for autism spectrum disorder in DSM-5?

A. Stereotyped or restricted patterns of interest.
B. Stereotyped and repetitive motor mannerisms.
C. Inflexible adherence to routines.
D. Persistent preoccupation with parts of objects.
E. None of the above.

Correct Answer: D. Persistent preoccupation with parts of objects.

Explanation: In DSM-5, the older requirement regarding objects was restated as follows: "Highly restricted, fixated interests that are abnormal in intensity or focus (e.g., strong attachment to or preoccupation with unusual objects, excessively circumscribed or perseverative interests)" in Criterion B3. In Criterion B4, DSM-5 mentions "fascination with lights or spinning objects." There is no mention of preoccupation with "parts of objects" in DSM-5 (Criterion A3d in DSM-IV autistic disorder).

1.17—Autism Spectrum Disorder / diagnostic criteria (p. 50)

1.18   A 7-year-old girl presents with a history of normal language skills (vocabulary and grammar intact) but is unable to use language in a socially pragmatic manner to share ideas and feelings. She has never made good eye contact, and she has difficulty reading social cues. Consequently, she has had difficulty making friends, which is further complicated by her being somewhat obsessed with cartoon characters, which she repetitively scripts. She tends to excessively smell objects. Because she insists on wearing the same shirt and shorts every day, regardless of the season, getting dressed is a difficult activity. These symptoms date from early childhood and cause significant impairment in her functioning. What diagnosis best fits this child's presentation?

A. Asperger's disorder.
B. Autism spectrum disorder.
C. Pervasive developmental disorder not otherwise specified (NOS).
D. Social (pragmatic) communication disorder.
E. Rett syndrome.

Correct Answer: B. Autism spectrum disorder.

Explanation: This child might have met criteria for Asperger's disorder or pervasive developmental disorder NOS in DSM-IV. Autism spectrum disorder in DSM-5 subsumed Asperger's disorder and pervasive developmental disorder NOS. Although the girl has intact formal language skills, it is the use of language for social communication that is particularly affected in autism spectrum disorder. A specific language delay is not required. She meets all three components of Criterion A (deficits in social-emotional reciprocity, deficits in nonverbal communicative behaviors used for social interaction, and deficits in developing, maintaining, and understanding relationships) and two components of Criterion B (highly restricted, fixated interests that are abnormal in intensity or focus; and hyper- or hyporeactivity to sensory input or unusual interest in sensory aspects of the environment).

1.18—Autism Spectrum Disorder / Diagnostic Features (p. 53)

1.19 A 15-year-old boy has a long history of nonverbal communication deficits. As an infant he was unable to follow someone else directing his attention by pointing. As a toddler he was not interested in sharing events, feelings, or games with his parents. From school age into adolescence, his speech was odd in tonality and phrasing, and his body language was awkward. What do these symptoms represent?

A. Stereotypies.
B. Restricted range of interests.
C. Developmental regression.
D. Prodromal schizophreniform symptoms.
E. Deficits in nonverbal communicative behaviors.

Correct Answer: E. Deficits in nonverbal communicative behaviors.

Explanation: These symptoms are examples of deficits in nonverbal communicative behavior, as described in Criterion A2 for autism spectrum disorder criteria in DSM-5.

1.19—Autism Spectrum Disorder / Diagnostic Features (p. 53)

1.20 A 10-year-old boy demonstrates hand-flapping and finger flicking, and he repetitively flips coins and lines up his trucks. He tends to "echo" the last several words of a question posed to him before answering, mixes up his pronouns (refers to himself in the second person), tends to repeat phrases in a perseverative fashion, and is quite fixated on routines related to dress, eating, travel, and play. He spends hours in his garage playing with his father's tools. What do these behaviors represent?

A. Restricted, repetitive patterns of behaviors, interests, or activities characteristic of autism spectrum disorder.
B. Symptoms of obsessive-compulsive disorder.
C. Prototypical manifestations of obsessive-compulsive personality.
D. Symptoms of pediatric acute-onset neuropsychiatric syndrome (PANS).
E. Complex tics.

Correct Answer: A. Restricted, repetitive patterns of behaviors, interests, or activities characteristic of autism spectrum disorder.

Explanation: In DSM-5, the symptoms in the category of "restrictive, repetitive patterns of behaviors, interests, or activities" (Criterion B) associated with autism spectrum disorder demonstrated by this patient include stereotyped or repetitive motor movements, use of objects, or speech; insistence on sameness, inflexible adherence to routines, or ritualized patterns of verbal or nonverbal behavior; and highly restricted, fixated interests that are abnormal in intensity or focus. He needs to have only two out of the four symptoms in this category (along with meeting Criterion A) to qualify for the autism spectrum disorder diagnosis. The fourth symptom in Criterion B (which this patient does not display) is hyper- or hyporeactivity to sensory input or unusual interest in sensory aspects of the environment.

1.20—Autism Spectrum Disorder / Diagnostic Features (p. 53)

1.21   A 25-year-old man presents with long-standing nonverbal communication deficits, inability to have a back-and-forth conversation or share interests in an appropriate fashion, and a complete lack of interest in having relationships with others. His speech reflects awkward phrasing and intonation and is mechanical in nature. He has a history of sequential fixations and obsessions with various games and objects throughout childhood; however, this is not currently a major issue for him. This patient meets criteria for autism spectrum disorder; true or false?

A. True.
B. False.

Correct Answer: A. True.

Explanation: This young man presents with all three symptoms in Criterion A; his symptoms satisfy Criterion C, which requires childhood onset; and he meets Criterion D, which requires clinically significant impairment in functioning. Although he has only one symptom in Criterion B (stereotyped or repetitive speech) and the diagnosis requires two, the fact that he has a history of fixations and obsessions satisfies the criteria, such that he does qualify for a diagnosis of autism spectrum disorder.

1.21—Autism Spectrum Disorder / diagnostic criteria (p. 50)

1.22   A 9-year-old girl presents with a history of intellectual impairment, a structural language impairment, nonverbal communication deficits, disinterest in peers, and inability to use language in a social manner. She has extreme food and tactile sensitivities. She is obsessed with one particular computer game that she plays for hours each day, and she scripts and imitates the characters in this game. She is clumsy, has an odd gait, and walks on her tiptoes. In the past year she has developed a seizure disorder and has begun to bang her wrists against the wall repetitively, causing bruising. On the other hand, she plays several musical instruments in an extremely precocious manner. Which feature of this child's clinical presentation fulfills a criterion symptom for DSM-5 autism spectrum disorder?

A. Motor abnormalities.
B. Seizures.
C. Structural language impairment.
D. Intellectual impairment.
E. Nonverbal communicative deficits.

Correct Answer: E. Nonverbal communicative deficits.

Explanation: Criterion A of autism spectrum disorder lists nonverbal communicative deficits as one of the symptoms. The rest of the options represent associated features supporting diagnosis, which according to the DSM-5 text notes that "the gap between intellectual and adaptive functional skills is often large."

1.22—Autism Spectrum Disorder / diagnostic criteria (p. 50); Associated Features Supporting Diagnosis (p. 55)

1.23 An 11-year-old girl with autism spectrum disorder displays no spoken language and is minimally responsive to overtures from others. She can be somewhat inflexible, which interferes with her ability to travel, do schoolwork, and be managed in the home; she has some difficulty transitioning; and she has trouble organizing and planning activities. These problems can usually be managed with incentives and reinforcers. What severity levels should be specified in the DSM-5 diagnosis?

A. Level 3 (requiring very substantial support) for social communication, and level 1 (requiring support) for restricted, repetitive behaviors.
B. Level 1 (requiring support) for social communication, and level 3 (requiring very substantial support) for restricted, repetitive behaviors.
C. Level 1 (requiring support) for social communication, and level 2 (requiring substantial support) for restricted, repetitive behaviors.
D. Level 3 (requiring very substantial support) for social communication, and level 1 (requiring support) for restricted, repetitive behaviors.
E. Level 2 (requiring substantial support) for social communication, and level 1 (requiring support) for restricted, repetitive behaviors.

Correct Answer: A. Level 3 (requiring very substantial support) for social communication, and level 1 (requiring support) for restricted, repetitive behaviors.

Explanation: In DSM-5, severity is noted separately for social communication impairments and for the restricted, repetitive patterns of behavior. In this case, the social communication deficits are quite severe, warranting a classification of level 3, but the restricted, repetitive behaviors are milder, reflecting the lowest classification of level 1. Level 2 is an intermediate category reflecting the need for "substantial support."

1.23—Autism Spectrum Disorder / Specifiers (p. 51)

1.24 Which of the following is *not* a specifier included in the diagnostic criteria for autism spectrum disorder?

A. With or without accompanying intellectual impairment.
B. With or without associated dementia.
C. With or without accompanying language impairment.
D. Associated with a known medical or genetic condition or environmental factor.
E. Associated with another neurodevelopmental, mental, or behavioral disorder.

Correct Answer: B. With or without associated dementia.

Explanation: The specifier "with or without associated dementia" is not included in the diagnostic criteria for autism spectrum disorder.

1.24—Autism Spectrum Disorder / diagnostic criteria (p. 51)

1.25 Which of the following is *not* characteristic of the developmental course of children diagnosed with autism spectrum disorder?

A. Behavioral features manifest before 3 years of age.
B. The full symptom pattern does not appear until age 2–3 years.
C. Developmental plateaus or regression in social-communicative behavior is frequently reported by parents.
D. Regression across multiple domains occurs after age 2–3 years.
E. First symptoms often include delayed language development, lack of social interest or unusual social behavior, odd play, and unusual communication patterns.

Correct Answer: D. Regression across multiple domains occurs after age 2–3 years.

Explanation: Regression across multiple domains after age 2–3 years may occur, but it is not typical of the developmental course in autism spectrum disorder. As noted in DSM-5, some children with autism spectrum disorder experience developmental plateaus or regression, with a gradual or relatively rapid deterioration in social behaviors or use of language, often during the first 2 years of life. Such losses are rare in other disorders and may be a useful "red flag" for autism spectrum disorder. Much more unusual and warranting more extensive medical investigation are losses of skills beyond social communication (e.g., loss of self-care, toileting, motor skills) or those occurring after the second birthday.

1.25—Autism Spectrum Disorder / Development and Course (pp. 55–56)

1.26   A 5-year-old girl has some mild food aversions. She enjoys having the same book read to her at night but does not become terribly upset if her mother asks her to choose a different book. She occasionally spins around excitedly when her favorite show is on. She generally likes her toys neatly arranged in bins but is only mildly upset when her sister leaves them on the floor. These behaviors should be considered suspicious for an autism spectrum disorder; true or false?

A. True.
B. False.

Correct Answer: B. False.

Explanation: The girl described in the question meets none of the criteria for autism spectrum disorder. Because many typically developing young children have strong preferences and enjoy repetition (e.g., eating the same foods, watching the same video multiple times), distinguishing restricted and repetitive behaviors that are diagnostic of autism spectrum disorder can be difficult in preschoolers. The clinical distinction is based on the type, frequency, and intensity of the behavior (e.g., a child who daily lines up objects for hours and is very distressed if any item is moved).

1.26—Autism Spectrum Disorder / Development and Course (p. 56)

1.27   Which of the following is *not* representative of the typical developmental course for autism spectrum disorder?

A. Lack of degenerative course.
B. Behavioral deterioration during adolescence.
C. Continued learning and compensation throughout life.
D. Marked presence of symptoms in early childhood and early school years, with developmental gains in later childhood in areas such as social interaction.
E. Good psychosocial functioning in adulthood, as indexed by independent living and gainful employment.

Correct Answer: B. Behavioral deterioration during adolescence.

Explanation: Most adolescents with autism spectrum disorder improve behaviorally; only a minority further deteriorates.

1.27—Autism Spectrum Disorder / Development and Course (pp. 55–56)

1.28   A 21-year-old man, not previously diagnosed with a developmental disorder, presents for evaluation after taking a leave from college for psychological reasons. He makes little eye contact, does not appear to pick up on social cues, has become disinterested in friends, spends hours each day on the computer surfing the Internet and playing games, and has become so sensitive to smells that he keeps multiple air fresheners in all locations of the home. He reports that he has had long-standing friendships dating from childhood and high school (corroborated by his parents). He reports making many friends in his fraternity at college. His parents report good social and communication skills in childhood, although he was quite shy and was somewhat inflexible and ritualistic at home. What is the *least likely* diagnosis?

A. Depression.
B. Schizophreniform disorder or schizophrenia.
C. Autism spectrum disorder.
D. Obsessive-compulsive disorder.
E. Social anxiety disorder (social phobia).

Correct Answer: C. Autism spectrum disorder.

Explanation: The history of good social and communication skills in childhood and long-standing friendships is not consistent with autism spectrum disorder. With respect to schizophrenia specifically, DSM-5 text notes that "schizophrenia with childhood onset usually develops after a period of normal, or near normal, development. A prodromal state has been described in which social impairment and atypical interests and beliefs occur, which could be confused with the social deficits seen in autism spectrum disorder. Hallucinations and delusions, which are defining features of schizophrenia, are not features of autism spectrum disorder."

1.28—Autism Spectrum Disorder / Differential Diagnosis (p. 58)

1.29   Which of the following characteristics is generally *not* associated with autism spectrum disorder?

A. Anxiety, depression, and isolation as an adult.
B. Catatonia.
C. Poor psychosocial functioning.
D. Insistence on routines and aversion to change.
E. Successful adaptation in regular school settings.

Correct Answer: E. Successful adaptation in regular school settings.

Explanation: In young children with autism spectrum disorder, lack of social and communication abilities may hamper learning, especially learning through social interaction or in settings with peers. In the home, insistence on routines and aversion to change, as well as sensory sensitivities, may interfere with eating and sleeping and make routine care (e.g., haircuts, dental work) extremely difficult. Adaptive skills are typically below measured IQ. Extreme difficulties in planning, organization, and coping with change negatively impact academic achievement, even for students with above-average intelligence.

During adulthood, these individuals may have difficulties establishing independence because of continued rigidity and difficulty with novelty.

1.29—Autism Spectrum Disorder / Functional Consequences of Autism Spectrum Disorder (p. 57)

1.30 Which of the following disorders is generally *not* comorbid with autism spectrum disorder (ASD)?

A. Attention-deficit/hyperactivity disorder (ADHD).
B. Rett syndrome.
C. Selective mutism.
D. Intellectual disability (intellectual developmental disorder).
E. Stereotypic movement disorder.

Correct Answer: C. Selective mutism.

Explanation: Children with selective mutism have appropriate communication skills in certain contexts and do not demonstrate severe impairments in social interaction and restricted patterns of behavior; in selective mutism, there are typically no abnormalities in early development, and no restricted and repetitive behavior or interests. ADHD can be comorbid with ASD in DSM-5 (unlike in DSM-IV); such comorbidity would be coded with the specifier "associated with another neurodevelopmental, mental, or behavioral disorder." ASD and Rett syndrome can be comorbid, with Rett syndrome similarly coded as the associated "known medical or genetic condition or environmental factor," as long as the child also meets criteria for autism spectrum disorder. ASD can be comorbid with intellectual developmental disorder when all criteria for both disorders are met, and "social communication and interaction are significantly impaired relative to the developmental level of the individual's nonverbal skills," that is, there is a discrepancy between social-communicative skills and nonverbal skills. ASD can be comorbid with stereotypic movement disorder if the repetitive movements cannot be accounted for as part of the autism spectrum disorder (e.g., hand flapping). In general, when criteria for another disorder are met along with meeting the criteria for ASD, both disorders are diagnosed. Comorbidity with additional diagnoses in ASD is common (about 70% of individuals with autism spectrum disorder have one comorbid mental disorder, and 40% have two or more comorbid mental disorders).

1.30—Autism Spectrum Disorder / Comorbidity (pp. 58–59)

1.31 Which of the following is *not* a criterion for the DSM-5 diagnosis of attention-deficit/hyperactivity disorder (ADHD)?

A. Onset of several inattentive or hyperactive-impulsive symptoms prior to age 12 years.

B. Manifestation of several inattentive or hyperactive-impulsive symptoms in two or more settings (e.g., at home, school, or work; with friends or relatives; in other activities).

C. Persistence of symptoms for at least 12 months.

D. Clear evidence that symptoms interfere with, or reduce the quality of, social, academic, or occupational functioning.

E. Inability to explain symptoms as a manifestation of another mental disorder (e.g., mood disorder, anxiety disorder, dissociative disorder, personality disorder, substance intoxication or withdrawal).

Correct Answer: C. Persistence of symptoms for at least 12 months.

Explanation: The essential feature of ADHD is a pervasive pattern of *inattention* and/or *hyperactivity-impulsivity* that interferes with functioning or development, with persistence of symptoms for at least 6 months to a degree that is inconsistent with developmental level and that negatively impacts directly on social and academic/occupational activities. ADHD begins in childhood. The requirement that several symptoms be present before age 12 years conveys the importance of a substantial clinical presentation during childhood. Manifestations of the disorder must be present in more than one setting (e.g., home and school, work). Confirmation of substantial symptoms across settings typically cannot be done accurately without consulting informants who have seen the individual in those settings.

1.31—Attention-Deficit/Hyperactivity Disorder / diagnostic criteria (p. 59); Diagnostic Features (p. 61)

1.32 The parents of a 15-year-old female tenth grader believe that she should be doing better in high school, given how bright she seems and the fact that she received mostly A's through eighth grade. Her papers are handed in late, and she makes careless mistakes on examinations. They have her tested, and the WAIS-IV results are as follows: Verbal IQ, 125; Perceptual Reasoning Index, 122; Full-Scale IQ, 123; Working Memory Index, 55th percentile; Processing Speed Index, 50th percentile. Weaknesses in executive function are noted. During a psychiatric evaluation, she reports a long history of failing to give close attention to details, difficulty sustaining attention while in class or doing homework, failing to finish chores and tasks, and significant difficulties with time management, planning, and organization. She is forgetful, often loses things, and is easily distracted. She has no history of restlessness or impulsivity, and she is well liked by her peers. What is the most likely diagnosis?

A. Adjustment disorder with anxiety.

B. Specific learning disorder.

C. Attention-deficit/hyperactivity disorder, predominantly inattentive.

D. Developmental coordination disorder.

E. Major depressive disorder.

Correct Answer: C. Attention-deficit/hyperactivity disorder, predominantly inattentive.

Explanation: The patient has six symptoms in the inattention cluster of attention-deficit/hyperactivity disorder (ADHD) and meets criteria for this disorder. She has common associated features of ADHD, including weaknesses in working memory and processing speed, and problems handing in her work (especially writing) on time. There is no evidence from the testing or history that her writing difficulty is secondary to a primary disorder involving writing or that she has any other specific learning disorder.

1.32—Attention-Deficit/Hyperactivity Disorder / Differential Diagnosis (p. 63)

1.33   A 7-year-old boy is having behavioral and social difficulties in his second-grade class. Although he seems to be able to attend and is doing "well" from an academic standpoint (though seemingly not what he is capable of), he is constantly interrupting, fidgeting, talking excessively, and getting out of his seat. He has friends, but he sometimes annoys his peers because of his difficulty sharing and taking turns and the fact that he is constantly talking over them. Although he seeks out play dates, his friends tire of him because he wants to play sports nonstop. At home, he can barely stay in his seat for a meal and is unable to play quietly. Although he shows remorse when the consequences of his behavior are pointed out to him, he can become angry in response and seems nevertheless unable to inhibit himself. What is the most likely diagnosis?

A. Bipolar disorder.
B. Autism spectrum disorder.
C. Generalized anxiety disorder.
D. Attention-deficit/hyperactivity disorder, predominantly hyperactive/impulsive.
E. Specific learning disorder.

Correct Answer: D. Attention-deficit/hyperactivity disorder, predominantly hyperactive/impulsive.

Explanation: This boy has all the cardinal features in the hyperactivity/impulsivity cluster of attention-deficit/hyperactivity disorder (ADHD). Although he is not currently displaying inattention or impairment in his academic functioning, it is quite likely that this will become more of an issue as schoolwork becomes more complex and tedious, and academic demands increase. His behaviors are somewhat alienating to peers, as is common in ADHD. There is no evidence that he has comorbid autism spectrum disorder, especially because he seeks out friendships. He meets Criterion C in that "several inattentive or hyperactive-impulsive symptoms are present in two or more settings (e.g., at home, school, or work; with friends or relatives; in other activities)" and Criterion D in that "there is clear evidence that the symptoms interfere with, or reduce the quality of, social, academic, or occupational functioning."

1.33—Attention-Deficit/Hyperactivity Disorder / Differential Diagnosis (p. 63)

1.34 A 37-year-old Wall Street trader schedules a visit after his 8-year-old son is diagnosed with attention-deficit/hyperactivity disorder (ADHD), combined inattentive and hyperactive. Although he does not currently note motor restlessness like his son, he recalls being that way when he was a boy, along with being quite inattentive, being impulsive, talking excessively, interrupting, and having problems waiting his turn. He was an underachiever in high school and college, when he inconsistently did his work and had difficulty following rules. Nevertheless, he never failed any classes, and he was never evaluated by a psychologist or psychiatrist. He works about 60–80 hours a week and often gets insufficient sleep. He tends to make impulsive business decisions, can be impatient and short-tempered, and notes that his mind tends to wander both in one-on-one interactions with associates and his wife and during business meetings, for which he is often late; he is forgetful and disorganized. Nevertheless, he tends to perform fairly well and is quite successful, although he can occasionally feel overwhelmed and demoralized. What is the most likely diagnosis?

A. Major depressive disorder.
B. Generalized anxiety disorder.
C. Specific learning disorder.
D. ADHD, in partial remission.
E. Oppositional defiant disorder.

Correct Answer: D. ADHD, in partial remission.

Explanation: This is a not uncommon story of a parent who presents to treatment after a son or daughter is diagnosed with ADHD, and the parent recognizes similarities from his or her own childhood. This man does present with a possible history of ADHD during childhood, along with a possible *prior* history of oppositional defiant disorder. Currently, there is no evidence that he has difficulty with rules, and the fact that he is no longer restless is common for the developmental course of ADHD. Currently, his ADHD symptoms include three symptoms in the inattention cluster (difficulty sustaining attention, difficulty organizing tasks and activities, forgetfulness), and only one clear symptom of impulsivity (impatience); since he has retained only some of the symptoms, a diagnosis of ADHD, *in partial remission,* is appropriate and provided for in DSM-5. It is unclear to what degree his work schedule and insufficient sleep are also contributing to his distress.

1.34—Attention-Deficit/Hyperactivity Disorder / Differential Diagnosis (p. 63)

1.35 A 5-year-old hyperactive, impulsive, and inattentive boy presents with hyper-telorism, highly arched palate, and low-set ears. He is uncoordinated and clumsy, he has no sense of time, and his toys and clothes are constantly strewn all over the house. He has recently developed what appears to be a motor tic involving blinking. He enjoys playing with peers, who tend to like him, al-though he seems to willfully defy all requests from his parents and kindergar-ten teacher, which does not seem to be due simply to inattention. He is delayed in beginning to learn how to read. What is the *least likely* diagnosis?

A. Autism spectrum disorder.
B. Developmental coordination disorder.
C. Oppositional defiant disorder (ODD).
D. Specific learning disorder.
E. Attention-deficit/hyperactivity disorder (ADHD).

Correct Answer: A. Autism spectrum disorder.

Explanation: There is no evidence that this boy has a disorder of relatedness, especially since he enjoys playing with peers, who like him. He has signs and symptoms of ADHD, along with some soft neurological signs and minor phys-ical anomalies that can be associated with ADHD (although genetic and neu-rological evaluations seem warranted). He may have an associated specific learning disorder in reading (which should also be evaluated by having him tested by a psychologist) and a comorbid diagnosis of ODD, since his opposi-tional behavior is not simply due to inattention.

1.35—Attention-Deficit/Hyperactivity Disorder / Differential Diagnosis (p. 63)

1.36 What is the prevalence of attention-deficit/hyperactivity disorder (ADHD) in children?

A. 8%.
B. 10%.
C. 2%.
D. 0.5%.
E. 5%.

Correct Answer: E. 5%.

Explanation: Population surveys suggest that ADHD occurs in most cultures in about 5% of children. Differences in ADHD prevalence rates across regions appear attributable mainly to different diagnostic and methodological prac-tices. However, there also may be cultural variation in attitudes toward or in-terpretations of children's behaviors. Clinical identification rates in the United States for African American and Latino populations tend to be lower than for

Caucasian populations. Informant symptom ratings may be influenced by the cultural group of the child and the informant, suggesting that culturally appropriate practices are relevant in assessing ADHD.

1.36—Attention-Deficit/Hyperactivity Disorder / Prevalence (p. 61); Culture-Related Diagnostic Issues (p. 62)

1.37   What is the prevalence of attention-deficit/hyperactivity disorder (ADHD) in adults?

A. 8%.
B. 10%.
C. 2.5%.
D. 0.5%.
E. 5%.

Correct Answer: C. 2.5%.

Explanation: Population surveys suggest that ADHD occurs in most cultures in about 2.5% of adults and about 5% of children.

1.37—Attention-Deficit/Hyperactivity Disorder / Prevalence (p. 61)

1.38   What is the gender ratio of attention-deficit/hyperactivity disorder (ADHD) in children?

A. Male:female ratio of 2:1.
B. Male:female ratio of 1:1.
C. Male:female ratio of 3:2.
D. Male:female ratio of 5:1.
E. Male:female ratio of 1:2.

Correct Answer: A. Male:female ratio of 2:1.

Explanation: ADHD is more prevalent in males than in females in the general population, with a gender ratio of approximately 2:1 in children and 1.6:1 in adults. Females are more likely than males to present primarily with inattentive features.

1.38—Attention-Deficit/Hyperactivity Disorder / Gender-Related Diagnostic Issues (p. 63)

1.39   Which of the following is a biological finding in individuals with attention-deficit/hyperactivity disorder (ADHD)?

A. Decreased slow-wave activity on electroencephalograms.
B. Reduced total brain volume on magnetic resonance imaging.

C. Early posterior to anterior cortical maturation.

D. Reduced thalamic volume.

E. Both B and C.

Correct Answer: B. Reduced total brain volume on magnetic resonance imaging.

Explanation: No biological marker is diagnostic for ADHD. As a group, compared with peers, children with ADHD display reduced total brain volume on magnetic resonance imaging, *increased* slow-wave electroencephalograms, and possibly *a delay in* posterior to anterior cortical maturation.

1.39—Attention-Deficit/Hyperactivity Disorder / Associated Features Supporting Diagnosis (p. 61)

1.40 Which of the following is *not* associated with attention-deficit/hyperactivity disorder (ADHD)?

A. Reduced school performance.

B. Poorer occupational performance and attendance.

C. Higher probability of unemployment.

D. Elevated interpersonal conflict.

E. Reduced risk of substance use disorders.

Correct Answer: E. Reduced risk of substance use disorders.

Explanation: Children with ADHD are significantly more likely than their peers without ADHD to develop conduct disorder in adolescence and antisocial personality disorder in adulthood, consequently increasing the likelihood for substance use disorders and incarceration. The risk of subsequent substance use disorders is elevated, especially when conduct disorder or antisocial personality disorder develops.

1.40—Attention-Deficit/Hyperactivity Disorder / Functional Consequences of Attention-Deficit/Hyperactivity Disorder (p. 63)

1.41 Which of the following is *not* associated with attention-deficit/hyperactivity disorder (ADHD)?

A. Social rejection.

B. Increased risk of developing conduct disorder in childhood and antisocial personality disorder in adulthood.

C. Increased risk of Alzheimer's disease.

D. Increased frequency of traffic accidents and violations.

E. Increased risk of accidental injury.

Correct Answer: C. Increased risk of Alzheimer's disease.

Explanation: The risk of Alzheimer's disease is not elevated in individuals with ADHD. Peer relationships in individuals with ADHD are often disrupted by peer rejection, neglect, or teasing. Children with ADHD are significantly more likely than their peers without ADHD to develop conduct disorder in adolescence and antisocial personality disorder in adulthood, consequently increasing the likelihood for substance use disorders and incarceration. Individuals with ADHD are more likely than peers to be injured. Traffic accidents and violations are more frequent in drivers with ADHD.

1.41—Attention-Deficit/Hyperactivity Disorder / Functional Consequences of Attention-Deficit/Hyperactivity Disorder (p. 63)

1.42 A 15-year-old boy has developed concentration problems in school that have been associated with a significant decline in grades. When interviewed, he explains that his mind is occupied with worrying about his mother, who has a serious autoimmune disease. As his grades falter, he becomes increasingly demoralized and sad, and he notices that his energy level drops, further compromising his ability to pay attention in school. At the same time, he complains of feeling restless and unable to sleep. What is the most likely diagnosis?

A. Bipolar disorder.
B. Specific learning disorder.
C. Attention-deficit/hyperactivity disorder (ADHD).
D. Adjustment disorder with mixed anxiety and depressed mood.
E. Separation anxiety disorder.

Correct Answer: D. Adjustment disorder with mixed anxiety and depressed mood.

Explanation: The inattention seen in this boy relates to anxiety and depressive symptoms that are in reaction to his mother's illness and his subsequent decline in grades. Inattention related to ADHD is not associated with worry and rumination, as would be the case in anxiety disorders.

1.42—Attention-Deficit/Hyperactivity Disorder / Differential Diagnosis (p. 64)

1.43 A 5-year-old boy is consistently moody, irritable, and intolerant of frustration. In addition, he is pervasively and chronically restless, impulsive, and inattentive. Which diagnosis best fits his clinical picture?

A. Attention-deficit/hyperactivity disorder (ADHD).
B. ADHD and disruptive mood dysregulation disorder (DMDD).
C. Bipolar disorder.
D. Oppositional defiant disorder (ODD).
E. Major depressive disorder (MDD).

Correct Answer: B. ADHD and DMDD.

Explanation: The boy's mood symptoms cannot be accounted for by ADHD alone, and they are characteristic of DMDD; ADHD is not associated with this level of affective symptoms on its own. A diagnosis of bipolar disorder in this age group should be made extremely cautiously, given that less than 1% of preadolescent referrals have this diagnosis, especially when the cycles of "mania" last less than a day. Young people with bipolar disorder may have increased activity, but this is episodic, varying with mood, and goal directed. Therefore, this child's irritability and hyperactivity do not qualify for bipolar disorder.

1.43—Attention-Deficit/Hyperactivity Disorder / Differential Diagnosis (p. 64)

1.44 Which of the following statements about comorbidity in attention-deficit/hyperactivity disorder (ADHD) is *true*?

A. Oppositional defiant disorder co-occurs with ADHD in about half of children with the combined presentation and about a quarter of those with the predominantly inattentive presentation.
B. Most children with disruptive mood dysregulation disorder do not also meet criteria for ADHD.
C. Fifteen percent of adults with ADHD have some type of anxiety disorder.
D. Intermittent explosive disorder occurs in about 5% of adults with ADHD.
E. Specific learning disorder very seldom co-occurs with ADHD.

Correct Answer: A. Oppositional defiant disorder co-occurs with ADHD in about half of children with the combined presentation and about a quarter of those with the predominantly inattentive presentation.

Explanation: In clinical settings, comorbid disorders are frequent in individuals whose symptoms meet criteria for ADHD. In the general population, oppositional defiant disorder co-occurs with ADHD in approximately half of children with the combined presentation and about a quarter with the predominantly inattentive presentation. Most children and adolescents with disruptive mood dysregulation disorder have symptoms that also meet criteria for ADHD; a lesser percentage of children with ADHD have symptoms that meet criteria for disruptive mood dysregulation disorder. Specific learning disorder commonly co-occurs with ADHD. Anxiety disorders and major depressive disorder occur in a minority of individuals with ADHD but more often than in the general population. Intermittent explosive disorder occurs in a minority of adults with ADHD, but at rates above population levels. In adults, antisocial and other personality disorders may co-occur with ADHD. Other disorders that may co-occur with ADHD include obsessive-compulsive disorder, tic disorders, and autism spectrum disorder.

1.44—Attention-Deficit/Hyperactivity Disorder / Comorbidity (p. 65)

1.45   Specific learning disorder is defined by persistent difficulties in learning academic skills, with onset during the developmental period. Which of the following statements about this disorder is *true*?

A. It is part of a more general learning impairment as manifested in intellectual disability (intellectual developmental disorder).
B. It can usually be attributed to a sensory, physical, or neurological disorder.
C. It involves pervasive and wide-ranging deficits across multiple domains of information processing.
D. It can be caused by external factors such as economic disadvantage or lack of education.
E. It replaces the DSM-IV diagnoses of reading disorder, mathematics disorder, disorder of written expression, and learning disorder not otherwise specified.

Correct Answer: E. It replaces the DSM-IV diagnoses of reading disorder, mathematics disorder, disorder of written expression, and learning disorder not otherwise specified.

Explanation: The DSM-5 diagnosis of specific learning disorder combines the DSM-IV diagnoses of reading disorder, mathematics disorder, disorder of written expression, and learning disorder not otherwise specified. The difficulties seen in specific learning disorder are considered "specific" for four reasons. First, they are not attributable to intellectual disabilities (intellectual disability [intellectual developmental disorder]); global developmental delay; hearing or vision disorders, or neurological or motor disorders) (Criterion D). Second, the learning difficulty cannot be attributed to more general external factors, such as economic or environmental disadvantage, chronic absenteeism, or lack of education as typically provided in the individual's community context. Third, the learning difficulty cannot be attributed to a neurological (e.g., pediatric stroke) or motor disorder or to vision or hearing disorders, which are often associated with problems learning academic skills but are distinguishable by presence of neurological signs. Finally, the learning difficulty may be restricted to one academic skill or domain (e.g., reading single words, retrieving or calculating number facts).

1.45—Specific Learning Disorder / diagnostic criteria (p. 66); Diagnostic Features (pp. 69–70)

1.46   In distinction to DSM-IV, DSM-5 classifies all learning disorders under the diagnosis of specific learning disorder, along with the requirement to "specify all academic domains and subskills that are impaired" at the time of assessment. Which of the following statements about specific learning disorder is *false*?

A. There are persistent difficulties in the acquisition of reading, writing, arithmetic, or mathematical reasoning skills during the formal years of schooling.
B. Current skills in one or more of these academic areas are well below the average range for the individual's age, gender, cultural group, and level of education.
C. There usually is a discrepancy of more than 2 standard deviations (SD) between achievement and IQ.
D. The learning difficulties significantly interfere with academic achievement, occupational performance, or activities of daily living that require these academic skills.
E. The learning difficulties cannot be acquired later in life.

Correct Answer: C. There usually is a discrepancy of more than 2 standard deviations (SD) between achievement and IQ.

Explanation: DSM-IV stipulated that the individual's achievement on standardized tests be "substantially below" that expected for age, schooling, and level of intelligence. DSM-5 text further clarifies that academic skills are distributed along a continuum, so there is no natural cutpoint that can be used to differentiate individuals with and without specific learning disorder. Thus, any threshold used to specify what constitutes significantly low academic achievement (e.g., academic skills well below age expectation) is to a large extent arbitrary. Low achievement scores on one or more standardized tests or subtests within an academic domain (i.e., at least 1.5 SD below the population mean for age, which translates to a standard score ≤78, which is below the 7th percentile) are needed for the greatest diagnostic certainty. However, precise scores will vary according to the particular standardized tests that are used. Based on clinical judgment, a more lenient threshold may be used (e.g., 1.0–2.5 SD below the population mean for age), when learning difficulties are supported by converging evidence from clinical assessment, academic history, school reports, or test scores. Moreover, since standardized tests are not available in all languages, the diagnosis may then be based in part on clinical judgment of scores on available test measures.

1.46—Specific Learning Disorder / Diagnostic Features (p. 68)

1.47   Which of the following statements about the diagnosis of specific learning disorder is *false*?

A. Specific learning disorder is distinct from learning problems associated with a neurodegenerative cognitive disorder.
B. If intellectual disability (intellectual developmental disorder) is present, the learning difficulties must be in excess of those expected.
C. An uneven profile of abilities is typical in specific learning disorder.

D. Attentional difficulties and motor clumsiness that are subthreshold for attention-deficit/hyperactivity disorder or developmental coordination disorder are frequently associated with specific learning disorder.

E. There are four formal subtypes of specific learning disorder.

Correct Answer: E. There are four formal subtypes of specific learning disorder.

Explanation: In DSM-5, there are no formal subtypes of specific learning disorder. Learning deficits in the areas of reading, written expression, and mathematics are coded as separate specifiers.

1.47—Specific Learning Disorder / Differential Diagnosis (p. 73)

1.48 Which of the following statements about prevalence rates for specific learning disorder is *false?*

A. Prevalence rates range from 5% to 15% among school-age children across languages and cultures.

B. Prevalence in adults is approximately 4%.

C. Specific learning disorder is equally common among males and females.

D. Prevalence rates vary according to the range of ages in the sample, selection criteria, severity of specific learning disorder, and academic domains investigated.

E. Gender ratios cannot be attributed to factors such as ascertainment bias, definitional or measurement variation, language, race, or socioeconomic status.

Correct Answer: C. Specific learning disorder is equally common among males and females.

Explanation: Specific learning disorder is more common in males than in females (ratios range from about 2:1 to 3:1 and cannot be attributed to factors such as ascertainment bias, definitional or measurement variation, language, race, or socioeconomic status). The prevalence of specific learning disorder across the academic domains of reading, writing, and mathematics is approximately 5%–15% among school-age children across different languages and cultures. Prevalence in adults is unknown but appears to be approximately 4%.

1.48—Specific Learning Disorder / Prevalence (p. 70); Gender-Related Diagnostic Issues (p. 73)

1.49 Which of the following statements about comorbidity in specific learning disorder is *true?*

A. Attention-deficit/hyperactivity disorder (ADHD) does not co-occur with specific learning disorder more frequently than would be expected by chance.
B. Speech sound disorder and specific language impairments are not commonly comorbid with specific learning disorder.
C. Identified clusters of co-occurrences include severe reading disorders; fine motor problems and handwriting problems; and problems with arithmetic, reading, and gross motor planning.
D. The co-occurrence of specific learning disorder and specific language impairments has been shown in up to 20% of children with language problems.
E. Co-occurring disorders generally do not influence the course or treatment of specific learning disorder.

Correct Answer: C. Identified clusters of co-occurrences include severe reading disorders; fine motor problems and handwriting problems; and problems with arithmetic, reading, and gross motor planning.

Explanation: Specific learning disorder commonly co-occurs with neurodevelopmental (e.g., ADHD, communication disorders, developmental coordination disorder, autistic spectrum disorder) or other mental disorders (e.g., anxiety disorders, depressive and bipolar disorders). These comorbidities do not necessarily exclude the diagnosis of specific learning disorder but may make testing and differential diagnosis more difficult, because each of the co-occurring disorders independently interferes with the execution of activities of daily living, including learning. Thus, clinical judgment is required to attribute such impairment to learning difficulties. If there is an indication that another diagnosis could account for the difficulties learning keystone academic skills described in Criterion A, specific learning disorder should not be diagnosed. Co-occurring disorders generally do influence the course or treatment, and when a child/adolescent is being evaluated, co-occurring disorders should be listed.

1.49—Specific Learning Disorder / Comorbidity (p. 74)

1.50 Which of the following statements about developmental coordination disorder (DCD) is *true*?

A. Some children with DCD show additional (usually suppressed) motor activity, such as choreiform movements of unsupported limbs or mirror movements.
B. The prevalence of DCD in children ages 5–11 years is 1%–3%.
C. In early adulthood, there is improvement in learning new tasks involving complex/automatic motor skills, including driving and using tools.
D. DCD has no association with prenatal exposure to alcohol or with low birth weight or preterm birth.

E. Impairments in underlying neurodevelopmental processes have not been found to primarily affect visuomotor skills.

Correct Answer: A. Some children with DCD show additional (usually suppressed) motor activity, such as choreiform movements of unsupported limbs or mirror movements.

Explanation: In regard to the choreiform or mirror movements seen in DCD, DSM-5 states, "these 'overflow' movements are referred to as *neurodevelopmental immaturities* or *neurological soft signs* rather than neurological abnormalities. In both current literature and clinical practice, their role in diagnosis is still unclear, requiring further evaluation." The prevalence of DCD in children ages 5–11 years is 5%–6% (in children age 7 years, 1.8% are diagnosed with severe DCD and 3% with probable DCD). In adulthood, there are often ongoing problems with learning new tasks involving complex/automatic motor skills. DCD is more common following prenatal exposure to alcohol and in preterm and low-birth-weight children. In DCD, deficits have been identified in both visuomotor perception and spatial mentalizing; these deficits affect the ability to make rapid motoric adjustments as the complexity of the required movements increases.

> 1.50—Developmental Coordination Disorder / Associated Features Supporting Diagnosis; Prevalence; Risk and Prognostic Factors (pp. 75, 76)

1.51 Which of the following statements about developmental coordination disorder (DCD) is *true?*

A. The disorder is usually not diagnosed before the age of 7 years.
B. Symptoms have usually improved significantly at 1-year follow-up.
C. In most cases, symptoms are no longer evident by adolescence.
D. DCD has no clear relationship with prenatal alcohol exposure, preterm birth, or low birth weight.
E. Cerebellar dysfunction is hypothesized to play a role in DCD.

Correct Answer: E. Cerebellar dysfunction is hypothesized to play a role in DCD.

Explanation: DCD is usually not diagnosed before 5 years of age, and the course has been demonstrated to be stable up to 1-year follow-up. In about 50%–70% of cases, symptoms continue into adolescence. Prenatal alcohol exposure, prematurity, and low birth weight may be risk factors.

> 1.51—Developmental Coordination Disorder / Development and Course (p. 75)

1.52   Which of the following is *not* a criterion for the DSM-5 diagnosis of stereotypic movement disorder?

A. Motor behaviors are present that are repetitive, seemingly driven, and apparently purposeless.
B. Onset of the behaviors is in the early developmental period.
C. The behaviors result in self-inflicted bodily injury that requires medical treatment.
D. The behaviors are not attributable to the physiological effects of a substance or neurological condition or better explained by another neurodevelopmental or mental disorder.
E. The behaviors interfere with social, academic, or other activities.

Correct Answer: C. The behaviors result in self-inflicted bodily injury that requires medical treatment.

Explanation: Although the repetitive behaviors *may* result in self-injury, that is not a criterion for the diagnosis. All of the other options represent criteria for the diagnosis of stereotypic movement disorder.

1.52—Stereotypic Movement Disorder / diagnostic criteria (p. 77)

1.53   Which of the following statements about the developmental course of stereotypic movement disorder is *false?*

A. The presence of stereotypic movements may indicate an undetected neurodevelopmental problem, especially in children ages 1–3 years.
B. Among typically developing children, the repetitive movements may be stopped when attention is directed to them or when the child is distracted from performing them.
C. In some children, the stereotypic movements would result in self-injury if protective measures were not used.
D. Whereas simple stereotypic movements (e.g., rocking) are common in young typically developing children, complex stereotypic movements are much less common (approximately 3%–4%).
E. Stereotypic movements typically begin within the first year of life.

Correct Answer: E. Stereotypic movements typically begin within the first year of life.

Explanation: The movements typically begin within the first 3 years of life. Simple stereotypic movements are common in infancy and may be involved in acquisition of motor mastery. In children who develop complex motor stereotypies, approximately 80% exhibit symptoms before 24 months of age, 12% between 24 and 35 months, and 8% at 36 months or older.

1.53—Stereotypic Movement Disorder / Development and Course (p. 79)

1.54   Which of the following is a DSM-5 diagnostic criterion for Tourette's disorder?

A. Tics occur throughout a period of more than 1 year, and during this period there was never a tic-free period of more than 3 consecutive months.
B. Onset is before age 5 years.
C. The tics may wax and wane in frequency but have persisted for more than 1 year since first tic onset.
D. Motor tics must precede vocal tics.
E. The tics may occur many times a day for at least 4 weeks, but no longer than 12 consecutive months.

Correct Answer: C. The tics may wax and wane in frequency but have persisted for more than 1 year since first tic onset.

Explanation: Only option C is a criterion for the DSM-5 diagnosis of Tourette's disorder. In DSM-IV, Criterion B specified that tics must have been present for "a period of more than 1 year, and during this period there was never a tic-free period of more than 3 consecutive months." In DSM-5 this criterion was simplified to the requirement that tics must have persisted for more than 1 year since first tic onset.

1.54—Tic Disorders / diagnostic criteria (p. 81)

1.55   At her child's third office visit, the mother of an 8-year-old boy with a 6-month history of excessive eye blinking and intermittent chirping says that she has noticed the development of grunting sounds since he started school this term. What is the most likely diagnosis?

A. Tourette's disorder.
B. Provisional tic disorder.
C. Temporary tic disorder.
D. Persistent (chronic) vocal tic disorder.
E. Transient tic disorder, recurrent.

Correct Answer: B. Provisional tic disorder.

Explanation: The presence of single or multiple motor and/or vocal tics for *less* than 1 year meets Criteria A and B for provisional tic disorder. This is in contrast to Tourette's disorder, where tics must be present for *more* than 1 year. Thus, option A is incorrect. There is no such disorder as temporary tic disorder (option C). Persistent (chronic) vocal tic disorder (option D) is incorrect because in this vignette the boy has *both* motor and vocal tics, and they have been present for less than 1 year. Transient tic disorder, recurrent (option E), would have been correct if the question were asking for a DSM-IV diagnosis; however, transient tic disorder has been revised and renamed provisional tic disorder in DSM-5.

1.55—Tic Disorders / diagnostic criteria (p. 81)

1.56   A 5-year-old girl is referred to your care with a DSM-IV diagnosis of chronic motor or vocal tic disorder. Under DSM-5, she would meet criteria for persistent (chronic) motor or vocal tic disorder. Which of the following statements about her new diagnosis under DSM-5 is *false?*

A. She may have single or multiple motor or vocal tics, but not both.
B. Her tics must persist for more than 1 year since first tic onset without a tic-free period for 3 consecutive months to meet diagnostic criteria.
C. Her tics may wax and wane in frequency but have persisted for more than 1 year since first tic onset.
D. She has never met criteria for Tourette's disorder.
E. A specifier may be added to the diagnosis of persistent (chronic) motor or vocal tic disorder to indicate whether the girl has motor or vocal tics.

Correct Answer: B. Her tics must persist for more than 1 year since first tic onset without a tic-free period for 3 consecutive months to meet diagnostic criteria.

Explanation: Under DSM-5 criteria for persistent (chronic) motor or vocal tic disorder, tics may wax and wane. There is also no longer a requirement for a tic-free period. Thus, option C is true, and option B is the false statement. Options A and D are diagnostic criteria that are true for this classification under both DSM-IV and DSM-5. Option E is true because in DSM-5, one can specify "motor tics only" or "vocal tics only."

1.56—Tic Disorders / diagnostic criteria (p. 81)

1.57   A highly functional 20-year-old college student with a history of anxiety symptoms and attention-deficit/hyperactivity disorder, for which she is prescribed lisdexamfetamine (Vyvanse), tells her psychiatrist that she has been researching the side effects of her medication for one of her class projects. In addition, she says that for the past week she has been feeling stressed by her schoolwork, and her friends have been asking her why she intermittently bobs her head up and down multiple times a day. What is the most likely diagnosis?

A. Provisional tic disorder.
B. Unspecified tic disorder.
C. Unspecified anxiety disorder.
D. Obsessive-compulsive personality disorder.
E. Unspecified stimulant-induced disorder.

Correct Answer: B. Unspecified tic disorder.

Explanation: Given the data provided by the vignette, unspecified tic disorder (option B) is the best answer. Included in this category are presentations in which there is uncertainty about whether the tic is attributable to medication versus primary. By definition, onset must be before age 18 years for all tic disorders. Tic onset after 18 years of age would be diagnosed as unspecified tic disorder. Option E is incorrect given that the student is highly functioning, lacks significant impairment in her life (based on the limited details provided in the vignette), and takes lisdexamfetamine (Vyvanse), which may have less abuse potential since it is a prodrug.

1.57—Tic Disorders / Differential Diagnosis (p. 84)

1.58 Which of the following is *not* a DSM-5 diagnostic criterion for language disorder?

A. Persistent difficulties in the acquisition and use of language across modalities due to deficits in comprehension or production.
B. Language abilities that are substantially and quantifiably below those expected for age.
C. Symptom onset in the early developmental period.
D. Inability to attribute difficulties to hearing or other sensory impairment, motor dysfunction, or another medical or neurological condition.
E. Failure to meet criteria for mixed receptive-expressive language disorder or a pervasive developmental disorder.

Correct Answer: E. Failure to meet criteria for mixed receptive-expressive language disorder or a pervasive developmental disorder.

Explanation: Options A through D constitute the DSM-5 diagnostic criteria for language disorder. This diagnosis replaced the DSM-IV diagnoses expressive language disorder and mixed receptive-expressive language disorder. Option E is a criterion for expressive language disorder in DSM-IV and is thus incorrect. In contrast to DSM-IV, in DSM-5 meeting criteria for pervasive developmental disorder does not preclude one from being diagnosed with language disorder.

1.58—Language Disorder / diagnostic criteria (p. 42)

1.59 Which of the following statements about speech sound disorder is *true*?

A. Speech sound production must be present by age 2 years.
B. "Failure to use developmentally expected speech sounds" is assessed by comparison of a child with his or her peers of the same age and dialect.
C. The difficulties in speech sound production need not result in functional impairment to meet diagnostic criteria.

D. Symptom onset is in the early developmental period.

E. Both A and C are true.

Correct Answer: D. Symptom onset is in the early developmental period.

Explanation: The diagnosis of speech sound disorder in DSM-5 replaces the diagnosis of phonological disorder in DSM-IV. According to DSM-IV, Criterion A in the classification of phonological disorder is the "failure to use developmentally expected speech sounds that are appropriate for age and dialect." This has been revised in DSM-5 such that presence of "persistent difficulties in speech sound production that interfere with communication" suffices for Criterion A. Thus, option B is incorrect. There is also no specific age at onset for symptoms in speech sound disorder, but Criterion C specifies that symptom onset must be in the early developmental period. Thus, options A and E are incorrect, and D is the correct answer. Option C is a false statement, because Criterion B of speech sound disorder *does* require that difficulties from speech sound production interfere with one's function in social, academic, and occupational performance.

1.59—Speech Sound Disorder / diagnostic criteria (p. 44)

1.60   A mother brings her 4-year-old son to you for an evaluation with concerns that her son has struggled with speech articulation since very young. He has not sustained any head injuries, is otherwise healthy, and has a normal IQ. His preschool teacher reports that she does not always understand what he is saying and that other children tease him by calling him a "baby" due to his difficulty with communication. He does not have trouble relating to other people or understanding nonverbal social cues. What is the most likely diagnosis?

A. Selective mutism.

B. Global developmental delay.

C. Speech sound disorder.

D. Avoidant personality disorder.

E. Unspecified anxiety disorder.

Correct Answer: C. Speech sound disorder.

Explanation: In this vignette, the child exhibits "persistent difficulty with speech sound production that interferes with speech intelligibility" leading to functional limitations in effective communication that interfere with social participation. Additionally, his symptoms are not attributable to a congenital or acquired medical condition and his symptom onset is in the early developmental period. These are the criteria for speech sound disorder. Option A is incorrect because the boy's difficulty in communication is in the sound production, rather than lack of communication during specific situations. Children who are selectively mute do not have difficulty with speech production. Option B is also incorrect because apart from difficulty with speech sound production, the boy relates well to other people and understands nonverbal cues. Option D is incorrect because the boy is too young to be diagnosed with an avoidant personality disorder; patterns of such behavior would be evident in early adulthood. Finally, although the boy may have some anxiety symptoms, this is difficult to assess without additional information. Thus, option E is incorrect.

1.60—Speech Sound Disorder / diagnostic criteria (p. 44)

1.61   A 6-year-old boy is failing school and continues to struggle significantly with grammar, sentence construction, and vocabulary. When he speaks, he also interjects "and" in between all his words. His teacher reports that he requires more verbal redirection than other students in order to stay on task. He is generally quiet and does not cause trouble otherwise. Which of the following diagnoses would be on your differential?

A. Language disorder.
B. Expressive language disorder.
C. Childhood-onset fluency disorder.
D. Attention-deficit/hyperactivity disorder (ADHD).
E. A and D.

Correct Answer: E. Language disorder and ADHD.

Explanation: This question asks for DSM-5 *diagnoses*, so option B is incorrect because expressive and mixed receptive-expressive language disorders are from DSM-IV. They are now consolidated into *language disorder* in DSM-5. Option A, language disorder, would be an important consideration in the differential diagnosis because the boy has persistent difficulties with both the production and possibly comprehension of language. The boy may need additional repetition to understand commands and may not interact with peers as readily due to communication difficulty, and thus appears quiet. Option C is incorrect because word interjections (e.g., "and") are no longer considered a type of speech disturbance in DSM-5. ADHD is a potential consideration given this boy's difficulty in staying on task and his poor academic performance. Thus, option E is the correct answer, and both language disorder and ADHD are diagnostic possibilities.

1.61—Language Disorder / Comorbidity (p. 44)

1.62   Which of the following types of disturbance in normal speech fluency/time patterning included in the DSM-IV criteria for stuttering was omitted in the DSM-5 criteria for childhood-onset fluency disorder (stuttering)?

A. Sound prolongation.
B. Circumlocution.
C. Interjections.

D. Words produced with an excess of physical tension.

E. Sound and syllable repetitions.

Correct Answer: C. Interjections.

Explanation: Criterion A for childhood-onset fluency disorder in DSM-5 requires the presence of one or more of seven types of disturbances, including those listed in options A, B, D, and E. The other speech fluency disturbances are broken words, audible or silent blocking, and monosyllabic whole-word repetitions. "Interjections" (option C) is the only fluency disturbance for stuttering in the DSM-IV criteria that was omitted in the DSM-5 criteria.

1.62—Childhood-Onset Fluency Disorder (Stuttering) / diagnostic criteria (p. 45)

1.63   A 14-year-old boy in regular education tells you that he thinks a girl in class likes him. His mother is surprised to hear this, because she reports that, since a young age, he has often struggled with making inferences or understanding nuances from what other people say. The teacher has also noticed that he sometimes misses nonverbal cues. He tends to get along better with adults, perhaps because they are not as likely to be put off by his overly formal speech. When he makes jokes, his peers do not always find the humor appropriate. Although he enjoys spending time with his best friend, he can be talkative and struggles with taking turns in conversation. What is the most likely diagnosis?

A. Social (pragmatic) communication disorder.

B. Asperger's disorder.

C. Autism spectrum disorder.

D. Social anxiety disorder.

E. Language disorder.

Correct Answer: A. Social (pragmatic) communication disorder.

Explanation: Social (pragmatic) communication disorder is a new DSM-5 diagnosis characterized by "persistent difficulties in the social use of verbal and nonverbal communication as manifested by all of the following: 1) deficits in using communication for social purposes…in a manner that is appropriate for the social context, 2) impairment in the ability to change communication to match context or needs of the listener, 3) difficulties following rules for conversation and storytelling…and knowing how to use verbal and nonverbal signals to regulate interaction, [and] 4) difficulties understanding what is not explicitly stated." These deficits present in the early development period and result in functional limitations. Options B and C are incorrect because, respectively, Asperger's disorder is no longer a classification in DSM-5, and if this boy had autism he would likely be more impaired and unable to sustain a conversation. Option D is incorrect because social anxiety disorder would not affect one's ability to understand nuances in verbal and nonverbal communication. Option E is incorrect because the boy does not have difficulty with the production or comprehension of language, but rather with the nuances and social appropriateness of language content.

1.63—Social (Pragmatic) Communication Disorder / Differential Diagnosis (p. 49)

1.64 A 15-year-old boy with a prior diagnosis of Tourette's disorder is referred to your care. His mother tells you that during middle school he was teased for having vocal and motor tics. Since starting ninth grade, his tics have become less frequent. Currently, only mild motor tics remain. What is the appropriate DSM-5 diagnosis?

A. Tourette's disorder.
B. Persistent (chronic) motor tic disorder.
C. Provisional tic disorder.
D. Unspecified tic disorder.
E. Persistent (chronic) vocal tic disorder.

Correct Answer: A. Tourette's disorder.

Explanation: There are four tic disorder diagnostic categories, and they follow a hierarchical order: 1) Tourette's disorder, 2) persistent (chronic) motor or vocal tic disorder, 3) provisional tic disorder, and 4) unspecified tic disorder. According to Criterion E for tic disorders in DSM-5, once someone is diagnosed with a tic disorder at one level of the hierarchy, a diagnosis that is lower in the hierarchy cannot be made. In this case, option A is the correct answer because the boy has already been previously diagnosed with Tourette's disorder, which is at the top of the tic disorder hierarchy. Thus, at this point, he can no longer be diagnosed with persistent (chronic) motor tic disorder (option B). Options C and D are incorrect.

1.64—Tic Disorders / diagnostic criteria (p. 81)

1.65 Tics typically present for the first time during which developmental stage?

A. Infancy.
B. Prepuberty.
C. Latency.
D. Adolescence.
E. Adulthood.

Correct Answer: B. Prepuberty.

Explanation: Although it is not uncommon for adolescents and adults to present for an initial diagnostic assessment for tics, the initial onset of tics generally occurs during the prepubertal stage (ages 4–6 years). Tics then reach peak severity around ages 10–12 years, followed by a decline during adolescence. The incidence of new tic disorders decreases during the teen years, and even more so during adulthood. Clinicians should be wary of new-onset abnormal movements suggestive of tics outside of the usual age range.

1.65—Tic Disorders / Development and Course (p. 83)

1.66   A 7-year-old boy who has speech delays presents with long-standing, repetitive hand waving, arm flapping, and finger wiggling. His mother reports that she first noticed these symptoms when he was a toddler and wonders whether they are tics. She says that he tends to flap more when he is engrossed in activities, such as while watching his favorite television program, but will stop when called or distracted. Based on the mother's report, which of the following conditions would be highest on your list of possible diagnoses?

A. Provisional tic disorder.
B. Persistent (chronic) motor or vocal tic disorder.
C. Chorea.
D. Dystonia.
E. Motor stereotypies.

Correct Answer: E. Motor stereotypies.

Explanation: The boy's movements are not tics, but stereotypies. *Motor stereotypies* are defined as involuntary rhythmic, repetitive, predictable movements that appear purposeful but serve no obvious adaptive function or purpose and stop with distraction. Motor stereotypies can be differentiated from tics based on the former's earlier age at onset (younger than 3 years), prolonged duration (seconds to minutes), constant repetitive fixed form and location, exacerbation when engrossed in activities, lack of a premonitory urge, and cessation with distraction (e.g., name called or touched). Clinical history is crucial for differentiation.

   Chorea represents rapid, random, continual, abrupt, irregular, unpredictable, nonstereotyped actions that are usually bilateral and affect all parts of the body (i.e., face, trunk, and limbs). The timing, direction, and distribution of movements vary from moment to moment, and movements usually worsen during attempted voluntary action. *Dystonia* is the simultaneous sustained contracture of both agonist and antagonist muscles, resulting in a distorted posture or movement of parts of the body. Dystonic postures are often triggered by attempts at voluntary movements and are not seen during sleep. The boy's movements do not fit these categories.

1.66—Stereotypic Movement Disorder / Differential Diagnosis (p. 84)

1.67   Assessment of co-occurring conditions is important for understanding the overall functional consequence of tics on an individual. Which of the following conditions has been associated with tic disorders?

A. Attention-deficit/hyperactivity disorder (ADHD).

B. Obsessive-compulsive and related disorders.

C. Other movement disorders.

D. Depressive disorders.

E. All of the above.

Correct Answer: E. All of the above.

Explanation: Many medical and psychiatric conditions have been described as co-occurring with tic disorders, with ADHD and obsessive-compulsive and related disorders being particularly common. Children with ADHD may demonstrate disruptive behavior, social immaturity, and learning difficulties that may interfere with academic progress and interpersonal relationships and lead to greater impairment than that caused by a tic disorder. Individuals with tic disorders can also have other movement disorders and other mental disorders, such as depressive, bipolar, or substance use disorders.

1.67—Tic Disorders / Comorbidity (p. 85)

1.68   By what age should most children have acquired adequate speech and language ability to understand and follow social rules of verbal and nonverbal communication, follow rules for conversation and storytelling, and change language according to the needs of the listener or situation?

A. Ages 2–3 years.

B. Ages 3–4 years.

C. Ages 4–5 years.

D. Ages 5–6 years.

E. Ages 6–7 years.

Correct Answer: C. Ages 4–5 years.

Explanation: Because social (pragmatic) communication depends on adequate developmental progress in speech and language, diagnosis of social (pragmatic) communication disorder is rare among children younger than 4 years. By age 4 or 5 years, most children should possess adequate speech and language abilities to permit identification of specific deficits in social communication. Milder forms of the disorder may not become apparent until early adolescence, when language and social interactions become more complex.

1.68—Social (Pragmatic) Communication Disorder / Development and Course (p. 48)

1.69   Having a family history of which of the following psychiatric disorders increases an individual's risk of social (pragmatic) communication disorder?

A. Social anxiety disorder (social phobia).

B. Autism spectrum disorder.

C. Attention-deficit/hyperactivity disorder (ADHD).

D. Specific learning disorder.

E. Either B or D.

Correct Answer: E. Either B or D.

Explanation: A family history of autism spectrum disorder, communication disorders, or specific learning disorder appears to increase the risk of social (pragmatic) communication disorder. Although deficits stemming from ADHD and social anxiety disorder (social phobia) may overlap with symptoms of social communication disorder and may represent important considerations in the differential diagnosis, their presence in an individual's family history is not currently known to increase that person's risk of social (pragmatic) communication disorder.

1.69—Social (Pragmatic) Communication Disorder / Development and Course (p. 48)

1.70   A 6-year-old boy with a history of mild language delay is brought to your office by his mother, who is concerned that he is being teased in school because he misinterprets nonverbal cues and speaks in overly formal language with his peers. She tells you that her son was in an early intervention program, but his written and spoken language is now at grade level. The boy does not have a history of repetitive movements, sensory issues, or ritualized behaviors. Although he prefers constancy, he adapts fairly well to new situations. Additionally, he has a long-standing interest in trains and cars and is able to recite for you all the car models he memorized from a book on the history of transportation. Which of the following disorders would be a primary consideration in the differential diagnosis?

A. Social (pragmatic) communication disorder.

B. Autism spectrum disorder.

C. Global developmental delay.

D. Language disorder.

E. A and B.

Correct Answer: A. Social (pragmatic) communication disorder.

Explanation: The presence of restricted interests and repetitive behaviors, interests, and activities beginning from early development is the primary diagnostic difference between autism spectrum disorder and social (pragmatic) communication disorder. In this vignette, the boy does not meet Criterion B for autism spectrum disorder, which requires evidence of at least two restricted, repetitive patterns of behavior, interests, or activities. Furthermore, although the boy has an interest in cars and trains, these are not necessarily atypical interests for boys at his age. Option E is also incorrect because in addition to the aforementioned reason, the two diagnoses are mutually exclusive. According to DSM-5, an individual who shows impairment in social communication and social interactions but does not show restricted and repetitive behavior or interests may meet criteria for social communication disorder instead of autism spectrum disorder. "The diagnosis of autism spectrum disorder supersedes that of social (pragmatic) communication disorder whenever the criteria for autism spectrum disorder are met, and care should be taken to enquire carefully regarding past or current restricted/repetitive behavior." Option D is incorrect because, from the limited data in the case, the mother suggests that his language is no longer a problem. Similarly, although option C would also be a consideration in the differential diagnosis, it is not the best answer given the data.

1.70—Social (Pragmatic) Communication Disorder / Differential Diagnosis (p. 49)

1.71 Below what age is it difficult to distinguish a language disorder from normal developmental variations?

A. Age 2 years.
B. Age 3 years.
C. Age 4 years.
D. Age 5 years.
E. Age 6 years.

Correct Answer: C. Age 4 years.

Explanation: During the early developmental period, there is significant variation in early language acquisition, and it may be difficult to distinguish normal variations from impairments. By the time a child is 4 years old, language ability becomes more stable.

1.71—Language Disorder / Differential Diagnosis (p. 43)

1.72 Which of the following psychiatric diagnoses is strongly associated with language disorder?

A. Attention-deficit/hyperactivity disorder.
B. Developmental coordination disorder.
C. Autism spectrum disorder.
D. Social (pragmatic) communication disorder.
E. All of the above.

Correct Answer: E. All of the above.

Explanation: Language disorder is strongly associated with other neurodevelopmental disorders in terms of specific learning disorder (literacy and numeracy), attention-deficit/hyperactivity disorder, autism spectrum disorder, and developmental coordination disorder. It is also associated with social (pragmatic) communication disorder. A positive family history of speech or language disorders is often present.

1.72—Language Disorder / Comorbidity (p. 44)

1.73 Which of the following statements about the development of speech as it applies to speech sound disorder is *false?*

A. Most children with speech sound disorder respond well to treatment.
B. Speech sound production should be mostly intelligible by age 3 years.
C. Most speech sounds should be pronounced clearly and accurately according to age and community norms before age 10 years.
D. Lisping may or may not be associated with speech sound disorder.
E. It is abnormal for children to shorten words when they are learning to talk.

Correct Answer: E. It is abnormal for children to shorten words when they are learning to talk.

Explanation: Speech sound production requires both phonological knowledge and the ability to coordinate movements of the jaw, tongue, lips, and breath. A speech sound disorder is diagnosed when the speech sound production is not what is expected based on the child's age and developmental stage. Developmentally, children often shorten words and syllables when they are learning to talk, but by age 3–4 years, most of their speech should be intelligible. By age 7, most speech sounds should be articulated clearly according to age and community norms. Lisping is common in speech sound disorder and may be associated with an abnormal tongue-thrust swallowing pattern.

1.73—Speech Sound Disorder (pp. 44–45)

1.74 Which of the following would likely *not* be an important condition to rule out in the differential diagnosis of speech sound disorder?

A. Normal variations in speech.
B. Hearing or other sensory impairment.
C. Dysarthria.
D. Depression.
E. Selective mutism.

Correct Answer: D. Depression.

Explanation: All of the options except option D are important considerations when making a diagnosis of speech sound disorder. Regional and cultural variations are important to consider, as well as abnormalities of speech due to hearing impairments. Dysarthria includes speech impairments due to a motor disorder and must also be considered, especially since this may be difficult to differentiate in young children. Selective mutism may be due to embarrassment or shyness.

1.74—Speech Sound Disorder / Differential Diagnosis (p. 45)

1.75 Which of the following statements about the development of childhood-onset fluency disorder (stuttering) is *true?*

A. Stuttering occurs by age 6 for 80%–90% of affected individuals.
B. Stuttering always begin abruptly and is noticeable to everyone.
C. Stress and anxiety do not exacerbate disfluency.
D. Motor movements are not associated with this disorder.
E. None of the above.

Correct Answer: A. Stuttering occurs by age 6 for 80%–90% of affected individuals.

Explanation: The key feature of childhood-onset fluency disorder is a disturbance in the normal fluency and time patterning of speech that is inappropriate for the individual's age. Age at onset ranges from 2 to 7 years and occurs by age 6 for 80%–90% of affected individuals. Disfluencies can be gradual or sudden, and even subtle (thus, option B is incorrect). Emotional stress or anxiety can exacerbate stuttering, and motor movements may sometimes accompany this disorder (thus, options C and D are incorrect).

1.75—Childhood-Onset Fluency Disorder (Stuttering) (pp. 45–47)

CHAPTER 2

Schizophrenia Spectrum and Other Psychotic Disorders

2.1   Criterion A for schizoaffective disorder requires an uninterrupted period of ill-
        ness during which Criterion A for schizophrenia is met. Which of the following
        additional symptoms must be present to fulfill diagnostic criteria for schizoaf-
        fective disorder?

        A. An anxiety episode—either panic or general anxiety.
        B. Rapid eye movement (REM) sleep behavior disorder.
        C. A major depressive or manic episode.
        D. Hypomania.
        E. Cyclothymia.

        Correct Answer: C. A major depressive or manic episode.

        Explanation: The diagnosis of schizoaffective disorder is based on the presence
        of an uninterrupted period of illness during which Criterion A for schizophre-
        nia is met. Criterion B (social dysfunction) and Criterion F (exclusion of autism
        spectrum disorder or other communication disorder of childhood onset) for
        schizophrenia do not have to be met. In addition to meeting Criterion A for
        schizophrenia, there must be a major mood episode (major depressive or
        manic) (Criterion A for schizoaffective disorder). Because loss of interest or
        pleasure is common in schizophrenia, to meet Criterion A for schizoaffective
        disorder, the major depressive episode must include pervasive depressed
        mood (i.e., the presence of markedly diminished interest or pleasure is not suf-
        ficient). The episodes of depression or mania must be present for the majority
        of the total duration of the illness (i.e., after Criterion A has been met) (Crite-
        rion C for schizoaffective disorder).

        2.1—Schizoaffective Disorder / Diagnostic Features (pp. 106–107)

2.2   There is a requirement for a major depressive episode or a manic episode to be
        part of the symptom picture for a DSM-5 diagnosis of schizoaffective disorder.
        In order to separate schizoaffective disorder from depressive or bipolar disor-
        der with psychotic features, which of the following symptoms must be present

for at least 2 weeks in the absence of a major mood episode at some point during the lifetime duration of the illness?

A. Delusions or hallucinations.
B. Delusions or paranoia.
C. Regressed behavior.
D. Projective identification.
E. Binge eating.

Correct Answer: A. Delusions or hallucinations.

Explanation: To separate schizoaffective disorder from a depressive or bipolar disorder with psychotic features, Criterion B for schizoaffective disorder specifies that delusions or hallucinations must be present for at least 2 weeks in the absence of a major mood episode (depressive or manic) at some point during the lifetime duration of the illness.

2.2—Schizoaffective Disorder / Diagnostic Features (p. 107)

2.3   A 27-year-old unmarried truck driver has a 5-year history of active and residual symptoms of schizophrenia. He develops symptoms of depression, including depressed mood and anhedonia, that last 4 months and resolve with treatment but do not meet criteria for major depression. Which diagnosis best fits this clinical presentation?

A. Schizoaffective disorder.
B. Unspecified schizophrenia spectrum and other psychotic disorder.
C. Unspecified depressive disorder.
D. Schizophrenia and unspecified depressive disorder.
E. Unspecified bipolar and related disorder.

Correct Answer: D. Schizophrenia and unspecified depressive disorder.

Explanation: The depressive and manic episodes, taken together, do not occupy more than 1 year during the 5-year history. Thus, the presentation does not meet Criterion C for schizoaffective disorder, and the diagnosis remains schizophrenia. The additional diagnosis of unspecified depressive disorder may be added to indicate the superimposed depressive episode.

2.3—Schizoaffective Disorder / Differential Diagnosis (pp. 109–110)

2.4   How common is schizoaffective disorder relative to schizophrenia?

A. Much more common.
B. Twice as common.
C. Equally common.

D. One-half as common.

E. One-third as common.

Correct Answer: E. One-third as common.

Explanation: Schizoaffective disorder appears to be about one-third as common as schizophrenia, with a lifetime prevalence of 0.3%.

2.4—Schizoaffective Disorder / Prevalence (p. 107)

2.5   A 30-year-old single woman reports having experienced auditory and persecutory delusions for 2 months, followed by a full major depressive episode with sad mood, anhedonia, and suicidal ideation lasting 3 months. Although the depressive episode resolves with pharmacotherapy and psychotherapy, the psychotic symptoms persist for another month before resolving. What diagnosis best fits this clinical picture?

A. Brief psychotic disorder.

B. Schizoaffective disorder.

C. Major depressive disorder.

D. Major depressive disorder with psychotic features.

E. Bipolar I disorder, current episode manic, with mixed features.

Correct Answer: B. Schizoaffective disorder.

Explanation: During this period of illness, the woman's symptoms concurrently met criteria for a major depressive episode and Criterion A for schizophrenia. Auditory hallucinations and delusions were present both before and after the depressive phase. The total period of illness lasted for about 6 months, with psychotic symptoms alone present during the initial 2 months, both depressive and psychotic symptoms present during the next 3 months, and psychotic symptoms alone present during the last month. The duration of the depressive episode was not brief relative to the total duration of the psychotic disturbance.

2.5—Schizoaffective Disorder / Diagnostic Features (pp. 106–107); Differential Diagnosis (pp. 109–110)

2.6   Which of the following statements about the incidence of schizoaffective disorder is *true?*

A. The incidence is equal in women and men.

B. The incidence is higher in men.

C. The incidence is higher in women.

D. The incidence rates are unknown.

E. The incidence rates vary based on seasonality of birth.

Correct Answer: C. The incidence is higher in women.

Explanation: The incidence of schizoaffective disorder is higher in women than in men, mainly due to an increased incidence of the depressive type among women.

2.6—Schizoaffective Disorder/ Prevalence (pp. 107–108)

2.7   Substance/medication-induced psychotic disorder cannot be diagnosed if the disturbance is better explained by an independent psychotic disorder that is not induced by a substance/medication. Which of the following psychotic symptom presentations would *not* be evidence of an independent psychotic disorder?

   A. Psychotic symptoms that precede the onset of severe intoxication or acute withdrawal.
   B. Psychotic symptoms that meet full criteria for a psychotic disorder and that persist for a substantial period after cessation of severe intoxication or acute withdrawal.
   C. Psychotic symptoms that are substantially in excess of what would be expected given the type or amount of the substance used or the duration of use.
   D. Psychotic symptoms that occur during a period of sustained substance abstinence.
   E. Psychotic symptoms that occur during a medical admission for substance withdrawal.

Correct Answer: E. Psychotic symptoms that occur during a medical admission for substance withdrawal.

Explanation: A substance/medication-induced psychotic disorder is distinguished from a primary psychotic disorder by considering the onset, course, and other factors. For drugs of abuse, there must be evidence from the history, physical examination, or laboratory findings of substance use, intoxication, or withdrawal. Substance/medication-induced psychotic disorders arise during or soon after exposure to a medication or after substance intoxication or withdrawal but can persist for weeks, whereas primary psychotic disorders may precede the onset of substance/medication use or may occur during times of sustained abstinence. Once initiated, the psychotic symptoms may continue as long as the substance/medication use continues. Another consideration is the presence of features that are atypical of a primary psychotic disorder (e.g., atypical age at onset or course). For example, the appearance of delusions de novo in a person older than 35 years without a known history of a primary psychotic disorder should suggest the possibility of a substance/medication-induced psychotic disorder. Even a prior history of a primary psychotic disorder does not rule out the possibility of a substance/medication-induced psychotic disorder. In contrast, factors that suggest that the psychotic symptoms are better accounted for by a primary psychotic disorder include persistence of psychotic symptoms for a substantial period of time (i.e., a month or more) after the end of substance intoxication or acute substance withdrawal or after cessation of medication use; or a history of prior recurrent primary psychotic disorders. Other causes of psychotic symptoms must be considered even in an individual with substance intoxication or withdrawal, because substance use problems are not uncommon among individuals with non-substance/medication-induced psychotic disorders.

2.7—Substance/Medication-Induced Psychotic Disorder / Diagnostic Features (p. 113)

2.8   A 55-year-old man with a known history of alcohol dependence and schizophrenia is brought to the emergency department because of frank delusions and visual hallucinations. Which of the following would *not* be a diagnostic possibility for inclusion in the differential diagnosis?

A. Schizophrenia.
B. Substance/medication-induced psychotic disorder.
C. Alcohol dependence.
D. Psychotic disorder due to another medical condition.
E. Borderline personality disorder with psychotic features.

Correct Answer: E. Borderline personality disorder with psychotic features.

Explanation: There is no evidence provided for a diagnosis of borderline personality disorder. A prior history of a primary psychotic disorder (schizophrenia) does not rule out the possibility of a substance/medication-induced psychotic disorder. The appearance of delusions de novo in a person older than 35 years without a known history of primary psychotic disorder should suggest the possibility of a substance/medication-induced psychotic disorder.

2.8—Substance/Medication-Induced Psychotic Disorder / Differential Diagnosis (pp. 109–110)

2.9   Which of the following sets of specifiers is included in the DSM-5 diagnostic criteria for substance/medication-induced psychotic disorder?

A. "With onset before intoxication" and "With onset before withdrawal."
B. "With onset during intoxication" and "With onset during withdrawal."
C. "With good prognostic features" and "Without good prognostic features."
D. "With onset prior to substance use" and "With onset after substance use."
E. "With catatonia" and 'Without catatonia."

Correct Answer: B. "With onset during intoxication" and "With onset during withdrawal."

Explanation: The specifier "with onset during intoxication" should be used if criteria for intoxication with the substance are met and the symptoms develop during intoxication. The specifier "with onset during withdrawal" should be used if criteria for withdrawal from the substance are met and the symptoms develop during, or shortly after, withdrawal.

2.9—Substance/Medication-Induced Psychotic Disorder / diagnostic criteria (p. 111)

2.10 A 65-year-old man with systemic lupus erythematosus who is being treated with corticosteroids witnesses a serious motor vehicle accident. He begins to have disorganized speech, which lasts for several days before resolving. What diagnosis best fits this clinical picture?

A. Schizophrenia.
B. Psychotic disorder associated with systemic lupus erythematosus.
C. Steroid-induced psychosis.
D. Brief psychotic disorder, with marked stressor.
E. Schizoaffective disorder.

Correct Answer: D. Brief psychotic disorder, with marked stressor.

Explanation: The essential features of psychotic disorder due to another medical condition are prominent delusions or hallucinations that are judged to be attributable to the physiological effects of another medical condition and are not better explained by another mental disorder (e.g., the symptoms are not a psychologically mediated response to a severe medical condition, in which case a diagnosis of brief psychotic disorder, with marked stressor, would be appropriate). In the vignette above, the symptoms are better understood as being a psychologically mediated response to the trauma of witnessing the accident.

2.10—Psychotic Disorder Due to Another Medical Condition / Diagnostic Features (p. 116)

2.11 Which of the following psychotic symptom presentations would *not* be appropriately diagnosed as "other specified schizophrenia spectrum and other psychotic disorder"?

A. Psychotic symptoms that have lasted for less than 1 month but have not yet remitted, so that the criteria for brief psychotic disorder are not met.
B. Persistent auditory hallucinations occurring in the absence of any other features.
C. Postpartum psychosis that does not meet criteria for a depressive or bipolar disorder with psychotic features, brief psychotic disorder, psychotic disorder due to another medical condition, or substance/medication-induced psychotic disorder.

D. Psychotic symptoms that are temporally related to use of a substance.

E. Persistent delusions with periods of overlapping mood episodes that are present for a substantial portion of the delusional disturbance.

Correct Answer: D. Psychotic symptoms that are temporally related to use of a substance.

Explanation: Psychotic symptoms that are temporally related to use of a substance would likely meet criteria for a DSM-5 substance/medication-induced psychotic disorder. The category *other specified schizophrenia spectrum and other psychotic disorder* applies to presentations in which symptoms characteristic of a schizophrenia spectrum and other psychotic disorder that cause clinically significant distress or impairment in social, occupational, or other important areas of functioning predominate but do not meet the full criteria for any of the disorders in the schizophrenia spectrum and other psychotic disorders diagnostic class. The other specified schizophrenia spectrum and other psychotic disorder category is used in situations in which the clinician chooses to communicate the specific reason that the presentation does not meet the criteria for any specific schizophrenia spectrum and other psychotic disorder. This is done by recording "other specified schizophrenia spectrum and other psychotic disorder" followed by the specific reason (e.g., "persistent auditory hallucinations").

2.11—Other Specified Schizophrenia Spectrum and Other Psychotic Disorder (p. 122)

2.12   Which of the following patient presentations would *not* be classified as psychotic for the purpose of diagnosing schizophrenia?

A. A patient is hearing a voice that tells him he is a special person.

B. A patient believes he is being followed by a secret police organization that is focused exclusively on him.

C. A patient has a flashback to a war experience that feels like it is happening again.

D. A patient cannot organize his thoughts and stops responding in the middle of an interview.

E. A patient presents wearing an automobile tire around his waist and gives no explanation.

Correct Answer: C. A patient has a flashback to a war experience that feels like it is happening again.

Explanation: Schizophrenia spectrum and other psychotic disorders are defined by abnormalities in one or more of the following five domains, the first four of which are considered to be psychotic symptoms: delusions, hallucinations, disorganized thinking (speech), grossly disorganized or abnormal motor behavior (including catatonia), and negative symptoms. A flashback to a traumatic experience is an intense, emotionally laden memory but does not reach the level of a psychotic symptom.

2.12—chapter intro; Key Features That Define the Psychotic Disorders (pp. 87–88)

2.13   In which of the following disorders can psychotic symptoms occur?

A. Bipolar and depressive disorders.
B. Substance use disorders.
C. Posttraumatic stress disorder.
D. Other medical conditions.
E. All of the above.

Correct Answer: E. All of the above.

Explanation: Mood disorders, substance use disorders, posttraumatic stress disorder, and other medical conditions all can include psychotic symptoms as part of their presentation. Thus, clinicians must consider these and other possibilities before concluding that a patient's psychosis to due to a primary psychotic disorder.

2.13—Brief Psychotic Disorder; Schizophrenia / Differential Diagnosis (pp. 96, 104–105)

2.14   A 32-year-old man presents to the emergency department distressed and agitated. He reports that his sister has been killed in a car accident on a trip to South America. When asked how he found out, he says that he and his sister were very close and he "just knows it." After putting him on the phone with his sister, who was comfortably staying with friends while on her trip, the man expressed relief that she was alive. Which of the following descriptions best fits this presentation?

A. He had a delusional belief, because he believed it was true without good warrant.
B. He did not have a delusional belief, because it changed in light of new evidence.
C. He had a grandiose delusion, because he believed he could know things happening far away.
D. He had a nihilistic delusion, because it involved an untrue, imagined catastrophe.
E. He did not have a delusion, because in some cultures people believe they can know things about family members outside of ordinary communications.

Correct Answer: B. He did not have a delusional belief, because it changed in light of new evidence.

Explanation: To be a delusion, a belief must be clearly false and must be fixed—that is, not amenable to change in light of additional information. This man's belief was false but held flexibly, and it was conditional on the evidence, such as talking to his living sister. Thus, it is not a delusion. Although cultural factors should be taken into account in determining whether a belief is delusional, that consideration is not relevant here, because the belief is not delusional independent of cultural background.

2.14—Key Features That Define the Psychotic Disorders / Delusions (p. 87)

2.15   Which of the following is *not* a commonly recognized type of delusion?

A. Persecutory.
B. Erotomanic.
C. Alien abduction.
D. Somatic.
E. Grandiose.

Correct Answer: C. Alien abduction.

Explanation: Commonly recognized delusion types include persecutory, referential, somatic, nihilistic, grandiose and erotomanic, as well as combinations of these types. A delusional belief in alien abduction may be grandiose and may involve somatic and/or erotomanic aspects, but it is not itself a major category of delusional thought.

2.15—Key Features That Define the Psychotic Disorders / Delusions (p. 87)

2.16   A 64-year-old man who had been a widower for 3 months presents to the emergency department on the advice of his primary care physician after he reports to the doctor that he hears his deceased wife's voice calling his name when he looks through old photos, and sometimes as he is trying to fall asleep. His primary care physician tells him he is having a psychotic episode and needs to get a psychiatric evaluation. Which of the following statements correctly explains why these experiences are not considered to be psychotic?

A. The voice he hears is from a family member.
B. The experience occurs as he is falling asleep.
C. He can invoke her voice with certain activities.
D. The voice calls his name.
E. Both B and C.

Correct Answer: E. Both B and C.

Explanation: If an auditory experience occurs only secondary to a controllable action (such as looking through highly affectively charged photos) or in an altered sensorial state, such as just before falling asleep (*hypnagogic*) or just as one is waking up (*hypnopompic*), it is not classified as a hallucination. Frank auditory hallucinations can involve the voice of someone known to the patient and often includes hearing one's name called.

2.16—Key Features That Define the Psychotic Disorders / Hallucinations (pp. 87–88)

2.17 A 19-year-old college student is brought by ambulance to the emergency department. His college dorm supervisor, who called the ambulance, reports that the student was isolating himself, was pacing in his room, and was not responding to questions. In the emergency department, the patient gets down in a crouching position and begins making barking noises at seemingly random times. His urine toxicology report is negative, and all labs are within normal limits. What is the best description of these symptoms?

A. An animal delusion—the patient believes he is a dog.
B. Intermittent explosive rage.
C. A paranoid stance leading to self-protective aggression.
D. Catatonic behavior.
E. Formal thought disorder.

Correct Answer: D. Catatonic behavior.

Explanation: Delusions involve beliefs, but we cannot assess the patient's belief structure or his formal thought patterns since he is not answering questions. Similarly, rage is an emotion that may result in intense motor activity, but we have not been able to assess the patient's thought content or his emotions. The patient is likely exhibiting psychomotor agitation but it is of a specific type, namely catatonic excitement that does not relate to the environment or to any goal-directed motivation. Mutism followed by catatonic excitement, such as stereotypic vocalizations, can occur in catatonia.

2.17—Key Features That Define the Psychotic Disorders / Grossly Disorganized or Abnormal Motor Behavior (Including Catatonia) (p. 88)

2.18 Which of the following does *not* represent a negative symptom of schizophrenia?

A. Affective flattening.
B. Decreased motivation.
C. Impoverished thought processes.
D. Sadness over loss of functionality.
E. Social disinterest.

Correct Answer: D. Sadness over loss of functionality.

Explanation: Patients with schizophrenia may be aware of their functional losses and may feel sadness about this. That emotional response would be the opposite of negative symptoms, because it would involve an active and expressive-emotional response. The other symptoms mentioned—affective flattening, decreased motivation, impoverished thought process, and social disinterest—are all part of the negative or deficit symptoms of schizophrenia. It is thus important to distinguish the uses of the word "negative." In reference to sad emotions it has one meaning, but the "negative" symptoms of schizophrenia mean deficits of normal psychological functioning, including absence of sad feelings.

2.18—Key Features That Define the Psychotic Disorders / Negative Symptoms (p. 88)

2.19   Schizophrenia spectrum and other psychotic disorders are defined by abnormalities in one or more of five domains, four of which are also considered psychotic symptoms. Which of the following is *not* considered a psychotic symptom?

A. Delusions.
B. Hallucinations.
C. Disorganized thinking.
D. Disorganized or abnormal motor behavior.
E. Avolition.

Correct Answer: E. Avolition.

Explanation: Avolition is a negative symptom of schizophrenia, not a positive (psychotic) symptom. Avolition is an absence of motivation for goal-oriented behaviors. The term *positive* refers not to something of positive valuation but rather to something that is present and existing, as opposed to a deficit symptom such as the negative symptoms of schizophrenia. The other symptom types listed are considered psychotic.

2.19—Key Features That Define the Psychotic Disorders / Negative Symptoms (p. 88)

2.20   What is the most common type of delusion?

A. Somatic delusion of distorted body appearance.
B. Grandiose delusion.
C. Thought insertion.
D. Persecutory delusion.
E. Former life regression.

Correct Answer: D. Persecutory delusion.

Explanation: Persecutory delusions are the most common form. This may be because such delusions are associated with a dysregulation of existing self-protective and/or social-psychological functionalities, but the reason that these are the most commonly encountered delusion is not yet well understood.

2.20—Key Features That Define the Psychotic Disorders / Delusions (p. 87)

2.21 Label each of the following beliefs as a bizarre delusion, a nonbizarre delusion, or a nondelusion.

A. A 25-year-old law student believes he has uncovered the truth about JFK's assassination and that CIA agents have been dispatched to follow him and monitor his Internet communications.

B. A 45-year-old homeless man presents to the psychiatric emergency room complaining of a skin rash. Upon removal of his clothes, it is seen that most of his body is wrapped in aluminum foil. The man explains that he is protecting himself from the electromagnetic ray guns that are constantly targeting him.

C. A 47-year-old unemployed plumber believes he has been elected to the House of Representatives. When the Capitol police evict him and bring him to the emergency department, he says that they are Tea Party activists who are merely impersonating police officers.

D. A 35-year-old high school physics teacher presents to your office with insomnia and tells you that he has discovered and memorized the formula for cold fusion energy, only to have the formula removed from his memory by telepathic aliens.

E. An 18-year-old recent immigrant from Eastern Europe believes that wearing certain colors will ward off the "evil eye" and prevent catastrophes that would otherwise occur.

Correct Answer: A, nonbizarre delusion; B, bizarre delusion; C, nonbizarre delusion; D, bizarre delusion; E, nondelusion.

Explanation: Delusions are deemed bizarre if they are clearly implausible and not understandable to same-culture peers and do not derive from ordinary life experiences. Thus, although it is probably untrue that the law student is being followed and that the plumber has been elected to Congress, these things *could* conceivably happen. By contrast, thought removal and external control by telepathically empowered aliens or electromagnetic ray guns is not in the realm of possibility by shared social consensus. The belief that use of colors or amulets will ward off bad events is an accepted part of many cultural belief systems and so is not classifiable as a delusion, even if it seems implausible to individuals from more secular backgrounds.

2.21—Key Features That Define the Psychotic Disorders / Delusions (p. 87); Schizophrenia / Culture-Related Diagnostic Issues (p. 103)

2.22   Which of the following presentations would *not* be classified as disorganized behavior for the purpose of diagnosing schizophrenia spectrum and other psychotic disorders?

A. Masturbating in public.
B. Wearing slacks on one's head.
C. Responding verbally to auditory hallucinations in a conversational mode.
D. Crouching on all fours and barking.
E. Turning to face 180 degrees away from the interviewer when answering questions.

Correct Answer: C. Responding verbally to auditory hallucinations in a conversational mode.

Explanation: Disorganized behavior including catatonic motor behavior is one of four categories of psychotic symptoms used to diagnose schizophrenia spectrum and other psychotic disorders. To fulfill diagnostic criteria, the behavior must be grossly disorganized or inappropriate. Masturbating in public is behavior that shows obliviousness to the environment and unconcern for the usual social norms of modesty and privacy. Wearing clothing in odd ways without justification is a disorganized form of behavior. Both barking like a dog and turning away in a bizarre fashion while conducting a conversation (if not induced by an expression of anger or other reasonable explanation) are grossly inappropriate behaviors. However, responding verbally to auditory hallucination is not in itself a disorganized behavior. Given the belief in the actuality of communication in an auditory hallucination, talking back is contingently a logical and goal-oriented behavior. Thus, this would count as one psychotic symptom (hallucination) but not as two symptoms (hallucination and grossly disorganized behavior).

> **2.22—Key Features That Define the Psychotic Disorders / Grossly Disorganized or Abnormal Motor Behavior (Including Catatonia) (p. 88)**

2.23   Which of the following statements about catatonic motor behaviors is *false?*

A. Catatonic motor behavior is a type of grossly disorganized behavior that has historically been associated with schizophrenia spectrum and other psychotic disorders.
B. Catatonic motor behaviors may occur in many mental disorders (such as mood disorders) and in other medical conditions.
C. A behavior is considered catatonic only if it involves motoric slowing or rigidity, such as mutism, posturing, or waxy flexibility.
D. Catatonia can be diagnosed independently of another psychiatric disorder.
E. Catatonic behaviors involve markedly reduced reactivity to the environment.

Correct Answer: C. A behavior is considered catatonic only if it involves motoric slowing or rigidity, such as mutism, posturing, or waxy flexibility.

Explanation: *Catatonic behavior* is a marked decrease in reactivity to the environment. This ranges from resistance to instructions (negativism); to maintaining a rigid, inappropriate or bizarre posture; to a complete lack of verbal and motor responses (mutism and stupor). It can also include purposeless and excessive motor activity without obvious cause (catatonic excitement). Other features are repeated stereotyped movements, staring, grimacing, mutism, and the echoing of speech. Although catatonia has historically been associated with schizophrenia, catatonic symptoms are nonspecific and may occur in other mental disorders (e.g., bipolar or depressive disorders with catatonia) and in medical conditions (catatonic disorder due to another medical condition).

2.23—Key Features That Define the Psychotic Disorders / Grossly Disorganized or Abnormal Motor Behavior (Including Catatonia) (p. 88); Catatonia (pp. 119–121)

2.24   Which of the following statements about negative symptoms of schizophrenia is *false*?

A. Negative symptoms are easily distinguished from medication side effects such as sedation.
B. Negative symptoms include diminished emotional expression.
C. Negative symptoms can be difficult to distinguish from medication side effects such as sedation.
D. Negative symptoms include reduced peer or social interaction.
E. Negative symptoms include decreased motivation for goal-directed activities.

Correct Answer: A. Negative symptoms are easily distinguished from medication side effects such as sedation.

Explanation: Negative symptoms of schizophrenia refer to the deficit aspects of the illness, in contrast to the "positive" symptoms (in the sense of being notable by their presence, not in the sense of being desirable). Positive symptoms include active hallucinations, delusions, disorganized behaviors, and disorganized thinking. Side effects of medication such as sedation and bradykinesia may mimic negative symptoms and be wrongly evaluated as primary negative symptomatology. The primary negative symptoms include diminished emotional expression, reduced interaction with others, and decreased motivation for goal-directed activities.

2.24—Key Features That Define the Psychotic Disorders / Negative Symptoms (p. 88)

2.25 Which of the following statements correctly describes a way in which schizoaffective disorder may be differentiated from bipolar disorder?

A. Schizoaffective disorder involves only depressive episodes, never manic or hypomanic episodes.
B. In bipolar disorder, psychotic symptoms do not last longer than 1 month.
C. In bipolar disorder, psychotic symptoms are always cotemporal with mood symptoms.
D. Schizoaffective disorder never includes full-blown episodes of major depression.
E. In bipolar disorder, psychotic symptoms are always mood congruent.

Correct Answer: C. In bipolar disorder, psychotic symptoms are always cotemporal with mood symptoms.

Explanation: Distinguishing schizoaffective disorder from depressive and bipolar disorders with psychotic features is often difficult. Schizoaffective disorder can be distinguished from a depressive or bipolar disorder with psychotic features by the presence of prominent delusions and/or hallucinations for at least 2 weeks in the absence of a major mood episode. In contrast, in depressive or bipolar disorders with psychotic features, the psychotic features primarily occur during the mood episode(s).

2.25—Schizoaffective Disorder / Differential Diagnosis (p. 109)

2.26 Which of the following symptom combinations, if present for 1 month, would meet Criterion A for schizophrenia?

A. Prominent auditory and visual hallucinations.
B. Grossly disorganized behavior and avolition.
C. Disorganized speech and diminished emotional expression.
D. Paranoid and grandiose delusions.
E. Avolition and diminished emotional expression.

Correct Answer: C. Disorganized speech and diminished emotional expression.

Explanation: To meet DSM-5 Criterion A, two (or more) of the following symptoms must be present for a significant portion of time during a 1-month period (or less if successfully treated): 1) delusions, 2) hallucinations, 3) disorganized speech (e.g., frequent derailment or incoherence), 4) grossly disorganized or catatonic behavior, 5) negative symptoms (i.e., diminished emotional expression or avolition). At least one of the two symptoms must be the clear presence of delusions (A1), hallucinations (A2), or disorganized speech (A3). Thus, two forms of hallucinations or two types of delusions alone in the absence of other symptoms would be insufficient to meet Criterion A. The combination of grossly disorganized behavior (although considered a psychotic symptom) with negative symptoms is also insufficient to meet Criterion A.

2.26—Schizophrenia / diagnostic criteria (p. 99)

2.27   Which of the following statements about violent or suicidal behavior in schizophrenia is *false?*

    A. About 5%–6% of individuals with schizophrenia die by suicide.
    B. Persons with schizophrenia frequently assault strangers in a random fashion.
    C. Compared with the general population, persons with schizophrenia are more frequently victims of violence.
    D. Command hallucinations to harm oneself sometimes precede suicidal behaviors.
    E. Youth, male gender, and substance abuse are factors that increase the risk for suicide among persons with schizophrenia.

Correct Answer: B. Persons with schizophrenia frequently assault strangers in a random fashion.

Explanation: Hostility and aggression can be associated with schizophrenia, although spontaneous or random assault is uncommon. Aggression is more frequent for younger males and for individuals with a past history of violence, nonadherence to treatment, substance abuse, and impulsivity. It should be noted that the vast majority of persons with schizophrenia are not aggressive and are more frequently victimized than are individuals in the general population.

Approximately 5%–6% of individuals with schizophrenia die by suicide, about 20% attempt suicide on one or more occasions, and many more have significant suicidal ideation. Suicidal behavior is sometimes in response to command hallucinations to harm oneself or others. Suicide risk remains high over the whole life span for males and females, although it may be especially high for younger males with comorbid substance use. Other risk factors include having depressive symptoms or feelings of hopelessness and being unemployed, and the risk is higher, also, in the period after a psychotic episode or hospital discharge.

2.27—Schizophrenia / Associated Features Supporting Diagnosis (p. 101); Suicide Risk (p. 104)

2.28   Which of the following statements about childhood-onset schizophrenia is *true?*

A. Childhood-onset schizophrenia tends to resemble poor-outcome adult schizophrenia, with gradual onset and prominent negative symptoms.
B. Disorganized speech patterns in childhood are usually indicative of schizophrenia.
C. Because of the childhood capacity for imagination, delusions and hallucinations in childhood-onset schizophrenia are more elaborate than those in adult-onset schizophrenia.
D. In a child presenting with disorganized behavior, schizophrenia should be ruled out before other childhood diagnoses are considered.
E. Visual hallucinations are extremely rare in childhood-onset schizophrenia.

Correct Answer: A. Childhood-onset schizophrenia tends to resemble poor-outcome adult schizophrenia, with gradual onset and prominent negative symptoms.

Explanation: The essential features of schizophrenia are the same in childhood, but it is more difficult to make the diagnosis. In children, delusions and hallucinations may be less elaborate than in adults, and visual hallucinations are more common and should be distinguished from normal fantasy play. Disorganized speech occurs in many disorders with childhood onset (e.g., autism spectrum disorder), as does disorganized behavior (e.g., attention-deficit/hyperactivity disorder). These symptoms should not be attributed to schizophrenia without due consideration of the more common disorders of childhood. Childhood-onset cases tend to resemble poor-outcome adult cases, with gradual onset and prominent negative symptoms. Children who later receive the diagnosis of schizophrenia are more likely to have experienced nonspecific emotional-behavioral disturbances and psychopathology, intellectual and language alterations, and subtle motor delays.

2.28—Schizophrenia / Development and Course (pp. 102–103)

2.29 Which of the following statements about gender differences in schizophrenia is *true?*

A. Women with schizophrenia tend to have fewer psychotic symptoms than do men over the course of the illness.
B. A first onset of schizophrenia after age 40 is more likely in women than in men.
C. Psychotic symptoms in women tend to burn out with age to a greater extent than they do in men.
D. Negative symptoms and affective flattening are more frequently observed in women with schizophrenia than in men with the disorder.
E. The overall incidence of schizophrenia is higher in women than it is in men.

Correct Answer: B. A first onset of schizophrenia after age 40 is more likely in women than in men.

Explanation: The lifetime prevalence of schizophrenia appears to be approximately 0.3%–0.7%, although there is reported variation by race/ethnicity, across countries, and by geographic origin for immigrants and children of immigrants. The sex ratio differs across samples and populations: for example, an emphasis on negative symptoms and longer duration of disorder (associated with poorer outcome) shows higher incidence rates for males, whereas definitions allowing for the inclusion of more mood symptoms and brief presentations (associated with better outcome) show equivalent risks for both sexes.

A number of features distinguish the clinical expression of schizophrenia in females and males. The general incidence of schizophrenia tends to be slightly lower in females, particularly among treated cases. The age at onset is later in females, with a second mid-life peak. Symptoms tend to be more affect-laden among females, and there are more psychotic symptoms, as well as a greater propensity for psychotic symptoms to worsen in later life. Other symptom differences include less frequent negative symptoms and disorganization. Finally, social functioning tends to remain better preserved in females. There are, however, frequent exceptions to these general caveats.

2.29—Schizophrenia / Prevalence (p. 102); Gender-Related Diagnostic Issues (pp. 103–104)

2.30 A 19-year-old female college student is brought to the emergency department by her family over her objections. Three months ago, she suddenly started feeling "odd," and she came home from college because she could not concentrate. Two weeks after she came home, she began hearing voices telling her that she is "a sinner" and must repent. Although never a religious person, she now believes she must repent, but she does not know how, and feels confused. She is managing her activities of daily living despite the ongoing auditory hallucinations and delusions, and she is affectively reactive on examination. Which diagnosis best fits this presentation?

A. Schizophreniform disorder, with good prognostic features, provisional.
B. Schizophreniform disorder, without good prognostic features, provisional.
C. Schizophreniform disorder, with good prognostic features.
D. Schizophreniform disorder, without good prognostic features.
E. Unspecified schizophrenia spectrum and other psychotic disorder.

Correct Answer: A. Schizophreniform disorder, with good prognostic features, provisional.

Explanation: Schizophreniform disorder is diagnosed under two conditions: 1) when an episode of illness lasts between 1 and 6 months and the individual has already recovered, and 2) when an individual is symptomatic for less than the 6 months' duration required for the diagnosis of schizophrenia but has not yet recovered (as in this vignette). One then adds the qualifier "provisional," because it is uncertain whether the individual will recover from the disturbance within the 6-month period. If the disturbance persists beyond 6 months, the diagnosis should be changed to schizophrenia. In either case, schizophreniform disorder takes the specifier "with good prognostic features" if at least two of the following features are present: 1) onset of prominent psychotic symptoms within 4 weeks of the first noticeable change in usual behavior or functioning; 2) confusion or perplexity; 3) good premorbid social and occupational functioning; and 4) absence of blunted or flat affect. This vignette demonstrates all four of these features. Because we have enough information to make the diagnosis of schizophreniform disorder, unspecified schizophrenia spectrum and other psychotic disorder would be incorrectly applied.

2.30—Schizophreniform Disorder / diagnostic criteria (pp. 96–97); Diagnostic Features (p. 97)

2.31   A 24-year-old male college student is brought to the emergency department by the college health service team. A few weeks ago he was involved in a car accident in which one of his friends was critically injured and died in his arms. The man has not come out of his room or showered for the last 2 weeks. He has eaten only minimally, claimed that aliens have targeted him for abduction, and asserted that he could hear their radio transmissions. Nothing seems to convince him that this abduction will not happen or that the transmissions are not real. Which of the following diagnoses (and justifications) is most appropriate for this man?

A. Brief psychotic disorder with a marked stressor, because the symptoms began after the tragic car accident.

B. Brief psychotic disorder without a marked stressor, because the content of the psychosis is unrelated to the accident.

C. Unspecified schizophrenia spectrum and other psychotic disorder, because more information is needed.

D. Schizophreniform disorder, because there are psychotic symptoms but not yet a full-blown schizophrenia picture.

E. Delusional disorder, because the central symptom is a delusion of persecution.

Correct Answer: C. Unspecified schizophrenia spectrum and other psychotic disorder, because more information is needed.

Explanation: The diagnosis of *brief psychotic disorder* requires that there be psychotic symptoms lasting more than 1 day but less than 1 month and that the patient has shown a full recovery. In this vignette, we do not know how long the symptoms will last or whether the patient will fully recover. If the patient's symptoms remit in less than 1 month and he shows full recovery, one could diagnose *brief psychotic disorder with a marked stressor*. There is no requirement that the content of the psychotic symptoms match the events that constitute the stressor, as long as the temporal sequence holds. The diagnosis of *delusional dis-*

order requires 1 month of symptoms and does not usually involve bizarre delusions, nor does it involve the functional deficits seen here. *Schizophreniform disorder* requires 1 month of symptoms. If these symptoms continue for a month and functional deficits persist, the diagnosis could be schizophreniform disorder, and possibly progress to schizophrenia after 6 months. We do not yet know the future trajectory of these psychotic symptoms and therefore can justify only the diagnosis of unspecified schizophrenia spectrum and other psychotic disorder. The unspecified schizophrenia spectrum and other psychotic disorder category is used in situations in which the clinician chooses not to specify the reason that the criteria are not met for a specific schizophrenia spectrum and other psychotic disorder, and includes presentations in which there is insufficient information to make a more specific diagnosis (e.g., in emergency room settings).

2.31—Unspecified Schizophrenia Spectrum and Other Psychotic Disorder (p. 122)

CHAPTER 3

Bipolar and Related Disorders

3.1 Which of the following statements accurately describes a change in DSM-5 from the DSM-IV criteria for bipolar disorders?

A. Diagnostic criteria for bipolar disorders now include both changes in mood and changes in activity or energy.
B. Diagnostic criteria for bipolar I disorder, mixed type, now require a patient to simultaneously meet full criteria for both mania and major depressive episode.
C. Subsyndromal hypomania has been removed from the allowed conditions under *other specified bipolar and related disorder.*
D. There is now a stipulation that manic or hypomanic episodes cannot be associated with recent administration of a drug known to cause similar symptoms.
E. The clinical symptoms associated with hypomanic episodes have been substantially changed.

Correct Answer: A. Diagnostic criteria for bipolar disorders now include both changes in mood and changes in activity or energy.

Explanation: Although the essential elements describing the clinical symptoms associated with depressive, manic, and hypomanic episodes have not substantially changed, there are a number of changes in the DSM-5 criteria for bipolar disorders. Diagnostic criteria for bipolar disorders now include both changes in mood and changes in activity or energy, with the addition of "and abnormally and persistently increased activity or energy" to Criterion A for manic and hypomanic episodes. The DSM-IV diagnosis of bipolar I disorder, mixed episodes—requiring that the individual simultaneously meet full criteria for both mania and major depressive episode—is replaced with a new specifier, "with mixed features." Particular conditions can now be diagnosed under *other specified bipolar and related disorder,* including categorization for individuals with a past history of a major depressive disorder who have too few symptoms of hypomania or too short a duration of a hypomanic episode to meet criteria for the full bipolar II disorder syndrome.

Mania or hypomania that emerges during antidepressant treatment (e.g., medication, electroconvulsive therapy) but persists at a fully syndromal level beyond the physiological effect of that treatment is considered to be sufficient evidence for a bipolar disorder diagnosis, not substance/medication-induced bipolar and related disorder.

3.1—Appendix / Highlights of Changes From DSM-IV to DSM-5 (p. 810); Substance/ Medication-Induced Bipolar and Related Disorder / Diagnostic Features (p. 144)

3.2   A 32-year-old man reports 1 week of feeling unusually irritable. During this time, he has increased energy and activity, sleeps less, and finds it difficult to sit still. He also is more talkative than usual and is easily distractible, to the point of finding it difficult to complete his work assignments. A physical examination and laboratory workup are negative for any medical cause of his symptoms and he takes no medications. What diagnosis best fits this clinical picture?

   A. Manic episode.
   B. Hypomanic episode.
   C. Bipolar I disorder, with mixed features.
   D. Major depressive episode.
   E. Cyclothymic disorder.

Correct Answer: A. Manic episode.

Explanation: In DSM-5, the definition of a manic episode has been broadened to include both an abnormal mood (elevated, expansive, or irritable) and increased activity for at least 1 week. The person must also experience at least three (four if the mood is irritable) of the following symptoms: 1) inflated self-esteem or grandiosity, 2) decreased need for sleep, 3) more talkative than usual or pressure to keep talking, 4) flight of ideas or subjective experience that thoughts are racing, 5) distractibility, 6) increase in goal-directed activity or psychomotor agitation, and 7) excessive involvement in activities that have a high potential for painful consequences.

3.2—Bipolar I Disorder / Manic Episode diagnostic criteria (p. 124); Appendix / Highlights of Changes From DSM-IV to DSM-5 (p. 810)

3.3   A 42-year-old man reports 1 week of increased activity associated with an elevated mood, a decreased need for sleep, and inflated self-esteem. Although the man does not object to his current state ("I'm getting a lot of work done!"), he is concerned because he recalls a similar episode 10 years ago during which he began to make imprudent business decisions. A physical examination and laboratory work are unrevealing for any medical cause of his symptoms. He had taken fluoxetine for a depressive episode but self-discontinued it 3 months ago because he felt that his mood was stable. Which diagnosis best fits this clinical picture?

A. Bipolar I disorder.
B. Bipolar II disorder.
C. Cyclothymic disorder.
D. Other specified bipolar disorder and related disorder.
E. Substance/medication-induced bipolar disorder.

Correct Answer: A. Bipolar I disorder.

Explanation: This patient most likely meets criteria for bipolar I disorder, current episode hypomanic, which is defined as a current hypomanic episode in an individual with a previous history of at least one manic episode. The history of a past manic episode rules out bipolar II disorder, and the time course and absence of numerous episodes of hypomania rule out cyclothymic disorder. Although antidepressants can precipitate manic episodes, the long period since medication discontinuation (more than 5 half-lives) makes this episode unlikely to be medication induced.

3.3—Bipolar I Disorder / Differential Diagnosis (pp. 131–132)

3.4 Approximately what percentage of individuals who experience a single manic episode will go on to have recurrent mood episodes?

A. 90%.
B. 50%.
C. 25%.
D. 10%.
E. 1%.

Correct Answer: A. 90%.

Explanation: Bipolar disorders are highly recurrent, and more than 90% of individuals who have a single manic episode go on to have recurrent mood episodes.

3.4—Bipolar I Disorder / Development and Course (p. 130)

3.5 Which of the following factors is most predictive of incomplete recovery between mood episodes in bipolar I disorder?

A. Being widowed.
B. Living in a higher-income country.
C. Being divorced.
D. Having a family history of bipolar disorder.
E. Having a mood episode accompanied by mood-incongruent psychotic symptoms.

Correct Answer: E. Having a mood episode accompanied by mood-incongruent psychotic symptoms.

Explanation: Incomplete interepisode recovery in bipolar I disorder is more common when the current episode is accompanied by mood-incongruent psychotic features. Being separated, divorced, or widowed and having a family history of bipolar disorder are risk factors for bipolar I disorder; however, they are not predictors of course. Bipolar I disorder is more common in high-income than in low-income countries (1.4% vs. 0.7%), but higher income does not predict incomplete interepisode recovery.

3.5—Bipolar I Disorder / Risk and Prognostic Factors (p. 130)

3.6   Which of the following is more common in men with bipolar I disorder than in women with the disorder?

A. Rapid cycling.
B. Alcohol abuse.
C. Eating disorders.
D. Anxiety disorders.
E. Mixed-state symptoms.

Correct Answer: B. Alcohol abuse.

Explanation: Although bipolar I disorder affects men and women equally, hypomanic, mixed-state, and rapid-cycling symptoms are more common in women. Alcohol abuse is higher in men than in women in all cases, although it should be noted that women with bipolar disorder have a higher rate of alcohol abuse than do women in the general population. Compared with bipolar men, bipolar women are more likely to experience rapid cycling and anxiety and have higher rates of lifetime comorbid eating disorders.

3.6—Bipolar I Disorder / Gender-Related Diagnostic Issues (pp. 130–131)

3.7   A patient with a history of bipolar I disorder presents with a new-onset manic episode and is successfully treated with medication adjustment. He notes chronic depressive symptoms that, on reflection, long preceded his manic episodes. He describes these symptoms as "feeling down," having decreased energy, and more often than not having no motivation. He denies other depressive symptoms but feels that these alone have been sufficient to negatively affect his marriage. Which diagnosis best fits this presentation?

A. Other specified bipolar and related disorder.
B. Bipolar I disorder, current or most recent episode depressed.
C. Cyclothymic disorder.
D. Bipolar I disorder and persistent depressive disorder (dysthymia).
E. Bipolar II disorder.

Correct Answer: D. Bipolar I disorder and persistent depressive disorder (dysthymia).

Explanation: This patient's presentation does not meet the full criteria for a major depressive episode and thus would not qualify for a diagnosis of bipolar I disorder, current or most recent episode depressed. If the patient meets criteria for persistent depressive disorder (dysthymia) *and* bipolar I disorder, both should be diagnosed. The presence of a manic episode makes bipolar II disorder, cyclothymic disorder, and other specified bipolar and related disorder inappropriate.

3.7—Bipolar I Disorder / Differential Diagnosis (pp. 131–132)

3.8   In which of the following ways do manic episodes differ from attention-deficit/hyperactivity disorder (ADHD)?

A. Manic episodes are more strongly associated with poor judgment.
B. Manic episodes are more likely to involve excessive activity.
C. Manic episodes have clearer symptomatic onsets and offsets.
D. Manic episodes are more likely to show a chronic course.
E. Manic episodes first appear at an earlier age.

Correct Answer: C. Manic episodes have clearer symptomatic onsets and offsets.

Explanation: ADHD and manic episodes are both characterized by poor judgment, excessive activity, impulsive behavior, and denial of problems. Patients with ADHD have an earlier onset of illness (i.e., before age 7 years), show a more chronic course (manic episodes are more episodic), and lack clear onsets and offsets of symptoms. In addition, ADHD patients tend not to have an unusually elevated mood or psychotic symptoms.

3.8—Bipolar I Disorder / Differential Diagnosis (pp. 131–132)

3.9   A patient with a history of bipolar disorder reports experiencing 1 week of elevated and expansive mood. Evidence of which of the following would suggest that the patient is experiencing a hypomanic, rather than manic, episode?

A. Irritability.
B. Decreased need for sleep.
C. Increased productivity at work.
D. Psychotic symptoms.
E. Good insight into the illness.

Correct Answer: C. Increased productivity at work.

Explanation: The primary factor that differentiates manic and hypomanic episodes is that manic episodes cause marked impairment in social or occupational functioning or necessitate hospitalization to prevent harm to self or others, or there are psychotic features (Criterion C of bipolar I disorder). In hypomania, "The episode is not severe enough to cause marked impairment in social or occupational functioning or to necessitate hospitalization" (Criterion E of bipolar II disorder). Both types of episodes can cause irritability or decreased need for sleep. Insight is not included in the diagnostic criteria.

3.9—Bipolar I and Bipolar II Disorder (pp. 123–136)

3.10   A 25-year-old graduate student presents to a psychiatrist complaining of feeling down and "not enjoying anything." Her symptoms began about a month ago, along with insomnia and poor appetite. She has little interest in activities and is having difficulty attending to her schoolwork. She recalls a similar episode 1 year ago that lasted about 2 months before improving without treatment. She also reports several episodes of increased energy in the past 2 years; these episodes usually last 1–2 weeks, during which time she is very productive, feels more social and outgoing, and tends to sleep less, although she feels energetic during the day. Friends tell her that she speaks more rapidly during these episodes but that they do not see it as off-putting and in fact think she seems more outgoing and clever. She has no medical problems and does not take any medications or abuse drugs or alcohol. What is the most likely diagnosis?

A. Bipolar I disorder, current episode depressed.
B. Bipolar II disorder, current episode depressed.
C. Bipolar I disorder, current episode unspecified.
D. Cyclothymic disorder.
E. Major depressive disorder.

Correct Answer: B. Bipolar II disorder, current episode depressed.

Explanation: With her current major depressive episode combined with a past history of elevated mood and activity, this patient likely has a bipolar disorder. Because her periods of mood elevation do not cause distress or impairment, they are probably hypomanic episodes, hence a diagnosis of bipolar II disorder. The lack of any current hypomanic symptoms rules out a mixed episode of the illness. The presence of major depressive episodes rules out cyclothymic disorder, and this patient's hypomanic episodes rule out major depressive disorder. This vignette is illustrative of the clinical observation that patients with bipolar II disorder generally present for treatment only when they experience depressive symptoms.

3.10—Bipolar II Disorder / Diagnostic Features (pp. 135–136)

3.11   How do the depressive episodes associated with bipolar II disorder differ from those associated with bipolar I disorder?

A. They are less frequent than those associated with bipolar I disorder.
B. They are lengthier than those associated with bipolar I disorder.
C. They are less disabling than those associated with bipolar I disorder.
D. They are less severe than those associated with bipolar I disorder.
E. They are rarely a reason for the patient to seek treatment.

Correct Answer: B. They are lengthier than those associated with bipolar I disorder.

Explanation: The recurrent major depressive episodes associated with bipolar II disorder are typically more frequent and lengthier than those associated with bipolar I disorder. The depressive episodes can be very severe and disabling; because of this, DSM-5 stresses that bipolar II disorder should not be considered a "milder" form of bipolar I disorder. Bipolar II patients are more likely to seek treatment when depressed than during hypomanic episodes.

3.11—Bipolar II Disorder / Diagnostic Features (p. 136)

3.12   How does the course of bipolar II disorder differ from the course of bipolar I disorder?

A. It is more chronic than the course of bipolar I disorder.
B. It is less episodic than the course of bipolar I disorder.
C. It involves longer asymptomatic periods than the course of bipolar I disorder.
D. It involves shorter symptomatic episodes than the course of bipolar I disorder.
E. It involves a much lower number of lifetime mood episodes than the course of bipolar I disorder.

Correct Answer: A. It is more chronic than the course of bipolar I disorder.

Explanation: Despite the substantial differences in duration and severity between manic and hypomanic episodes, bipolar II disorder is not a "milder form" of bipolar I disorder. Compared with individuals with bipolar I disorder, individuals with bipolar II disorder have greater chronicity of illness and spend, on average, more time in the depressive phase of their illness, which can be severe and/or disabling.

The number of lifetime episodes (both hypomanic and major depressive episodes) tends to be higher for bipolar II disorder than for major depressive disorder or bipolar I disorder. The interval between mood episodes in the course of bipolar II disorder tends to decrease as the individual ages. While the hypomanic episode is the feature that defines bipolar II disorder, depressive episodes are more enduring and disabling over time.

3.12—Bipolar II Disorder / Diagnostic Features; Development and Course (p. 136)

3.13 Which of the following features confers a worse prognosis for a patient with bipolar II disorder?

A. Younger age.
B. Higher educational level.
C. Rapid-cycling pattern.
D. "Married" marital status.
E. Less severe depressive episodes.

Correct Answer: C. Rapid-cycling pattern.

Explanation: A rapid-cycling pattern is associated with a poorer prognosis. Return to previous level of social function for individuals with bipolar II disorder is more likely for individuals of younger age and with less severe depression, suggesting adverse effects of prolonged illness on recovery. More education, fewer years of illness, and being married are independently associated with functional recovery in individuals with bipolar disorder, even after diagnostic type (I vs. II), current depressive symptoms, and presence of psychiatric comorbidity are taken into account.

3.13—Bipolar II Disorder / Risk and Prognostic Factors (p. 137)

3.14 The course of bipolar II disorder would likely be worse for individuals who have an onset of the disorder at which of the following ages?

A. Age 10 years.
B. Age 20 years.
C. Age 40 years.
D. Age 70 years.
E. None of the above; there is no association between onset age and course.

Correct Answer: A. Age 10 years.

Explanation: Compared with adult onset of bipolar II disorder, childhood or adolescent onset of bipolar II disorder may be associated with a more severe lifetime course. The 3-year incidence rate of first-onset bipolar II disorder in adults older than 60 years is 0.34%. However, distinguishing individuals older than 60 years with bipolar II disorder by late versus early onset does not appear to have any clinical utility.

3.14—Bipolar II Disorder / Development and Course (p. 137)

3.15   Which of the following statements about postpartum hypomania is *true?*

    A. It tends to occur in the late postpartum period.
    B. It occurs in less than 1% of postpartum women.
    C. It is a risk factor for postpartum depression.
    D. It is easily distinguished from the normal adjustments to childbirth.
    E. It is more common in multiparous women.

Correct Answer: C. It is a risk factor for postpartum depression.

Explanation: Childbirth may be a specific trigger for a hypomanic episode, which can occur in 10%–20% of females in nonclinical populations and most typically in the early postpartum period. Distinguishing hypomania from the elated mood and reduced sleep that normally accompany the birth of a child may be challenging. Postpartum hypomania may foreshadow the onset of a depression that occurs in about half of females who experience postpartum "highs." Accurate detection of bipolar II disorder may help in establishing appropriate treatment of the depression, which may reduce the risk of suicide and infanticide.

3.15—Bipolar II Disorder / Gender-Related Diagnostic Issues (p. 137)

3.16   For an adolescent who presents with distractibility, which of the following additional features would suggest an association with bipolar II disorder rather than attention-deficit/hyperactivity disorder (ADHD)?

    A. Rapid speech noted on examination.
    B. A report of less need for sleep.
    C. Complaints of racing thoughts.
    D. Evidence that the symptoms are episodic.
    E. Evidence that the symptoms represent the individual's baseline behavior.

Correct Answer: D. Evidence that the symptoms are episodic.

Explanation: ADHD may be misdiagnosed as bipolar II disorder, especially in adolescents and children. Many symptoms of ADHD, such as rapid speech, racing thoughts, distractibility, and less need for sleep, overlap with the symptoms of hypomania. The double counting of symptoms toward both ADHD and bipolar II disorder can be avoided if the clinician clarifies whether the symptoms represent a distinct episode and if the noticeable increase over baseline required for the diagnosis of bipolar II disorder is present.

3.16—Bipolar II Disorder / Differential Diagnosis (pp. 138–139)

3.17   A 50-year-old man with a history of a prior depressive episode is given an antidepressant by his family doctor to help with his depressive symptoms. Two weeks later, his doctor contacts you for a consultation because the patient now is euphoric, has increased energy, racing thoughts, psychomotor agitation, poor concentration and attention, pressured speech, and a decreased need to sleep. These symptoms began with the initiation of the patient's new medication. The patient stopped the medication after 2 days, as he no longer felt depressed; however, the symptoms have continued ever since. What is the patient's diagnosis?

A. Substance/medication-induced bipolar and related disorder.
B. Bipolar I disorder.
C. Bipolar II disorder.
D. Cyclothymic disorder.
E. Major depressive disorder.

Correct Answer: B. Bipolar I disorder.

Explanation: Manic symptoms or syndromes that are attributable to the physiological effects of a drug of abuse (e.g., in the context of cocaine or amphetamine intoxication), the side effects of medications or treatments (e.g., steroids, L-dopa, antidepressants, stimulants), or another medical condition do not count toward the diagnosis of bipolar I disorder. However, a fully syndromal manic episode that arises during treatment (e.g., with medications, electroconvulsive therapy, light therapy) or drug use and persists beyond the physiological effect of the inducing agent (i.e., after a medication is fully out of the individual's system or the effects of electroconvulsive therapy would be expected to have dissipated completely) is sufficient evidence for a manic episode diagnosis (Criterion D). The diagnostic features of substance/medication-induced bipolar and related disorder are essentially the same as those for mania, hypomania, or depression. A key exception to the diagnosis of substance/medication-induced bipolar and related disorder is the case of hypomania or mania that occurs after antidepressant medication use or other treatments and persists beyond the physiological effects of the medication. This condition is considered an indicator of true bipolar disorder, not substance/medication-induced bipolar and related disorder.

3.17—Bipolar I Disorder / Diagnostic Features (pp. 127–129); Substance/Medication-Induced Bipolar and Related Disorder / Diagnostic Features (p. 144)

3.18   In which of the following aspects does cyclothymic disorder differ from bipolar I disorder?

A. Duration.
B. Severity.
C. Age at onset.
D. Pervasiveness.
E. All of the above.

Correct Answer: B. Severity.

Explanation: The essential feature of cyclothymic disorder is a chronic, fluctuating mood disturbance involving numerous periods of hypomanic symptoms and periods of depressive symptoms that are distinct from each other (Criterion A). The hypomanic symptoms are of insufficient number, severity, pervasiveness, or duration to meet full criteria for a hypomanic episode, and the depressive symptoms are of insufficient number, severity, pervasiveness, or duration to meet full criteria for a major depressive episode. During the initial 2-year period (1 year for children or adolescents), the symptoms must be persistent (present more days than not), and any symptom-free intervals must last no longer than 2 months (Criterion B). The diagnosis of cyclothymic disorder is made only if the criteria for a major depressive, manic, or hypomanic episode have never been met (Criterion C).

3.19—Cyclothymic Disorder / Diagnostic Features (p. 140)

CHAPTER 4

Depressive Disorders

4.1   How does DSM-5 differ from DSM-IV in its classification of mood disorders?

A. There is no difference between the two editions.
B. DSM-IV separated mood disorders into different sections; DSM-5 consolidates mood disorders into one section.
C. DSM-IV included all mood disorders in a single section; DSM-5 places depressive and bipolar mood disorders in separate sections.
D. DSM-IV placed mood and anxiety disorders in separate sections; DSM-5 consolidates mood and anxiety disorders within a single section.
E. DSM-IV placed mood disorders with psychotic features in the same section as other mood disorders; DSM-5 places mood disorders with psychosis in a separate section.

Correct Answer: C. DSM-IV included all mood disorders in a single section; DSM-5 places depressive and bipolar mood disorders in separate sections.

Explanation: Unlike DSM-IV, DSM-5 separates depressive disorders from bipolar and related disorders, and several new disorders have been added. "With psychotic features" is a specifier for bipolar and depressive disorders; there is no separate diagnostic section for mood disorders with psychotic symptoms.

4.1—chapter intro (p. 155)

4.2   How does DSM-5 differ from DSM-IV in its classification of premenstrual dysphoric disorder (PMDD)?

A. PMDD was in the Appendix in DSM-IV and remains in this location in DSM-5.
B. PMDD was not included in DSM-IV but is in the Appendix of DSM-5.
C. PMDD is no longer considered a valid psychiatric diagnosis.
D. PMDD is included in the "Depressive Disorders" chapter of DSM-5 but was not included in the "Mood Disorders" chapter of DSM-IV.
E. PMDD is included in DSM-5 but the name of the diagnosis has been changed.

Correct Answer: D. PMDD is included in the "Depressive Disorders" chapter of DSM-5 but was not included in the "Mood Disorders" chapter of DSM-IV.

Explanation: After careful scientific review of the evidence, PMDD has been moved from Appendix B ("Criteria Sets and Axes Provided for Further Study") of DSM-IV to Section II of DSM-5. Almost 20 years of additional research on this condition has confirmed a specific and treatment-responsive form of depressive disorder that begins sometime following ovulation and remits within a few days of menses and has a marked impact on functioning.

4.2—chapter intro (p. 155)

4.3   What DSM-5 diagnostic provision is made for depressive symptoms following the death of a loved one?

A. Depressive symptoms lasting less than 2 months after the loss of a loved one are excluded from receiving a diagnosis of major depressive episode.
B. To qualify for a diagnosis of major depressive episode, the depression must start no less than 12 weeks following the loss.
C. To qualify for a diagnosis of major depressive episode, the depressive symptoms in such individuals must include suicidal ideation.
D. Depressive symptoms following the loss of a loved one are not excluded from receiving a major depressive episode diagnosis if the symptoms otherwise fulfill the diagnostic criteria.
E. Depressive symptoms following the loss of a loved one are excluded from receiving a major depressive episode diagnosis; however, a proposed diagnostic category for postbereavement depression is included in "Conditions for Further Study" (DSM-5 Appendix) pending further research.

Correct Answer: D. Depressive symptoms following the loss of a loved one are not excluded from receiving a major depressive episode diagnosis if the symptoms otherwise fulfill the diagnostic criteria.

Explanation: In DSM-IV, there was an exclusion criterion for a major depressive episode that was applied to depressive symptoms lasting less than 2 months following the death of a loved one (i.e., the bereavement exclusion). This exclusion is omitted in DSM-5 for several reasons, including the recognition that bereavement is a severe psychosocial stressor that can precipitate a major depressive episode in a vulnerable individual, generally beginning soon after the loss, and can add an additional risk of suffering, feelings of worthlessness, suicidal ideation, poorer medical health, and worse interpersonal and work functioning. It was critical to remove the implication that bereavement typically lasts only 2 months, when both physicians and grief counselors recognize that the duration is more commonly 1–2 years. A detailed footnote has replaced the more simplistic DSM-IV exclusion to aid clinicians in making the critical distinction between the symptoms characteristic of bereavement and those of a major depressive disorder.

4.3—Appendix / Highlights of Changes From DSM-IV to DSM-5 / Depressive Disorders (p. 811)

4.4   Which of the following statements about how grief differs from a major depressive episode (MDE) is *false?*

A. In grief the predominant affect is feelings of emptiness and loss, while in MDE it is persistent depressed mood and the inability to anticipate happiness or pleasure.
B. The pain of grief may be accompanied by positive emotions and humor that are uncharacteristic of the pervasive unhappiness and misery characteristic of MDE.
C. The thought content associated with grief generally features a preoccupation with thoughts and memories of the deceased, rather than the self-critical or pessimistic ruminations seen in MDE.
D. In grief, feelings of worthlessness and self-loathing are common; in MDE, self-esteem is generally preserved.
E. If a bereaved individual thinks about death and dying, such thoughts are generally focused on the deceased and possibly about "joining" the deceased, whereas in MDE such thoughts are focused on ending one's own life because of feeling worthless, undeserving of life, or unable to cope with the pain of depression.

Correct Answer: D. In grief, feelings of worthlessness and self-loathing are common; in MDE, self-esteem is generally preserved.

Explanation: In distinguishing grief from an MDE, it is useful to consider that in grief the predominant affect is feelings of emptiness and loss, while in MDE it is persistent depressed mood and the inability to anticipate happiness or pleasure. The dysphoria in grief is likely to decrease in intensity over days to weeks and occurs in waves, the so-called pangs of grief. These waves tend to be associated with thoughts or reminders of the deceased. The depressed mood of MDE is more persistent and not tied to specific thoughts or preoccupations. The pain of grief may be accompanied by positive emotions and humor that are uncharacteristic of the pervasive unhappiness and misery characteristic of MDE. The thought content associated with grief generally features a preoccupation with thoughts and memories of the deceased, rather than the self-critical or pessimistic ruminations seen in MDE. In grief, self-esteem is generally preserved, whereas in MDE feelings of worthlessness and self-loathing are common. If self-derogatory ideation is present in grief, it typically involves perceived failings vis-à-vis the deceased (e.g., not visiting frequently enough, not telling the deceased how much he or she was loved). If a bereaved individual thinks about death and dying, such thoughts are generally focused on the deceased and possibly about "joining" the deceased, whereas in MDE such thoughts are focused on ending one's own life because of feeling worthless, undeserving of life, or unable to cope with the pain of depression.

4.4—Major Depressive Episode / diagnostic criteria (p. 161)

4.5   How do individuals with substance/medication-induced depressive disorder differ from individuals with major depressive disorder who do not have a substance use disorder?

A. They are more likely to be female.
B. They are more likely to have graduate school education.
C. They are more likely to be male.
D. They are more likely to be white.
E. They are less likely to report suicidal thoughts/attempts.

Correct Answer: C. They are more likely to be male.

Explanation: In a representative U.S. adult population, compared with individuals with major depressive disorder who did not have a substance use disorder, individuals with substance-induced depressive disorder were more likely to be male, to be black, to have at most a high school diploma, to lack insurance, and to have lower family income. They were also more likely to report higher family history of substance use disorders and antisocial behavior, higher 12-month history of stressful life events, a greater number of DSM-IV major depressive disorder criteria, and feelings of worthlessness, insomnia/hypersomnia, and thoughts of death and suicide attempts.

4.5—Substance/Medication-Induced Depressive Disorder / Risk and Prognostic Factors (Course modifiers) (p. 179)

4.6   A 50-year-old man presents with persistently depressed mood for several weeks that interferes with his ability to work. He has insomnia and fatigue, feels guilty, has thoughts he would be better off dead, and has thought about how he could die without anyone knowing it was a suicide. His wife informs you that he requests sex several times a day and that she thinks he may be going to "massage parlors" regularly, both of which are changes from his typical behavior. He has told her he has ideas for a "better Internet," and he has invested thousands of dollars in software programs that he cannot use. She notes that he complains of fatigue but sleeps only 1 or 2 hours each night and seems to have tremendous energy during the day. Which diagnosis best fits this patient?

A. Manic episode.
B. Hypomanic episode.
C. Major depressive episode.
D. Major depressive episode, with mixed features.
E. Major depressive episode, with atypical features.

Correct Answer: D. Major depressive episode, with mixed features.

Explanation: The specifier "with mixed features" now denotes the coexistence of at least three manic symptoms insufficient to satisfy criteria for a manic episode, within a major depressive episode. This change is based on findings from studies of family history and diagnostic stability showing that the presence of mixed features in an episode of major depressive disorder increases the likelihood that the illness exists in a bipolar spectrum. This likelihood was judged insufficient to assign such individuals a diagnosis of bipolar disorder. The presence of a full manic syndrome within a depressive episode will continue to be an exclusion criterion for a depressive disorder diagnosis, and individuals with this pattern will be considered to have a manic episode.

4.6—Specifiers for Depressive Disorders / With mixed features (pp. 184–185)

4.7 A 45-year-old man with classic features of schizophrenia has always experienced co-occurring symptoms of depression—including feeling "down in the dumps," having a poor appetite, feeling hopeless, and suffering from insomnia—during his episodes of active psychosis. These depressive symptoms occurred only during his psychotic episodes and only during the 2-year period when the patient was experiencing active symptoms of schizophrenia. After his psychotic episodes were successfully controlled by medication, no further symptoms of depression were present. The patient has never met full criteria for major depressive disorder at any time. What is the appropriate DSM-5 diagnosis?

A. Schizophrenia.
B. Schizoaffective disorder.
C. Persistent depressive disorder (dysthymia).
D. Schizophrenia and persistent depressive disorder (dysthymia).
E. Unspecified schizophrenia spectrum and other psychotic disorder.

Correct Answer: A. Schizophrenia.

Explanation: Depressive symptoms are a common associated feature of chronic psychotic disorders (e.g., schizoaffective disorder, schizophrenia, delusional disorder). A separate diagnosis of persistent depressive disorder is not made if the symptoms occur only during the course of the psychotic disorder (including residual phases).

4.7—Persistent Depressive Disorder (Dysthymia) / Differential Diagnosis (pp. 170–171)

4.8 What are the new depressive disorder diagnoses in DSM-5?

A. Subsyndromal depressive disorder, premenstrual dysphoric disorder, and mixed anxiety and depressive disorder.
B. Disruptive mood dysregulation disorder, premenstrual dysphoric disorder, and persistent depressive disorder (dysthymia).
C. Disruptive mood dysregulation disorder, premenstrual dysphoric disorder, and subsyndromal depressive disorder.

D. Disruptive mood dysregulation disorder, postmenopausal dysphoric disorder, and persistent depressive disorder (dysthymia).

E. Mixed anxiety and depressive disorder, bereavement-induced major depressive disorder, and postmenopausal dysphoric disorder.

Correct Answer: B. Disruptive mood dysregulation disorder, premenstrual dysphoric disorder, and persistent depressive disorder (dysthymia).

Explanation: Several new diagnoses appear in the DSM-5 "Depressive Disorders" chapter. After careful scientific review of the evidence, premenstrual dysphoric disorder (PMDD) has been moved from Appendix B ("Criteria Sets and Axes Provided for Further Study") of DSM-IV to Section II of DSM-5. Almost 20 years of additional research on this condition has confirmed a specific and treatment-responsive form of depressive disorder that begins sometime following ovulation and remits within a few days of menses and has a marked impact on functioning.

In order to address concerns about the potential for the overdiagnosis of and treatment for bipolar disorder in children, a new diagnosis, disruptive mood dysregulation disorder (DMDD), referring to the presentation of children with persistent irritability and frequent episodes of extreme behavioral dyscontrol, is added to the depressive disorders for children up to 12 years of age. Its placement in this chapter reflects the finding that children with this symptom pattern typically develop unipolar depressive disorders or anxiety disorders, rather than bipolar disorders, as they mature into adolescence and adulthood.

A more chronic form of depression, persistent depressive disorder (dysthymia), can be diagnosed when the mood disturbance continues for at least 2 years in adults or 1 year in children. This diagnosis, new in DSM-5, includes the DSM-IV diagnostic categories of chronic major depression and dysthymia.

4.8—chapter intro (p. 155)

4.9   A depressed patient reports that he experiences no pleasure from his normally enjoyable activities. Which of the following additional symptoms would be required for this patient to qualify for a diagnosis of major depressive disorder with melancholic features?

A. Despondency, depression that is worse in the morning, and inability to fall asleep.

B. Depression that is worse in the evening, psychomotor agitation, and significant weight loss.

C. Inappropriate guilt, depression that is worse in the morning, and early-morning awakening.

D. Significant weight gain, depression that is worse in the evening, and excessive guilt.

E. Despondency, significant weight gain, and psychomotor retardation.

Correct Answer: C. Inappropriate guilt, depression that is worse in the morning, and early-morning awakening.

Explanation: Two criteria must be met to qualify for the specifier "with melancholic features" for major depressive disorder. Criterion A specifies that one of the following must be present during the most severe period of the current episode: 1) loss of pleasure in all, or almost all, activities; 2) lack of reactivity to usually pleasurable stimuli (does not feel much better, even temporarily, when something good happens). Criterion B specifies that three (or more) of the following must be present: 1) a distinct quality of depressed mood characterized by profound despondency, despair, and/or moroseness or by so-called empty mood; 2) depression that is regularly worse in the morning; 3) early-morning awakening (i.e., at least 2 hours before usual awakening); 4) marked psychomotor agitation or retardation; 5) significant anorexia or weight loss; 6) excessive or inappropriate guilt. The specifier "with melancholic features" can be applied to the current (or, if the full criteria are not currently met for major depressive episode, to the most recent) major depressive episode in major depressive disorder or in bipolar I or II disorder only if it is the most recent type of mood episode.

4.9—Specifiers for Depressive Disorders / With melancholic features (p. 185)

4.10   A 39-year-old woman reports that she became quite depressed in the winter last year when her company closed for the season, but she felt completely normal in the spring. She recalls experiencing several other episodes of depression over the past 5 years (for which she cannot identify a seasonal pattern) that would have met criteria for major depressive disorder. Which of the following correctly summarizes this patient's eligibility for a diagnosis of "major depressive disorder, with seasonal pattern"?

   A. She does *not* qualify for this diagnosis: the episode must start in the fall, and the patient must have no episodes that do not have a seasonal pattern.
   B. She *does* qualify for this diagnosis: the single episode described started in the winter and ended in the spring.
   C. She does *not* qualify for this diagnosis: the patient must have had two episodes with a seasonal relationship in the past 2 years and no nonseasonal episodes during that period.
   D. She *does* qualify for this diagnosis: the symptoms described are related to psychosocial stressors.
   E. She *does* qualify for this diagnosis: the symptoms are not related to bipolar I or bipolar II disorder.

Correct Answer: C. She does *not* qualify for this diagnosis: the patient must have had two episodes with a seasonal relationship in the past 2 years and no nonseasonal episodes during that period.

Explanation: The "with seasonal pattern" specifier requires a regular temporal relationship between the onset of major depressive episodes (MDEs) in major depressive disorder or in bipolar I or bipolar II disorder and a particular time of the year (e.g., in the fall or winter). The diagnosis excludes cases in which there is an obvious effect of seasonal-related psychosocial stressors (e.g., regularly being unemployed every winter). Full remissions (or a change from major depression to mania or hypomania) also occur at a characteristic time of the year (e.g., depression disappears in the spring). In the past 2 years, two MDEs must have occurred that demonstrate the temporal seasonal relationships defined above, and no nonseasonal MDEs must have occurred during that same period. Seasonal MDEs must substantially outnumber the nonseasonal MDEs that may have occurred over the individual's lifetime. The specifier "with seasonal pattern" can be applied to the pattern of MDEs in bipolar I disorder, bipolar II disorder, or major depressive disorder, recurrent.

4.10—Specifiers for Depressive Disorders / With seasonal pattern (pp. 187–188)

4.11 Which of the following statements about the prevalence of major depressive disorder in the United States is *true?*

A. The 12-month prevalence is 17%.
B. Females and males have equal prevalence at all ages.
C. Females have increased prevalence at all ages.
D. The prevalence in 18- to 29-year-olds is three times higher than that in 60-year-olds.
E. The prevalence in 60-year-olds is three times higher than that in 18- to 29-year-olds.

Correct Answer: D. The prevalence in 18- to 29-year-olds is three times higher than that in 60-year-olds.

Explanation: The 12-month prevalence of major depressive disorder in the United States is 7%, with marked differences by age group such that the prevalence in 18- to 29-year-old individuals is threefold higher than the prevalence in individuals age 60 years or older. Females experience 1.5- to 3-fold higher rates than males beginning in early adolescence.

4.11—Major Depressive Disorder / Prevalence (p. 165)

4.12 Which of the following statements about the heritability of major depressive disorder (MDD) is *true?*

A. Nearly 100% of people with genetic liability can be accounted for by the personality trait of dogmatism.
B. The heritability is approximately 40%, and the personality trait of neuroticism accounts for a substantial portion of this genetic liability.

C. Less than 10% of people with genetic liability can be accounted for by the personality trait of perfectionism.
D. Nearly 50% of people with genetic liability can be accounted for by the personality trait of aggressiveness.
E. The heritability of MDD depends on whether the individual's mother or father had MDD.

Correct Answer: B. The heritability is approximately 40%, and the personality trait of neuroticism accounts for a substantial portion of this genetic liability.

Explanation: First-degree family members of individuals with major depressive disorder have a risk of major depressive disorder two- to fourfold higher than that of the general population. Relative risks appear to be higher for early-onset and recurrent forms. Heritability is approximately 40%, and the personality trait neuroticism accounts for a substantial portion of this genetic liability. Neuroticism (negative affectivity) is a well-established risk factor for the onset of major depressive disorder, and high levels appear to render individuals more likely to develop depressive episodes in response to stressful life events.

4.12—Major Depressive Disorder / Risk and Prognostic Factors (p. 166)

4.13 Which of the following statements about diagnostic markers for major depressive disorder (MDD) is *true?*

A. No laboratory test has demonstrated sufficient sensitivity and specificity to be used as a diagnostic tool for MDD.
B. Several diagnostic laboratory tests exist, but no commercial enterprise will offer them to the public.
C. Diagnostic laboratory tests have been withheld for fear that people testing positive for MDD may attempt suicide.
D. Tests that exist are adequate diagnostically but are not covered by health insurance.
E. Only functional magnetic resonance imaging (fMRI) provides absolute diagnostic reliability for MDD.

Correct Answer: A. No laboratory test has demonstrated sufficient sensitivity and specificity to be used as a diagnostic tool for MDD.

Explanation: Although an extensive literature exists describing neuroanatomical, neuroendocrinological, and neurophysiological correlates of MDD, no laboratory test has yielded results of sufficient sensitivity and specificity to be used as a diagnostic tool for this disorder. Until recently, hypothalamic-pituitary-adrenal axis hyperactivity had been the most extensively investigated abnormality associated with major depressive episodes, and it appears to be associated with melancholia, psychotic features, and risks for eventual suicide.

Molecular studies have also implicated peripheral factors, including genetic variants in neurotrophic factors and pro-inflammatory cytokines. Additionally, fMRI studies provide evidence for functional abnormalities in specific neural systems supporting emotion processing, reward seeking, and emotion regulation in adults with major depression.

4.13—Major Depressive Disorder / Associated Features Supporting Diagnosis (p. 165)

4.14 Which of the following statements about gender differences in suicide risk and suicide rates in major depressive disorder (MDD) is *true?*

A. The risk of suicide attempts and completions is higher for women.
B. The risk of suicide attempts and completions is higher for men.
C. The risk of suicide attempts and completions is equal for men and women.
D. The disparity in suicide rate by gender is much greater in individuals with MDD than in the general population.
E. The risk of suicide attempts is higher for women, but the risk of suicide completions is lower.

Correct Answer: E. The risk of suicide attempts is higher for women, but the risk of suicide completions is lower.

Explanation: In women, the risk of suicide attempts is higher, and the risk of suicide completions is lower. The disparity in suicide rate by gender is not as great among those with depressive disorders as it is in the population as a whole.

4.14—Major Depressive Disorder / Gender-Related Diagnostic Issues (p. 167)

4.15 A 12-year-old boy begins to have new episodes of temper outbursts that are out of proportion to the situation. Which of the following is *not* a diagnostic possibility for this patient?

A. Disruptive mood dysregulation disorder.
B. Bipolar disorder.
C. Oppositional defiant disorder.
D. Conduct disorder.
E. Attention-deficit/hyperactivity disorder.

Correct Answer: A. Disruptive mood dysregulation disorder.

Explanation: Criteria G and H of disruptive mood dysregulation disorder state that the chronological age at onset is at least 6 years (or equivalent developmental level) and the onset is before 10 years.

4.15—Disruptive Mood Dysregulation Disorder / diagnostic criteria (p. 156)

4.16   Which of the following features distinguishes disruptive mood dysregulation disorder (DMDD) from bipolar disorder in children?

   A. Age at onset.
   B. Gender of the child.
   C. Irritability.
   D. Chronicity.
   E. Severity.

Correct Answer: D. Chronicity.

Explanation: The core feature of DMDD is chronic, severe, persistent irritability. This severe irritability has two prominent clinical manifestations, the first of which is frequent temper outbursts. These outbursts typically occur in response to frustration and can be verbal or behavioral (the latter in the form of aggression against property, self, or others).

   The clinical presentation of DMDD must be carefully distinguished from presentations of other, related conditions, particularly pediatric bipolar disorder. DMDD was added to DSM-5 to address the considerable concern about the appropriate classification and treatment of children who present with chronic, persistent irritability relative to children who present with classic (i.e., episodic) bipolar disorder.

   In DSM-5, the term *bipolar disorder* is explicitly reserved for episodic presentations of bipolar symptoms. DSM-IV did not include a diagnosis designed to capture youths whose hallmark symptoms consisted of very severe, nonepisodic irritability, whereas DSM-5, with the inclusion of DMDD, provides a distinct category for such presentations.

4.16—Disruptive Mood Dysregulation Disorder / Diagnostic Features (pp. 156–157)

4.17   Children with disruptive mood dysregulation disorder are most likely to develop which of the following disorders in adulthood?

   A. Bipolar I disorder.
   B. Schizophrenia.
   C. Bipolar II disorder.
   D. Borderline personality disorder.
   E. Unipolar depressive disorders.

Correct Answer: E. Unipolar depressive disorders.

Explanation: Approximately half of children with severe, chronic irritability will have a presentation that continues to meet criteria for the condition 1 year later. Rates of conversion from severe, nonepisodic irritability to bipolar disorder are very low. Instead, children with chronic irritability are at risk to develop unipolar depressive and/or anxiety disorders in adulthood.

4.17—Disruptive Mood Dysregulation Disorder / Development and Course (p. 157)

4.18   An irritable 8-year-old child has a history of temper outbursts both at home and at school. What characteristic mood feature must be also present to qualify him for a diagnosis of disruptive mood dysregulation disorder?

A. The child's mood between outbursts is typically euthymic.
B. The child's mood between outbursts is typically hypomanic.
C. The child's mood between outbursts is typically depressed.
D. The child's mood between outbursts is typically irritable or angry.
E. The mood symptoms and temper outbursts must not have persisted for more than 6 months.

Correct Answer: D. The child's mood between outbursts is typically irritable or angry.

Explanation: Criterion D of disruptive mood dysregulation disorder requires that the child's mood between temper outbursts be persistently irritable or angry most of the day, nearly every day, and observable by others (e.g., parents, teachers, peers).

4.18—Disruptive Mood Dysregulation Disorder / diagnostic criteria (p. 156)

4.19   Children with disruptive mood dysregulation disorder (DMDD) often meet criteria for what additional DSM-5 diagnosis?

A. Pediatric bipolar disorder.
B. Oppositional defiant disorder.
C. Schizophrenia.
D. Intermittent explosive disorder.
E. Major depressive disorder.

Correct Answer: B. Oppositional defiant disorder.

Explanation: Because chronically irritable children and adolescents typically present with complex histories, the diagnosis of DMDD must be made while considering the presence or absence of multiple other conditions. The differential diagnosis of DMDD from both bipolar disorder and oppositional defiant disorder requires careful consideration. DMDD differs from bipolar disorder in that the former is chronic, whereas the latter is episodic. DMDD differs from oppositional defiant disorder in that very severe irritability is required in the former but not the latter. For this reason, while most children who meet criteria for DMDD will also meet criteria for oppositional defiant disorder, the reverse is not the case.

4.19—Disruptive Mood Dysregulation Disorder / Differential Diagnosis (pp. 158–159)

4.20 The diagnostic criteria for disruptive mood dysregulation disorder (DMDD) state that the diagnosis should not be made for the first time before age 6 years or after 18 years (Criterion G). Which of the following statements best describes the rationale for this age range restriction?

A. Validity of the diagnosis has been established only in the age group 7–18 years.
B. The restriction represents an attempt to differentiate DMDD from bipolar disorder.
C. The restriction is based on existing genetic data.
D. The restriction represents an attempt to differentiate DMDD from intermittent explosive disorder.
E. The restriction represents an attempt to differentiate DMDD from autism spectrum disorder.

Correct Answer: A. Validity of the diagnosis has been established only in the age group 7–18 years.

Explanation: By definition, the onset of DMDD (by history or observation) must be before age 10 years (Criterion H), and the diagnosis should not be applied to children with a developmental age of less than 6 years. It is unknown whether the condition presents only in this age-delimited fashion. Because the symptoms of disruptive mood dysregulation disorder are likely to change as children mature, use of the diagnosis should be restricted to age groups similar to those in which validity has been established (7–18 years). Approximately half of children with severe, chronic irritability will have a presentation that continues to meet criteria for the condition 1 year later. Rates of conversion from severe, nonepisodic irritability to bipolar disorder are very low. Instead, children with chronic irritability are at risk to develop unipolar depressive and/or anxiety disorders in adulthood.

4.20—Disruptive Mood Dysregulation Disorder / Development and Course (p. 157)

4.21 A 9-year-old boy is brought in for evaluation because of explosive outbursts when he is frustrated with schoolwork. The parents report that their son is well behaved and pleasant at other times. Which diagnosis best fits this clinical picture?

A. Disruptive mood dysregulation disorder.
B. Pediatric bipolar disorder.
C. Intermittent explosive disorder.
D. Major depressive disorder.
E. Persistent depressive disorder (dysthymia).

Correct Answer: C. Intermittent explosive disorder.

Explanation: Children with intermittent explosive disorder present with instances of severe temper outbursts much like those in children with disruptive mood dysregulation disorder. However, unlike children with disruptive mood dysregulation disorder, children with intermittent explosive disorder do not exhibit persistent disruption in mood between outbursts. Thus, the two diagnoses are mutually exclusive and cannot be made in the same child. For children with outbursts and intercurrent, persistent irritability, the diagnosis of disruptive mood dysregulation disorder should be made. For children with outbursts but no such irritability, the diagnosis of intermittent explosive disorder should be made.

4.21—Disruptive Mood Dysregulation Disorder / Differential Diagnosis (p. 160)

4.22   A 14-year-old boy describes himself as feeling "down" all of the time for the past year. He remembers feeling better while he was at camp for 4 weeks during the summer; however, the depressed mood returned when he came home. He reports poor concentration, feelings of hopelessness, and low self-esteem but denies suicidal ideation or changes in his appetite or sleep. What is the most likely diagnosis?

A. Major depressive disorder.
B. Disruptive mood dysregulation disorder.
C. Depressive episodes with short-duration hypomania.
D. Persistent depressive disorder (dysthymia), with early onset.
E. Schizoaffective disorder.

Correct Answer: D. Persistent depressive disorder (dysthymia), with early onset.

Explanation: The essential feature of persistent depressive disorder (dysthymia) is a depressed mood that occurs for most of the day, for more days than not, for at least 2 years, or at least 1 year for children and adolescents (Criterion A). This disorder represents a consolidation of DSM-IV-defined chronic major depressive disorder and dysthymic disorder. Major depression may precede persistent depressive disorder, and major depressive episodes may occur during persistent depressive disorder. Individuals whose symptoms meet major depressive disorder criteria for 2 years should be given a diagnosis of persistent depressive disorder as well as major depressive disorder.

Individuals with persistent depressive disorder describe their mood as sad or "down in the dumps." During periods of depressed mood, at least two of the six symptoms from Criterion B are present. Because these symptoms have become a part of the individual's day-to-day experience, particularly in the case of early onset (e.g., "I've always been this way"), they may not be reported unless the individual is directly prompted. During the 2-year period (1 year for children or adolescents), any symptom-free intervals last no longer than 2 months (Criterion C).

4.22—Persistent Depressive Disorder (Dysthymia) / Diagnostic Features (pp. 169–170)

4.23   A 30-year-old woman reports 2 years of persistently depressed mood, accompanied by loss of pleasure in all activities, ruminations that she would be better off dead, feelings of guilt about "bad things" she has done, and thoughts about quitting work because of her inability to make decisions. Although she has never been treated for depression, she feels so distressed at times that she wonders if she should be hospitalized. She experiences an increased need for sleep but still feels fatigued during the day. Her overeating has led to a 12-kg weight gain. She denies drug or alcohol use, and her medical workup is completely normal, including laboratory tests for vitamins. The consultation was prompted by her worsened mood for the past several weeks. What is the most appropriate diagnosis?

A. Major depressive disorder (MDD).
B. Persistent depressive disorder (dysthymia), with persistent major depressive episode.
C. Cyclothymia.
D. Bipolar II disorder.
E. MDD, with melancholic features.

Correct Answer: B. Persistent depressive disorder (dysthymia), with persistent major depressive episode.

Explanation: The essential feature of persistent depressive disorder (dysthymia) is a depressed mood that occurs for most of the day, for more days than not, for at least 2 years. This disorder represents a consolidation of DSM-IV-defined chronic major depressive disorder and dysthymic disorder. Major depression may precede persistent depressive disorder, and major depressive episodes may occur during persistent depressive disorder. Individuals whose symptoms meet major depressive disorder criteria for 2 years should be given a diagnosis of persistent depressive disorder as well as major depressive disorder.

If there is a depressed mood plus two or more symptoms meeting criteria for a persistent depressive episode for 2 years or more, then the diagnosis of persistent depressive disorder is made. The diagnosis depends on the 2-year duration, which distinguishes it from episodes of depression that do not last 2 years. If the symptom criteria are sufficient for a diagnosis of a major depressive episode at any time during this period, then the diagnosis of major depression should be noted, but it is coded not as a separate diagnosis but rather as a specifier with the diagnosis of persistent depressive disorder. If the individual's symptoms currently meet full criteria for a major depressive episode, then the specifier "with intermittent major depressive episodes, with current episode" would be applied. If—as in the patient described in the above vignette—the major depressive episode has persisted for at least a 2-year duration and remains present, then the specifier "with persistent major depressive episode" is used. When full major depressive episode criteria are not currently met but there has been at least one previous episode of major depression in the context of at least 2 years of persistent depressive symptoms, then the specifier "with intermittent major depressive episodes, without current episode" is used. If the individual has not experienced an episode of major depression in the past 2 years, then the specifier "with pure dysthymic syndrome" is used.

4.23—Persistent Depressive Disorder (Dysthymia) / diagnostic criteria (pp. 168–169); Diagnostic Features (pp. 169–170); Differential Diagnosis (Major depressive disorder) (pp. 170–171)

4.24 A 45-year-old woman with multiple sclerosis was treated with interferon beta-1a a year ago, which resolved her physical symptoms. She now presents with depressed mood (experienced daily for the past several months), middle insomnia (of recent onset), poor appetite, trouble concentrating, and lack of interest in sex. Although she has no physical symptoms, she is frequently absent from work. She denies any active plans to commit suicide but admits that she often thinks about it, as her mood has worsened. What is the most likely diagnosis?

A. Major depressive disorder.
B. Persistent depressive disorder (dysthymia).
C. Depressive disorder due to another medical condition.
D. Substance/medication-induced depressive disorder.
E. Persistent depressive disorder (dysthymia) and multiple sclerosis.

Correct Answer: C. Depressive disorder due to another medical condition.

Explanation: The essential feature of depressive disorder due to another medical condition is a prominent and persistent period of depressed mood or markedly diminished interest or pleasure in all, or almost all, activities that predominates in the clinical picture and that is thought to be related to the direct physiological effects of another medical condition. In determining whether the mood disturbance is due to another medical condition, the clinician must first establish the presence of such a condition. Furthermore, the clinician must establish that the mood disturbance is etiologically related to the other medical condition through a physiological mechanism. A careful and comprehensive assessment of multiple factors is necessary to make this judgment.

4.24—Depressive Disorder Due to Another Medical Condition / Diagnostic Features (p. 181)

4.25 An 18-year-old college student, recently arrived in the United States from Beijing, complains to her gynecologist of irritability, problems with her roommates, increased appetite, feeling bloated, and feeling depressed for 3–4 days prior to the onset of menses. She reports that these symptoms have been present since she reached menarche at age 12 (although she has never kept a mood log). The gynecologist calls you for a consultation about the correct diagnosis, because she is as yet unfamiliar with the new DSM-5 diagnostic criteria. What is your response?

A. The patient has premenstrual syndrome because she does not meet criteria for premenstrual dysphoric disorder.
B. The patient would qualify for a provisional diagnosis of premenstrual dysphoric disorder; however, the diagnosis does not exist in DSM-5.
C. The patient would qualify for a provisional diagnosis of premenstrual dysphoric disorder.
D. The patient would qualify for a provisional diagnosis of premenstrual dysphoric disorder if the diagnosis had been validated in Asian women.
E. The patient has no DSM-5 diagnosis.

Correct Answer: C. The patient would qualify for a provisional diagnosis of premenstrual dysphoric disorder.

Explanation: Premenstrual dysphoric disorder is not a culture-bound syndrome and has been observed in individuals in the United States, Europe, India, and Asia. It is unclear as to whether rates differ by race.

The essential features of premenstrual dysphoric disorder are the expression of mood lability, irritability, dysphoria, and anxiety symptoms that occur repeatedly during the premenstrual phase of the cycle and remit around the onset of menses or shortly thereafter. These symptoms may be accompanied by behavioral and physical symptoms. Symptoms must have occurred in most of the menstrual cycles during the past year and must have an adverse effect on work or social functioning.

Typically, symptoms peak around the time of the onset of menses. While the core symptoms include mood and anxiety symptoms, behavioral and somatic symptoms commonly also occur. In order to confirm a provisional diagnosis, daily prospective symptom ratings are required for at least two symptomatic cycles.

4.25—Premenstrual Dysphoric Disorder / Diagnostic Features; Culture-Related Diagnostic Issues (pp. 172–173)

4.26 What is the appropriate method of confirming a diagnosis of premenstrual dysphoric disorder?

A. Laboratory tests.
B. Family history.
C. Neuropsychological testing.
D. Two or more months of prospective symptom ratings on validated scales.
E. One month of scoring high on the Daily Rating of Severity of Problems or 1 month of scoring high on the Visual Analogue Scales for Premenstrual Mood Symptoms.

Correct Answer: D. Two or more months of prospective symptom ratings on validated scales.

Explanation: The diagnosis of premenstrual dysphoric disorder is appropriately confirmed by 2 months of prospective symptom ratings. (Note: The diagnosis may be made provisionally prior to this confirmation.) A number of scales, including the Daily Rating of Severity of Problems and the Visual Analogue Scales for Premenstrual Mood Symptoms, have undergone validation and are commonly used in clinical trials for premenstrual dysphoric disorder. The Premenstrual Tension Syndrome Rating Scale has a self-report and an observer version, both of which have been validated and used widely to measure illness severity in women who have premenstrual dysphoric disorder.

4.26—Premenstrual Dysphoric Disorder / Diagnostic Markers (pp. 173–174)

4.27   A 29-year-old woman complains of sad mood every month in anticipation of her very painful menses. The pain begins with the start of her flow and continues for several days. She does not experience pain during other times of the month. She has tried a variety of treatments, none of which have given her relief. What is the appropriate diagnosis?

A. Premenstrual dysphoric disorder.
B. Premenstrual syndrome.
C. Dysmenorrhea.
D. Factitious disorder.
E. Persistent depressive disorder (dysthymia).

Correct Answer: C. Dysmenorrhea.

Explanation: Dysmenorrhea is a syndrome of painful menses, but this is distinct from a syndrome characterized by affective changes. Symptoms of dysmenorrhea begin with the onset of menses, whereas symptoms of premenstrual dysphoric disorder, by definition, begin before the onset of menses, even if they linger into the first few days of menses.

4.27—Premenstrual Dysphoric Disorder / Differential Diagnosis (p. 174)

4.28   Which of the following symptoms must be present for a woman to meet criteria for premenstrual dysphoric disorder?

A. Marked affective lability.
B. Decreased interest in usual activities.
C. Physical symptoms such as breast tenderness.
D. Marked change in appetite.
E. A sense of feeling overwhelmed or out of control.

Correct Answer: A. Marked affective lability.

Explanation: Of the 11 symptoms in the premenstrual dysphoric disorder diagnostic criteria, patients must have a total of at least 5 symptoms. One of the 5 must be one of the following symptoms: 1) marked affective lability; 2) marked irritability or anger or increased interpersonal conflicts; 3) marked depressed mood, feelings of hopelessness, or self-deprecating thoughts; 4) marked anxiety, tension, and/or feelings of being keyed up or on edge.

4.28—Premenstrual Dysphoric Disorder / diagnostic criteria (pp. 171–172)

4.29   A 23-year-old woman reports that during every menstrual cycle she experiences breast swelling, bloating, hypersomnia, an increased craving for sweets, poor concentration, and a feeling that she cannot handle her normal responsibilities. She notes that she also feels somewhat more sensitive emotionally and may become tearful when hearing a sad story. She takes no oral medication but does use a drospirenone/ethinyl estradiol patch. What diagnosis best fits this clinical picture?

    A. Premenstrual dysphoric disorder (PMDD).
    B. Dysthymia.
    C. Dysmenorrhea.
    D. Premenstrual syndrome.
    E. Substance/medication-induced depressive disorder.

Correct Answer: D. Premenstrual syndrome.

Explanation: Premenstrual syndrome differs from PMDD in that a minimum of five symptoms is not required and there is no stipulation of affective symptoms for individuals who suffer from premenstrual syndrome. This condition may be more common than PMDD, although the estimated prevalence of premenstrual syndrome varies. Premenstrual syndrome shares with PMDD the feature of symptom expression during the premenstrual phase of the menstrual cycle, but it is generally considered to be less severe than PMDD. Individuals who experience physical or behavioral symptoms in the premenstruum, without the required affective symptoms, likely meet criteria for premenstrual syndrome and not for PMDD.

4.29—Premenstrual Dysphoric Disorder / Differential Diagnosis (p. 174)

4.30   A 31-year-old woman with no history of mood symptoms reports that she experiences distressing mood lability and irritability starting about 4 days before the onset of menses. She feels "on edge," cannot concentrate, has little enjoyment from any of her activities, and experiences bloating and swelling of her breasts. The patient reports that these symptoms started 6 months ago when she began taking oral contraceptives for the first time. If she stops the oral contraceptives and her symptoms remit, what would the diagnosis be?

A. Premenstrual dysphoric disorder.

B. Dysthymia.

C. Major depressive episode.

D. Substance/medication-induced depressive disorder.

E. Premenstrual syndrome.

Correct Answer: D. Substance/medication-induced depressive disorder.

Explanation: If the woman stops the hormones and her symptoms disappear, this is consistent with substance/medication-induced depressive disorder. Some women who present with moderate to severe premenstrual symptoms may be using hormonal contraceptives. If such symptoms occur after initiation of exogenous hormone use, the symptoms may be due to the use of hormones rather than the underlying condition of premenstrual dysphoric disorder.

4.30—Premenstrual Dysphoric Disorder / Differential Diagnosis (pp. 174–175)

4.31   A 45-year-old man is admitted to the hospital with profound hypothyroidism. He is depressed but does not meet full criteria for major depressive disorder (MDD), the diagnosis given to him by his internist. The patient has no prior history of a mood disorder, and all of the depressive symptoms are temporally related to the hypothyroidism. Based on this information, you determine that a change in diagnosis—to depressive disorder due to another medical condition—is warranted, as well as a specifier to indicate that full criteria for MDD are not met. How would the full diagnosis be recorded?

A. Hypothyroidism would be coded on Axis III in DSM-5.

B. There is no special coding procedure in DSM-5.

C. Hypothyroidism would be recorded as the name of the "other medical condition" in the DSM-5 diagnosis.

D. Medical disorders are not coded as part of a mental disorder diagnosis in DSM-5.

E. A revision to DSM-5 is planned to deal with this issue.

Correct Answer: C. Hypothyroidism would be recorded as the name of the "other medical condition" in the DSM-5 diagnosis.

Explanation: In recording a diagnosis of depressive disorder due to another medical condition, the name of the other medical condition is inserted in the mental disorder diagnosis (i.e., "depressive disorder due to hypothyroidism"). In addition, the other medical condition should be coded and listed separately immediately before the depressive disorder due to the medical condition. In this vignette, the full coding would be "244.9 [E03.9] hypothyroidism; 293.83 [F06.31] depressive disorder due to hypothyroidism, with depressive features." (The "with depressive features" specifier denotes that full criteria are not met for a major depressive episode.) There is no longer an Axis III in DSM-5.

4.31—Depressive Disorder Due to Another Medical Condition / diagnostic criteria (p. 181)

CHAPTER 5

Anxiety Disorders

5.1   Which of the following disorders is included in the "Anxiety Disorders" chapter of DSM-5?

A. Obsessive-compulsive disorder.
B. Posttraumatic stress disorder.
C. Acute stress disorder.
D. Panic disorder with agoraphobia.
E. Separation anxiety disorder.

Correct Answer: E. Separation anxiety disorder.

Explanation: The DSM-5 "Anxiety Disorders" chapter contains a number of additions and deletions when compared with the prior edition. A number of anxiety disorders classified by DSM-IV as disorders usually first diagnosed in infancy, childhood, or adolescence are now included among the DSM-5 anxiety disorders, including separation anxiety disorder and selective mutism. Several DSM-IV disorders from the "Anxiety Disorders" chapter, including obsessive-compulsive disorder, posttraumatic stress disorder, and acute stress disorder, were removed from that section in DSM-5. This reorganization was the result of a scientific review that concluded that these were distinct disorders that were not sufficiently described by the presence of anxiety symptoms. Agoraphobia has been separated from panic disorder as a distinct disorder in DSM-5, which includes a panic attack specifier when they co-occur.

5.1—chapter intro (pp. 189–190)

5.2   A 9-year-old boy cannot go to sleep without having a parent in his room. While falling asleep, he frequently awakens to check that a parent is still there. One parent usually stays until the boy falls asleep. If he wakes up alone during the night, he starts to panic and gets up to find his parents. He also reports frequent nightmares in which he or his parents are harmed. He occasionally calls out that he saw a strange figure peering into his dark room. The parents usually wake in the morning to find the boy asleep on the floor of their room. They once tried to leave him with a relative so they could go on a vacation; however, he became so distressed in anticipation of this that they canceled their plans. What is the most likely diagnosis?

A. Specific phobia.
B. Nightmare disorder.

C. Delusional disorder.
D. Separation anxiety disorder.
E. Agoraphobia.

Correct Answer: D. Separation anxiety disorder.

Explanation: The essential feature of separation anxiety disorder is excessive anxiety about being separated from home or attachment figures, beyond what would be expected for the person's developmental stage. By definition, it firsts presents before age 18; however, it may continue into adulthood. Typical presentations include reluctance to leave home or even stay in a room without a parent. In the latter case, children frequently have difficulty at bedtime and may insist that a parent stay with them. They frequently express fear of harm or untoward events that may prevent them from being with a loved one, and they may have nightmares regarding these fears as well as unusual perceptual experiences, particularly at night or in the dark. Although the other disorders listed should be ruled out, the child's focus on a fear of being left alone makes separation anxiety disorder the most likely diagnosis.

5.2—Separation Anxiety Disorder / Diagnostic Features (p. 191)

5.3   Which of the following is considered a culture-specific symptom of panic attacks?

A. Derealization.
B. Headaches.
C. Fear of going crazy.
D. Shortness of breath.
E. Heat sensations.

Correct Answer: B. Headaches.

Explanation: All of the symptoms listed may occur as part of a panic attack. Culture-specific symptoms (e.g., tinnitus, neck soreness, headache, and uncontrollable screaming or crying) may be seen; however, such symptoms should not count as one of the four required symptoms. Frequency of each of the 13 symptoms varies cross-culturally (e.g., higher rates of paresthesias in African Americans and of dizziness in several Asian groups). Cultural syndromes also influence the cross-cultural presentation of panic attacks, resulting in different symptom profiles across different cultural groups. Examples include *khyâl* (wind) attacks, a Cambodian cultural syndrome involving dizziness, tinnitus, and neck soreness; and *trúng gió* (wind-related) attacks, a Vietnamese cultural syndrome associated with headaches.

5.3—Panic Attack Specifier / Culture-Related Diagnostic Issues (p. 216)

5.4   Which of the following statements best describes how panic attacks differ from panic disorder?

   A. Panic attacks require fewer symptoms for a definitive diagnosis.
   B. Panic attacks are discrete, occur suddenly, and are usually less severe.
   C. Panic attacks are invariably unexpected.
   D. Panic attacks represent a syndrome that can occur with a variety of other disorders.
   E. Panic attacks cannot be secondary to a medical condition.

Correct Answer: D. Panic attacks represent a syndrome that can occur with a variety of other disorders.

Explanation: Panic attacks are abrupt surges of intense fear or intense discomfort that reach a peak within minutes, accompanied by physical and/or cognitive symptoms. Panic attacks may be either *expected* (e.g., in response to a typically feared object or situation) or *unexpected* (meaning that the panic attack occurs for no apparent reason). Although DSM-5 defines symptoms for the purpose of identifying a panic attack, panic attack is not a mental disorder and cannot be coded. Panic attacks can occur in the context of any anxiety disorder as well as other mental disorders (e.g., depressive disorders, posttraumatic stress disorder, substance use disorders) and some medical conditions (e.g., cardiac, respiratory, vestibular, gastrointestinal). When the presence of a panic attack is identified, it should be noted as a specifier (e.g., "posttraumatic stress disorder with panic attacks"). For panic disorder, the presence of panic attack is contained within the criteria for the disorder, and panic attack is not used as a specifier.

5.4—chapter intro (p. 190); Panic Attack Specifier / diagnostic criteria (p. 214); Features (pp. 214–215)

5.5   The determination of whether a panic attack is expected or unexpected is ultimately best made by which of the following?

   A. Careful clinical judgment.
   B. Whether the patient associates it with external stress.
   C. The presence or absence of nocturnal panic attacks.
   D. Ruling out possible culture-specific syndromes.
   E. 24-Hour electroencephalographic monitoring.

Correct Answer: A. Careful clinical judgment.

Explanation: It can be difficult to determine whether panic attacks are expected (i.e., triggered by some external stress or situation). Patients (particularly older individuals) may retrospectively attribute panic attacks to certain stressful situations even if they were unexpected in the moment. Laboratory testing may rule out other potential medical causes. Agents with disparate mechanisms of action, such as sodium lactate, caffeine, isoproterenol, yohimbine, carbon dioxide, or cholecystokinin, provoke panic attacks in individuals with panic disorder to a much greater extent than in healthy control subjects (and in some cases, than in individuals with other anxiety, depressive, or bipolar disorders without panic attacks). In a proportion of individuals with panic disorder, panic attacks are related to hypersensitive medullary carbon dioxide detectors, resulting in hypocapnia and other respiratory irregularities; however, none of these laboratory findings are considered diagnostic of panic disorder. There is no definitive test; ultimately the determination is based on a clinical judgment that takes into account the sequence of events leading to the attack, the patient's own sense of whether triggers are present, and potential cultural factors that may influence a determination of cause.

5.5—Panic Attack Specifier / Features (p. 215)

5.6   A 50-year-old man reports episodes in which he suddenly and unexpectedly awakens from sleep feeling a surge of intense fear that peaks within minutes. During this time, he feels short of breath and has heart palpitations, sweating, and nausea. His medical history is significant only for hypertension, which is well controlled with hydrochlorothiazide. As a result of these symptoms, he has begun to have anticipatory anxiety associated with going to sleep. What is the most likely explanation for his symptoms?

A. Anxiety disorder due to another medical condition (hypertension).
B. Substance/medication-induced anxiety disorder.
C. Panic disorder.
D. Sleep terrors.
E. Panic attacks.

Correct Answer: C. Panic disorder.

Explanation: Panic disorder involves recurrent, unexpected panic attacks. Panic attacks are a syndrome, not a disorder, and can occur with a variety of disorders. Other medical conditions, substance-related disorders, and other psychiatric disorders must be ruled out; in this vignette, the patient's well-controlled hypertension and use of a diuretic are unlikely to be the cause of his attacks. Nocturnal panic attacks associated with sleep are an example of an unexpected panic attack. Although sleep-related disorders should be ruled out, this classic presentation makes panic disorder the most likely explanation.

5.6—Panic Disorder / diagnostic criteria; Diagnostic Features (pp. 209–201)

5.7   A 32-year-old woman reports sudden, unexpected episodes of intense anxiety, accompanied by headaches, a rapid pulse, nausea, and shortness of breath. During the episodes she fears that she is dying, and she has presented several times to emergency departments. Each time she has been told that she is medically healthy; she is usually reassured for a time, but on the occurrence of a new episode she again becomes concerned that she has some severe medical problem. She was given lorazepam once but disliked the sedating effect and has not taken it again. She abstains from all medications and alcohol in an attempt to minimize potential causes for her attacks. What is the most likely explanation for her symptoms?

A. Panic disorder.
B. Somatic symptom disorder.
C. Anxiety due to another medical condition.
D. Illness anxiety disorder.
E. Specific phobia.

Correct Answer: A. Panic disorder.

Explanation: The presence of sudden, unexpected panic attacks in the absence of a medical disorder is the main feature of panic disorder. In addition to worries about the attacks, many individuals report broader concerns about health and mental health outcomes. In a search for an explanation for their symptoms, they may worry about having a major disease. This differs from illness anxiety disorder in that the concern with panic attacks stems from what might be seen as a reasonable concern over their dramatic and unexplained symptoms; patients with panic attacks do not show the preoccupation with having a feared disease that is typical of illness anxiety disorder (or hypochondriasis in DSM-IV). Specific phobia refers to anxiety centered on a specific trigger.

5.7—Panic Disorder / Differential Diagnosis (pp. 212–213)

5.8   A 65-year-old woman reports being housebound despite feeling physically healthy. Several years ago, she fell while shopping; although she sustained no injuries, the situation was so upsetting that she became extremely nervous when she had to leave her house unaccompanied. Because she has no children and few friends whom she can ask to accompany her, she is very distressed that she has few opportunities to venture outside her home. What is the most likely diagnosis?

A. Specific phobia, situational type.
B. Social anxiety disorder (social phobia).
C. Posttraumatic stress disorder.
D. Agoraphobia.
E. Adjustment disorder.

Correct Answer: D. Agoraphobia.

Explanation: The essential feature of agoraphobia is marked fear or anxiety triggered by real or anticipated exposure to a variety of situations (e.g., using public transportation, going to open or public spaces) from which escape or help might not be available. DSM-IV treated agoraphobia as a feature of panic disorder, and individuals do frequently report a fear of having a panic attack in the dreaded situations; however, there are other incapacitating situations that could cause similar fear, including a fear of falling or of incontinence. This disorder can be very similar to other phobias such as social anxiety disorder (social phobia) and specific phobia, situational type; however, the focus of the fear is not the situation itself, but rather the fear that an incapacitating event may occur during the situation. Agoraphobia does not have the cluster of symptoms associated with posttraumatic stress disorder and is not merely indicative of poor adjustment to a uniquely stressful situation.

5.8—Agoraphobia / diagnostic criteria; Diagnostic Features (pp. 217–219)

5.9   A 32-year-old man has regularly experienced panic attacks when out of his home alone and when on the bus. He now avoids leaving home for fear of experiencing these attacks. What is the most appropriate diagnosis?

   A. Panic disorder with agoraphobia.
   B. Agoraphobia with panic attacks.
   C. Specific phobia, situational type.
   D. Two separate disorders: panic disorder and agoraphobia.
   E. Delusional disorder.

Correct Answer: D. Two separate disorders: panic disorder and agoraphobia.

Explanation: This man has panic disorder, not just panic attacks, and he also has agoraphobia. Whereas DSM-IV considered the co-occurrence of panic and agoraphobia as a subtype of panic attacks, agoraphobia with or without panic is now a separate diagnosis; the presence of panic attacks can be indicated by a specifier. In specific phobia, the fear would be of the situation itself rather than the possibility of having a panic attack.

5.9—Agoraphobia / diagnostic criteria / Diagnostic Features (pp. 217–219)

5.10   A 35-year-old man is in danger of losing his job because it requires frequent long-range traveling and for the past year he has avoided flying. Two years earlier he was on a particularly turbulent flight, and although he was not in any real danger, he was convinced that the pilot minimized the risk and that the plane almost crashed. He flew again 1 month later and, despite having a smooth flight, the anticipation of turbulence was so distressing that he experienced a panic attack during the flight; he has not flown since. What is the most appropriate diagnosis?

A. Agoraphobia.

B. Acute stress disorder.

C. Specific phobia, situational type.

D. Social anxiety disorder (social phobia).

E. Panic disorder.

Correct Answer: C. Specific phobia, situational type.

Explanation: Specific phobia is characterized by the marked fear or anxiety of a specific object or situation, which is perceived as being dangerous. This differs from agoraphobia, in which the focus of the anxiety is on the possibility of having panic or other incapacitating symptoms, or social anxiety disorder in which the focus is on being scrutinized by others. Trauma-related disorders should be considered in the differential diagnosis; however, the lack of any real danger makes this unlikely, and the time course is not compatible with the criteria for acute stress disorder. Although the man did experience a panic attack, patients with many disorders, including specific phobia, can experience such attacks. Panic disorder should be diagnosed only when the attacks are unexpected and not otherwise explained by other disorders.

5.10—Specific Phobia / diagnostic criteria; Diagnostic Features (pp. 197–199)

5.11   Which of the following types of specific phobia is most likely to be associated with vasovagal fainting?

A. Animal type.

B. Natural environment type.

C. Blood-injection-injury type.

D. Situational type.

E. Other (e.g.,. in children, loud sounds or costumed characters).

Correct Answer: C. Blood-injection-injury type.

Explanation: Whereas most phobias show a profile of sympathetic nervous system arousal, individuals with blood-injection-injury phobias often demonstrate vasovagal fainting or near-fainting marked by brief increases in heart rate and blood pressure, followed by subsequent rapid decreases of both.

5.11—Specific Phobia / Associated Features Supporting Diagnosis (p. 199)

5.12   Which of the following most accurately describes people with specific phobias?

A. The average individual with a phobia has fears of only one object or situation.

B. The fear is usually quite mild in intensity.

C. Fewer than 10% of people fear more than one object or situation.
D. The fear occurs almost every time the person encounters the object or situation.
E. The fear is exactly the same in intensity each time the object or situation is encountered.

Correct Answer: D. The fear occurs almost every time the person encounters the object or situation.

Explanation: A key feature of specific phobia is that the fear or anxiety is circumscribed to the presence of a particular situation or object (Criterion A), which may be termed the *phobic stimulus*. Categories of feared situations or objects (i.e., *phobic stimuli*) are provided as specifiers in the diagnostic criteria. Many individuals fear objects or situations from more than one category. For the diagnosis of specific phobia, the response must differ from normal, transient fears that commonly occur in the population. To meet the criteria for a diagnosis, the fear or anxiety must be intense or severe (i.e., "marked"; Criterion A). The amount of fear experienced may vary with proximity to the feared object or situation and may occur in anticipation of or in the actual presence of the object or situation. Also, the fear or anxiety may take the form of a full or limited-symptom panic attack (i.e., expected panic attack). Another characteristic of specific phobias is that fear or anxiety is evoked nearly every time the individual comes into contact with the phobic stimulus (Criterion B). Thus, an individual who becomes anxious only occasionally upon being confronted with the situation or object (e.g., becomes anxious when flying only on one out of every five airplane flights) would not be diagnosed with specific phobia. However, the degree of fear or anxiety expressed may vary (from anticipatory anxiety to a full panic attack) across different occasions of encountering the phobic object or situation because of various contextual factors, such as the presence of others, duration of exposure, and other threatening elements such as turbulence on a flight for individuals who fear flying.

5.12—Specific Phobia / Specifiers; Diagnostic Features (pp. 198–199)

5.13   Although onset of a specific phobia can occur at any age, specific phobia most typically develops during which age period?

A. Childhood.
B. Late adolescence to early adulthood.
C. Middle age.
D. Old age.
E. Any age.

Correct Answer: A. Childhood.

Explanation: Specific phobia usually develops in early childhood, with the majority of cases developing prior to age 10 years. The median age at onset is between 7 and 11 years, with the mean at about 10 years. *Situational* specific phobias tend to have a later age at onset than do *natural environment, animal,* or *blood-injection-injury* specific phobias. Specific phobias that develop in childhood and adolescence are likely to wax and wane during that period. However, phobias that persist into adulthood are unlikely to remit for the majority of individuals.

When specific phobia is being diagnosed in children, two issues should be considered. First, young children may express their fear and anxiety by crying, tantrums, freezing, or clinging. Second, young children typically are not able to understand the concept of avoidance. Therefore, the clinician should assemble additional information from parents, teachers, or others who know the child well.

5.13—Specific Phobia / Development and Course (p. 200)

5.14   In social anxiety disorder (social phobia), the object of an individual's fear is the potential for which of the following?

A. Social or occupational impairment.
B. Harm to self or others.
C. Embarrassment.
D. Separation from objects of attachment.
E. Incapacitating symptoms.

Correct Answer: C. Embarrassment.

Explanation: The anxiety disorders differ in the object or cause of an individual's fear. In the case of social anxiety disorder, an individual experiences fear or anxiety in situations in which he or she is exposed to scrutiny; the fear is that this may result in humiliation, embarrassment, or offense to others. In contrast, individuals with specific phobia fear harmful objects, animals, or situations; individuals with separation anxiety fear being away from home or loved ones; and individuals with agoraphobia avoid situations in which the individual might have panic-like or other incapacitating symptoms. In all cases, the disorders cause significant social or occupational impairment; however, this impairment is the result rather than the object of the fear.

5.14—Social Anxiety Disorder (Social Phobia) / diagnostic criteria (pp. 202–203)

5.15   When called on at school, a 7-year-old boy will only nod or write in response. The family of the child is surprised to hear this from the teacher, because the boy speaks normally when at home with his parents. The child has achieved appropriate developmental milestones, and a medical evaluation indicates that he is healthy. The boy is unable to give any explanation for his behavior, but the parents are concerned that it will affect his school performance. What diagnosis best fits this child's symptoms?

A. Separation anxiety disorder.
B. Autism spectrum disorder.
C. Agoraphobia.
D. Selective mutism.
E. Communication disorder.

Correct Answer: D. Selective mutism.

Explanation: When encountering other individuals in social interactions, children with selective mutism do not initiate speech or reciprocally respond when spoken to. Lack of speech occurs in social interactions with children or adults. Children with selective mutism will speak in their home in the presence of immediate family members but often not even in front of close friends or second-degree relatives, such as grandparents or cousins. The disturbance is often marked by high social anxiety. Children with selective mutism often refuse to speak at school, leading to academic or educational impairment, as teachers often find it difficult to assess skills such as reading. The lack of speech may interfere with social communication, although children with this disorder sometimes use nonspoken or nonverbal means (e.g., grunting, pointing, writing) to communicate and may be willing or eager to perform or engage in social encounters when speech is not required (e.g., nonverbal parts in school plays).

5.15—Selective Mutism / Diagnostic Features (p. 195)

5.16   Social anxiety disorder (social phobia) differs from normative shyness in that the disorder leads to which of the following?

A. Social or occupational dysfunction.
B. Marked social reticence.
C. Avoidance of social situations.
D. Derealization or depersonalization.
E. Pervasive social deficits with poor insight.

Correct Answer: A. Social or occupational dysfunction.

Explanation: Shyness (i.e., social reticence) is a common personality trait and is not by itself pathological. In some societies, shyness is even evaluated positively. However, when there is a significant adverse impact on social, occupational, and other important areas of functioning, a diagnosis of social anxiety disorder should be considered, and when full diagnostic criteria for social anxiety disorder are met, the disorder should be diagnosed. Only a minority (12%) of self-identified shy individuals in the United States have symptoms that meet diagnostic criteria for social anxiety disorder.

5.16—Social Anxiety Disorder (Social Phobia) / Differential Diagnosis (p. 206)

5.17 In addition to feeling restless or "keyed up," individuals with generalized anxiety disorder are most likely to experience which of the following symptoms?

A. Panic attacks.
B. Obsessions.
C. Muscle tension.
D. Multiple somatic complaints.
E. Social anxiety.

Correct Answer: C. Muscle tension.

Explanation: Generalized anxiety disorder is defined as excessive anxiety and worry that occurs more days than not, lasts for at least 6 months, and is associated with restlessness or feeling keyed up or on edge and muscle tension. The anxiety cannot be due to other anxiety disorders; the symptoms listed in the other options suggest other disorders that would be part of the differential diagnosis (i.e., panic disorder [option A], obsessive-compulsive disorder [option B], somatic symptom disorder [option D], and social anxiety disorder [social phobia] [option E]).

5.17—Generalized Anxiety Disorder / diagnostic criteria (p. 222)

5.18 Which of the following characteristics of generalized anxiety disorder is especially common in children who have the disorder?

A. Complaining of physical aches and pains.
B. Excessively preparing for activities.
C. Avoiding activities that may provoke anxiety.
D. Seeking frequent reassurance from others.
E. Delaying or procrastinating before activities.

Correct Answer: D. Seeking frequent reassurance from others.

Explanation: All of the behaviors listed are typical of generalized anxiety disorder; however, seeking reassurance from others (i.e., friends, family, practitioners) is especially common in children.

5.18—Generalized Anxiety Disorder / Development and Course (p. 224)

5.19 What is the primary difference in the clinical expression of generalized anxiety disorder across age groups?

A. Content of worry.
B. Degree of worry.
C. Patterns of comorbidity.
D. Predominance of cognitive versus somatic symptoms.
E. Severity of impairment.

Correct Answer: A. Content of worry.

Explanation: The clinical expression of generalized anxiety disorder is relatively consistent across the life span and the primary difference across age groups is the content of an individual's worry. Children and adolescents tend to worry about school or sports performance, whereas adults are more likely to be concerned about their personal health or the well-being of their family.

5.19—Generalized Anxiety Disorder / Development and Course (pp. 223–224)

5.20 In what aspect of generalized anxiety disorder do men and women most commonly differ?

A. Course.
B. Symptom profile.
C. Degree of impairment.
D. Patterns of comorbidity.
E. Age at onset.

Correct Answer: D. Patterns of comorbidity.

Explanation: Women and men with generalized anxiety disorder tend to have similar symptoms and presentation; however, they have different patterns of comorbidity consistent with gender differences in the prevalence of mental disorders.

5.20—Generalized Anxiety Disorder / Gender-Related Diagnostic Issues (pp. 224–225)

5.21 Which of the following is more suggestive of anxiety that is not pathological than of anxiety that qualifies for a diagnosis of generalized anxiety disorder?

A. Anxiety and worry that interferes significantly with functioning.
B. Anxiety and worry that lasts for months to years.
C. Anxiety and worry in response to a clear precipitant.
D. Anxiety and worry focused on a wide range of life circumstances.
E. Anxiety and worry accompanied by physical symptoms.

Correct Answer: C. Anxiety and worry in response to a clear precipitant.

Explanation: Several features distinguish generalized anxiety disorder from anxiety that is not pathological. First, the worries associated with generalized anxiety disorder are more pervasive, pronounced, and distressing; have longer duration; and frequently occur without precipitants. Second, the worries associated with generalized anxiety disorder are excessive and typically interfere significantly with psychosocial functioning, whereas the worries of everyday life are not excessive and are perceived as more manageable and may be put off when more pressing matters arise. The greater the range of life circumstances about which a person worries (e.g., finances, children's safety, job performance), the more likely his or her symptoms are to meet criteria for generalized anxiety disorder. Third, everyday worries are much less likely to be accompanied by physical symptoms (e.g., restlessness or feeling keyed up or on edge). Individuals with generalized anxiety disorder report subjective distress due to constant worry and related impairment in social, occupational, or other important areas of functioning.

5.21—Generalized Anxiety Disorder / Diagnostic Features (pp. 222–223)

5.22 A 26-year-old man is brought to the emergency department suffering from a sudden, severe surge of panic. He has no history of panic disorder, but he reports taking several doses of an over-the-counter cold medication earlier that day. Which of the following clinical features, if present in this case, would help to confirm a diagnosis of substance/medication-induced anxiety disorder?

A. Symptoms that are mild and do not impair functioning.
B. Symptoms that persist for a long time after substance/medication use.
C. Symptoms that are in excess of what would be expected for the substance/medication.
D. Presence of a delirium or gross confusion.
E. Lack of any history of anxiety disorder or panic symptoms.

Correct Answer: E. Lack of any history of anxiety disorder or panic symptoms.

Explanation: Many substances can potentially cause anxiety symptoms, and it can sometimes be difficult to determine whether medication use is etiologically related to the onset of anxiety symptoms. Evidence to support the presence of a substance/medication-induced anxiety disorder includes temporal associations and symptoms that are consistent with the medication and dose. By definition, a substance/medication-induced anxiety disorder must cause significant distress or impairment in functioning, and it cannot occur exclusively during the course of a delirium.

5.22—Substance/Medication-Induced Anxiety Disorder / diagnostic criteria; Diagnostic Features (pp. 226–228)

5.23   In which of the following circumstances would a diagnosis of substance/medication-induced anxiety disorder be appropriate for an individual who stopped taking benzodiazepines the previous day?

A. Significant anxiety symptoms are present.
B. Anxiety is present that is clearly related to the withdrawal state.
C. Anxiety is present that is sufficiently severe to warrant independent clinical attention.
D. Anxiety is present only during bouts of delirium.
E. Never: the diagnosis of substance withdrawal would supersede the anxiety disorder diagnosis.

Correct Answer: C. Anxiety is present that is sufficiently severe to warrant independent clinical attention.

Explanation: Anxiety symptoms commonly occur in substance intoxication and substance withdrawal. The diagnosis of the substance-specific intoxication or substance-specific withdrawal will usually suffice to categorize the symptom presentation. A diagnosis of substance/medication-induced anxiety disorder should be made in addition to substance intoxication or substance withdrawal only when the panic or anxiety symptoms are predominant in the clinical picture and are sufficiently severe to warrant independent clinical attention.

5.23—Substance/Medication-Induced Anxiety Disorder / Differential Diagnosis (p. 229)

5.24   A 60-year-old man has just been diagnosed with congestive heart failure. He is intensely anxious and reports feeling as if he cannot breathe, which causes him to panic. Which of the following features, if present in this case, would tend to support a diagnosis of anxiety disorder due to another medical condition rather than adjustment disorder with anxiety?

A. The patient says that he is relieved to know his diagnosis.
B. The patient has no anxiety-associated physical symptoms.
C. The patient is focused on the reasons he has a cardiac disorder.
D. The patient is delirious.
E. The patient is extremely concerned that he will not be able to return to work.

Correct Answer: A. The patient says that he is relieved to know his diagnosis.

Explanation: The essential feature of anxiety disorder due to another medical condition is clinically significant anxiety that is judged to be best explained as a physiological effect of another medical condition. Symptoms can include prominent anxiety symptoms or panic attacks (Criterion A). The judgment that the symptoms are best explained by the associated physical condition must be based on evidence from the history, physical examination, or laboratory findings. In individuals who have serious medical illness and comorbid anxiety symptoms, anxiety disorder due to another medical condition is a potential cause. Anxiety disorder due to another medical condition is more likely to have a physical component of the anxiety than are the adjustment disorders. Anxiety disorder due to another medical condition should be distinguished from adjustment disorders, with anxiety, or with anxiety and depressed mood. Adjustment disorder is warranted when individuals experience a maladaptive response to the stress of having another medical condition. The reaction to stress usually concerns the meaning or consequences of the stress, as compared with the experience of anxiety or mood symptoms that occur as a physiological consequence of the other medical condition. In adjustment disorder, the anxiety symptoms are typically related to coping with the stress of having a general medical condition, whereas in anxiety disorder due to another medical condition, individuals are more likely to have prominent physical symptoms and to be focused on issues other than the stress of the illness itself.

5.24—Anxiety Disorder Due to Another Medical Condition / Diagnostic Features; Differential Diagnosis (pp. 230, 232)

CHAPTER 6

Obsessive-Compulsive and Related Disorders

6.1   Which of the following statements about compulsive behaviors in obsessive-compulsive disorder (OCD) is *true?*

    A. Compulsions in OCD are best understood as a form of addictive behavior.
    B. Compulsive behaviors in OCD are aimed at reducing the distress triggered by obsessions.
    C. Examples of compulsive behaviors include paraphilias (sexual compulsions), gambling, and substance use.
    D. Compulsions involve repetitive and persistent thoughts (e.g., of contamination), images (e.g., of violent or horrific scenes), or urges (e.g., to stab someone).
    E. Compulsive behaviors in OCD are typically goal directed, fulfilling a realistic purpose.

Correct Answer: B. Compulsive behaviors in OCD are aimed at reducing the distress triggered by obsessions.

Explanation: *Obsessions* are repetitive and persistent thoughts (e.g., of contamination), images (e.g., of violent or horrific scenes), or urges (e.g., to stab someone). *Compulsions* (or rituals) are repetitive behaviors (e.g., washing, checking) or mental acts (e.g., counting, repeating words silently) that the individual feels driven to perform in response to an obsession or according to rules that must be applied rigidly. Most individuals with OCD have both obsessions and compulsions. Compulsions are typically performed in response to an obsession (e.g., thoughts of contamination leading to washing rituals or that something is incorrect leading to repeating rituals until it feels "just right"). The aim is to reduce the distress triggered by obsessions or to prevent a feared event (e.g., becoming ill). However, these compulsions either are not connected in a realistic way to the feared event (e.g., arranging items symmetrically to prevent harm to a loved one) or are clearly excessive (e.g., showering for hours each day). Compulsions are not done for pleasure, although some individuals experience relief from anxiety or distress.

    Certain behaviors are sometimes described as "compulsive," including sexual behavior (in the case of paraphilias), gambling (i.e., gambling disorder), and substance use (e.g., alcohol use disorder). However, these behaviors differ from the compulsions of OCD in that the person usually derives pleasure from the activity and may wish to resist it only because of its deleterious consequences.

6.1—Obsessive-Compulsive Disorder / diagnostic criteria (p. 237); Diagnostic Features (p. 238); Differential Diagnosis (Other compulsive-like behaviors) (pp. 241–242)

6.2 A 52-year-old man with raw, chapped hands is referred to a psychiatrist by his primary care doctor. The man reports that he washes his hands repeatedly, spending up to 4 hours a day, using abrasive cleansers and scalding hot water. Although he admits that his hands are uncomfortable, he is entirely convinced that unless he washes in this manner he will become gravely ill. A medical workup is unrevealing, and the man takes no medications. What is the most appropriate diagnosis?

    A. Delusional disorder, somatic type.
    B. Illness anxiety disorder.
    C. Obsessive-compulsive disorder, with absent insight.
    D. Obsessive-compulsive personality disorder.
    E. Generalized anxiety disorder.

Correct Answer: C. Obsessive-compulsive disorder, with absent insight.

Explanation: DSM-5 has added an insight specifier to the diagnosis of obsessive-compulsive disorder (OCD) to acknowledge that persons with the disorder can range from having good insight into the irrationality of their behaviors to having no insight (i.e., being delusional). In DSM-5, if the delusional belief is limited to the obsessions and compulsions, a separate psychotic disorder diagnosis is not required. Individuals with illness anxiety disorder worry about having an illness; however, they do not have the classic obsessions and compulsions found in OCD. Individuals with generalized anxiety disorder may constantly worry; however, their worries are usually about real-life concerns. Obsessive-compulsive personality disorder is not characterized by intrusive thoughts, images, or urges or by repetitive behaviors that are performed in response to these intrusions; instead, it involves an enduring and pervasive maladaptive pattern of excessive perfectionism and rigid control.

6.2—Obsessive-Compulsive Disorder / diagnostic criteria (p. 237); Differential Diagnosis (p. 242)

6.3 Men with obsessive-compulsive disorder (OCD) differ from women with the disorder in which of the following ways?

    A. Men tend to get OCD later in life.
    B. Men are more likely to have comorbid tics.
    C. Men are more likely to be obsessed with cleaning.
    D. Men are more likely to spontaneously recover.
    E. Men have much higher rates of OCD.

Correct Answer: B. Men are more likely to have comorbid tics.

Explanation: Males have an earlier age at onset of OCD than females and are more likely to have comorbid tic disorders. Gender differences in the pattern of symptom dimensions have been reported, with, for example, females more likely to have symptoms in the cleaning dimension and males more likely to have symptoms in the forbidden thoughts and symmetry dimensions.

The 12-month prevalence of OCD in the United States is 1.2%, with a similar prevalence internationally (1.1%–1.8%). Females are affected at a slightly higher rate than males in adulthood, although males are more commonly affected in childhood. For both genders, the course of OCD is usually chronic, often with waxing and waning symptoms. Without treatment, remission rates in adults are low (e.g., 20% for those reevaluated 40 years later).

6.3—Obsessive-Compulsive Disorder / Prevalence (p. 239); Development and Course (p. 239); Gender-Related Diagnostic Issues (p. 240)

6.4   A 63-year-old woman has been saving financial documents and records for many years, placing papers in piles throughout her apartment to the point where it has become unsafe. She acknowledges that the piles are a concern; however, she says that the papers include important documents and she is afraid to throw them away. She recalls several instances in which her taxes were audited and she needed certain documents to avoid a penalty. She is concerned because her landlord is threatening to evict her unless she removes the piles of papers. What is the most likely diagnosis?

A. Obsessive-compulsive disorder.
B. Hoarding disorder.
C. Delusional disorder.
D. Nonpathological collecting behavior.
E. Dementia (major neurocognitive disorder).

Correct Answer: A. Obsessive-compulsive disorder.

Explanation: Although hoarding shares some features with obsessive-compulsive disorder (OCD), research suggests that it is an independent disorder. DSM-5 recognizes hoarding disorder as a diagnosis; however, distinguishing individuals with hoarding disorder from those with OCD (who may hoard as a result of their disorder) can be difficult. This woman is worried about the harm that may ensue should she discard potentially important information. The focus on performing a ritual to prevent harm is more typical of OCD, whereas persons with hoarding disorder simply have difficulty discarding items that they have accumulated (i.e., the focus is on the hoarding itself). This woman appears to have insight into her behavior; thus, it is not delusional. However, it is clearly pathological because it is causing distress and potential harm (i.e., eviction from her apartment). Patients with major neurocognitive disorder may develop symptoms characteristic of OCD as a result of the dementia, and this presentation would receive a diagnosis of obsessive-compulsive and related disorder due to another medical condition. However, the patient in this vignette shows no evidence of cognitive decline.

6.4—Obsessive-Compulsive Disorder / Differential Diagnosis (Other obsessive-compulsive and related disorders) (p. 241)

6.5   Although gambling can seem compulsive, gambling disorder is not considered a type of obsessive-compulsive disorder (OCD) for which of the following reasons?

    A. A person with gambling disorder derives direct pleasure from the behavior.
    B. Individuals with gambling disorder have poorer insight into their irrational behavior.
    C. Gambling disorder is better conceived of as a personality trait.
    D. The repetitive behavior associated with gambling is meant to avoid anxiety.
    E. In gambling disorder, individuals have control over their repetitive behaviors.

Correct Answer: A. A person with gambling disorder derives direct pleasure from the behavior.

Explanation: Although a number of behaviors, such as gambling or sexual behavior, can seem compulsive, gambling disorder and sexual paraphilias differ from OCD in that the compulsive behaviors associated with OCD are meant to decrease anxiety, whereas in the other disorders they are a source of direct pleasure. Individuals with gambling disorder seek treatment mainly out of concern for the deleterious consequences of their behavior. In both gambling disorder and OCD, the level of insight into the behavior can vary, but like individuals with OCD, those with gambling disorder cannot control their gambling.

6.5—Obsessive-Compulsive Disorder / Differential Diagnosis (Other compulsive-like behaviors) (pp. 241–242)

6.6   In addition to preoccupations with a perceived body flaw, which of the following behaviors would be most suggestive of a diagnosis of body dysmorphic disorder (BDD)?

    A. Repetitive mirror checking in response to the preoccupation.
    B. Consulting a psychiatrist because of the distress caused by the preoccupation.
    C. Losing an unhealthy amount of weight in order to improve one's appearance.

D. Having a related preoccupation with having or acquiring a disfiguring illness.

E. Experiencing discomfort with one's primary or secondary sex characteristics.

Correct Answer: A. Repetitive mirror checking in response to the preoccupation.

Explanation: People with BDD are excessively preoccupied with perceived defects in their appearance that are either not apparent or only slightly apparent to other individuals. In addition to the preoccupation, individuals engage in excessive and repetitive behaviors and/or mental acts associated with the preoccupation, including repetitive checking of their appearance in a mirror, excessive grooming, and comparing their appearance with that of others. BDD does not include a primary preoccupation with weight, which is instead associated with eating disorders. Insight varies, but individuals with BDD are not likely to see it as a psychiatric disorder. Concerns about having a medical illness are rare, and the rate of somatization is not usually increased in this group.

6.6—Body Dysmorphic Disorder / Differential Diagnosis (pp. 245–247)

6.7 A 25-year-old man is concerned that he looks "weak" and "puny" despite the fact that to neutral observers he appears very muscular. When confronted about his belief he believes he is being humored and that people are in fact making fun of his small size behind his back. He has tried a number of strategies to increase muscle mass, including exercising excessively and using anabolic steroids; however, he remains dissatisfied with his appearance. What is the most likely diagnosis?

A. Delusional disorder, somatic type.
B. Narcissistic personality disorder.
C. Body identity integrity disorder.
D. Body dysmorphic disorder, with muscle dysmorphia.
E. *Koro.*

Correct Answer: D. Body dysmorphic disorder, with muscle dysmorphia.

Explanation: Muscle dysmorphia is a form of body dysmorphic disorder (BDD) in which an individual—usually a male—is preoccupied with the idea that his body build is too small or insufficiently muscular. Although insight may be so poor as to be considered delusional, the focus on body appearance alone warrants the BDD diagnosis, and the sole focus on perceived appearance differentiates this disorder from personality disorders. Body identity integrity disorder (apotemnophilia) (which is not a DSM-5 disorder) involves a desire to have a limb amputated to correct an experience of mismatch between a person's sense of body identity and his or her actual anatomy. However, the concern does not focus on the limb's appearance, as it would in BDD. *Koro*, a culturally related disorder that usually occurs in epidemics in Southeastern Asia, consists of a fear that the penis (labia, nipples, or breasts in females) is shrinking or retracting and will disappear into the abdomen, often accompanied by a belief that death will result. *Koro* differs from BDD in several ways, including a focus on death rather than preoccupation with perceived ugliness.

6.7—Body Dysmorphic Disorder / Differential Diagnosis (Other disorders and symptoms) (pp. 245–247)

6.8   A 19-year-old woman is referred to a psychiatrist by her internist after she admits to him that she recurrently pulls hair from her eyebrows to the point that she has scarring and there is little or no eyebrow hair left. She states that her natural eyebrows are "bushy" and "repulsive" and that she "looks like a caveman." A photograph of the woman before she began pulling her eyebrow hair shows a normal-looking teenager. What is the most appropriate diagnosis?

A. Trichotillomania (hair-pulling disorder).
B. Body dysmorphic disorder.
C. Delusional disorder, somatic type.
D. Normal age-appropriate appearance concerns.
E. Obsessive-compulsive disorder.

Correct Answer: B. Body dysmorphic disorder.

Explanation: There can be a variety of causes for hair pulling. Individuals with trichotillomania pull hair out of anxiety or boredom; the behavior provides distraction, pleasure, or a relief from anxiety. When hair pulling is purely for the purpose of improving a perceived defect in appearance, the behavior is better conceptualized as symptomatic of body dysmorphic disorder (BDD). As with other presentations of BDD, insight into the behavior can be poor, and the belief can reach delusional levels. If the delusions are limited to the appearance concerns, an additional diagnosis is not necessary. The behavior is similar to obsessive-compulsive disorder; however, the focus on appearance is diagnostic for BDD. It may be normal for teenagers to be concerned about their appearance; however, the fact that this patient has pulled her hair to the point of causing scarring makes this a pathological behavior.

6.8—Body Dysmorphic Disorder / Differential Diagnosis (Other obsessive-compulsive and related disorders) (p. 246)

6.9   A 48-year-old man presents to a psychiatrist, stating that he was pressured by his wife to seek help. He explains that he likes to collect wine, and he does not see a problem with this; he claims that many of the wines are quite valuable and a potential investment. On further questioning, he admits that he rarely drinks the wines, because it "never seems the right time." He has never sold or given away any wine because he finds it hard to part with the bottles. He has had to use increasing portions of his house for storage of the wine, which, along with the financial hardship, is his wife's primary concern. He admits that many of the wine bottles have probably spoiled because he cannot afford to properly store the wine and the bottles have sat for years on shelves. What is the most appropriate diagnosis?

A. Normal collecting behavior.
B. Hoarding disorder, excessive acquisition type.
C. Obsessive-compulsive disorder.
D. Delusional disorder.
E. Narcissistic personality disorder.

Correct Answer: B. Hoarding disorder, excessive acquisition type.

Explanation: Although wine collecting is not in itself pathological, in this case the patient's difficulty parting with or drinking the wine, the fact that his acquisition exceeds his ability to store the wine, and his wife's distress (along with a possible financial impact) make hoarding disorder the most likely diagnosis. Hoarding disorder describes a syndrome in which an individual has difficulty parting with possessions, to the point that the possessions present an unsafe or unhygienic situation. Approximately 80%–90% of individuals with hoarding disorder also display excessive acquisition in which they collect, buy, or steal objects that are not needed and for which there is no space. In such cases, this is indicated with a specifier. Although persons with obsessive-compulsive disorder may hoard items, they usually experience distress at their inability to throw the objects away, or their storage of the possessions serves some other purpose related to their obsessions (e.g., worrying that they will throw out something important).

6.9—Hoarding Disorder / diagnostic criteria (p. 247)

6.10   Which of the following statements about risk and prognostic factors in hoarding disorder is *true?*

A. About 10% of individuals who hoard report having a relative who also hoards.
B. Approximately half of the variability in hoarding behavior is due to genetic factors.
C. Separation insecurity is a prominent temperamental feature of individuals with hoarding disorder and their first-degree relatives.
D. Hoarding disorder has been associated with high rates of childhood neglect and abuse.
E. Stressful or traumatic life events play no role in the onset or exacerbation of hoarding disorder.

Correct Answer: B. Approximately half of the variability in hoarding behavior is due to genetic factors.

Explanation: Hoarding behavior is familial, with about 50% of individuals who hoard reporting having a relative who also hoards. Twin studies indicate that approximately 50% of the variability in hoarding behavior is attributable to additive genetic factors.

Indecisiveness is a prominent temperamental feature of individuals with hoarding disorder and their first-degree relatives. Individuals with hoarding disorder often retrospectively report stressful and traumatic life events preceding the onset of the disorder or causing an exacerbation.

6.10—Hoarding Disorder / Risk and Prognostic Factors (p. 249)

6.11 Which of the following statements about the course of hoarding disorder is *true?*

A. Hoarding behavior tends to wax and wane in severity throughout an individual's life.
B. Hoarding behavior peaks in young adulthood and subsequently lessens in severity.
C. Hoarding behavior tends to become more severe with increasing age.
D. Hoarding disorder begins in childhood, is chronic, and tends not to change in severity.
E. Hoarding disorder has a worse course when it begins in later adulthood or old age.

Correct Answer: C. Hoarding behavior tends to become more severe with increasing age.

Explanation: Hoarding tends to begin early in life and is generally chronic throughout a person's life. The severity of the behavior increases with each decade of life.

6.11—Hoarding Disorder / Development and Course (p. 249)

6.12 What is the most common site of hair pulling in trichotillomania?

A. Scalp.
B. Axillary area.
C. Facial area.
D. Pubic area.
E. Perirectal area.

Correct Answer: A. Scalp.

Explanation: Trichotillomania can involve any area of the body, but the most common sites are scalp, eyebrows, and eyelids.

6.12—Trichotillomania (Hair-Pulling Disorder) / Diagnostic Features (pp. 251–252)

6.13 Although microscopic examination of hair can aid the diagnosis of trichotillomania (hair-pulling disorder), such examination is rarely performed, for which of the following reasons?

A. Patients generally admit to the hair pulling.
B. The effects on hair are easily observed macroscopically.
C. Patients generally have a long medical history of the disorder.
D. Patients rarely consent to the examination.
E. Microscopic examination is prohibitively expensive.

Correct Answer: A. Patients generally admit to the hair pulling.

Explanation: Although patients with hair-pulling disorder often carry out their behaviors when others are not looking, they usually admit to the behavior, and dermatopathological diagnosis is rarely required. When performed, dermoscopy shows decreased hair density, short vellus hair, broken hairs with different shaft lengths, coiled hairs, trichoptilosis, sparse yellow dots, and absence of "exclamation mark" hairs.

6.13—Trichotillomania (Hair-Pulling Disorder) / Diagnostic Markers (p. 253)

6.14 A 25-year-old man is referred to a psychiatrist by his primary care doctor after mentioning to the doctor that he routinely spends a lot of time pulling out facial hair with tweezers, even after carefully shaving. On evaluation, he admits to frequent pulling of his facial hair, consuming significant amount of time; he explains that he becomes anxious when looking at himself because his moustache, hairline, and sideburns are asymmetrical. He pulls out hairs in an effort to make them more symmetrical, but is rarely satisfied with the results. He finds this very upsetting but cannot resist the urge to try and "fix" his facial hair. What is the most appropriate diagnosis?

A. Trichotillomania (hair-pulling disorder).
B. Body dysmorphic disorder (BDD).
C. Delusional disorder, somatic type.
D. Normal age-appropriate appearance concerns.
E. Obsessive-compulsive disorder (OCD).

Correct Answer: E. Obsessive-compulsive disorder (OCD).

Explanation: In the case of repetitive hair pulling, distinguishing among trichotillomania, BDD, and OCD can sometimes be difficult. The differential diagnosis rests on the reasons for the pulling. Trichotillomania generally stems from boredom or anxiety, whereas BDD-related hair pulling is generally associated with perceived ugliness of the hair. When the pulling is in the service of symmetry, OCD is the more appropriate diagnosis. Further examination of the individual would likely reveal additional examples of his preoccupation with symmetry. Although some amount of hair pulling may be normal, the degree and the distress caused make normal age-appropriate appearance concerns an unlikely explanation in this case. Psychotic disorders should be ruled out—in this vignette, the patient's symptoms appear to be more a preoccupation than a delusion.

6.14—Trichotillomania (Hair-Pulling Disorder) / Differential Diagnosis (pp. 253–254)

6.15 To fulfill diagnostic criteria for excoriation (skin-picking) disorder, the picking must be severe enough to result in which of the following?

A. Itching.
B. Skin lesions.
C. An infection.
D. Medical attention.
E. Permanent deformity.

Correct Answer: B. Skin lesions.

Explanation: Individuals with excoriation disorder have recurrent skin-picking behaviors that are severe enough to cause skin lesions. It is not necessary that the behavior cause deformity.

6.15—Excoriation (Skin-Picking) Disorder / diagnostic criteria (p. 254)

6.16 Which of the following statements about the course of excoriation (skin-picking) disorder is *true?*

A. Skin-picking behavior tends to wax and wane in severity throughout an individual's life.
B. Skin-picking behavior peaks in young adulthood and subsequently lessens in severity.
C. Excoriation disorder tends to become more severe with increasing age.
D. Skin-picking behavior begins in childhood, is chronic, and tends not to change in severity.
E. Excoriation disorder has a worse course when it begins in later adulthood or old age.

Correct Answer: A. Skin-picking behavior tends to wax and wane in severity throughout an individual's life.

Explanation: Although it can begin at any age, excoriation disorder usually begins during adolescence, coincident with the onset of puberty, and is frequently triggered by skin conditions such as acne. The disorder usually has a chronic course with some waxing and waning if untreated. In some cases, the disorder may come and go for weeks, months, or even years at a time.

6.16—Excoriation (Skin-Picking) Disorder / Development and Course (p. 255)

6.17 In excoriation (skin-picking) disorder, which of the following is the most typical motivation for the skin-picking behavior?

    A. Inflicting pain that brings relief by reaffirming one's ability to feel.
    B. Appearance concerns.
    C. Symmetry concerns.
    D. Boredom.
    E. Fear of infection.

Correct Answer: D. Boredom.

Explanation: Individuals with excoriation disorder usually pick their skin out of anxiety or boredom. Skin picking to fix imaginary defects in appearance would suggest body dysmorphic disorder, and picking to fix defects in symmetry or to prevent infection would suggest obsessive-compulsive disorder. Skin picking in excoriation disorder is not comparable to self-mutilative behavior that occurs in the context of dissociative experiences or borderline personality disorder.

6.17—Excoriation (Skin-Picking) Disorder / Associated Features Supporting Diagnosis (p. 255)

6.18 A 55-year-old retail worker believes that he has "chronic halitosis" and fears that his bad breath is "scaring away shoppers." He is in danger of losing his job because he so frequently absents himself from the sales floor to brush his teeth and use mouthwash. He constantly chews mint gum, even though his employer has asked him not to. His coworkers regularly reassure him that his breath is fine, but he is convinced that they are just being polite. Although the possibility of losing his job causes him concern, he finds his worries about his breath to be intolerable. He has seen his doctor and dentist, both of whom tell him that he is healthy and does not have malodorous breath. What is the most appropriate diagnosis?

    A. Social anxiety disorder (social phobia).
    B. Obsessive-compulsive disorder.
    C. Body dysmorphic disorder.
    D. Other specified obsessive-compulsive and related disorder.
    E. Illness anxiety disorder.

Correct Answer: D. Other specified obsessive-compulsive and related disorder.

Explanation: Olfactory reference syndrome is characterized by excessive odor-related preoccupations and repetitive behaviors designed to address the odor sufficient to cause distress or impairment. Currently this disorder is provisional and classified under *other specified obsessive-compulsive and related disorder.* When the individual lacks any insight, a delusional disorder should be diagnosed as well. Although the other disorders listed could cause repetitive behaviors, the focus on an imaginary odor is diagnostic for olfactory reference syndrome.

6.18—Other Specified Obsessive-Compulsive and Related Disorder (pp. 263–264)

6.19   Which of the following substances, when abused, is most likely to cause symptoms mimicking obsessive-compulsive disorder?

A. Heroin.
B. Cocaine.
C. Alprazolam.
D. Marijuana.
E. Lysergic acid diethylamide (LSD).

Correct Answer: B. Cocaine.

Explanation: Drugs that most commonly cause obsessive-compulsive and related disorder include amphetamines and related substances, cocaine, and some heavy metals and toxins (e.g., carbon monoxide).

6.19—Substance/Medication-Induced Obsessive-Compulsive and Related Disorder / Associated Features Supporting Diagnosis (p. 259)

CHAPTER 7

Trauma- and Stressor-Related Disorders

7.1 How does DSM-5 differ from DSM-IV in its classification of posttraumatic stress disorder (PTSD)?

A. In DSM-5, PTSD has been placed with the dissociative disorders.
B. In DSM-5, PTSD has been placed with the depressive disorders.
C. In DSM-5, PTSD has been placed in a newly created chapter.
D. In DSM-5, PTSD has been placed with "Other Conditions That May Be a Focus of Clinical Attention."
E. In DSM-5, PTSD has been placed with "Conditions for Further Study" in Section III.

Correct Answer: C. In DSM-5 PTSD has been placed in a newly created chapter.

Explanation: The establishment of a separate chapter for trauma- and stressor-related disorders is based on strong evidence that the clinical expression of psychological distress following exposure to a traumatic or stressful event is quite variable. In some cases, symptoms can be understood within an anxiety-based or fear-based context. This was the rationale for designating acute stress disorder and posttraumatic stress disorder as anxiety disorders in DSM-IV. Many individuals exhibit a phenotype in which, rather than anxiety- or fear-based symptoms, the most prominent clinical characteristics are anhedonic and dysphoric symptoms, externalizing angry and aggressive symptoms, or dissociative symptoms. These individuals are better grouped under a separate category: trauma- and stressor-related disorders.

> **7.1—chapter intro (p. 265); Appendix / Highlights of Changes From DSM-IV to DSM-5 (p. 812)**

7.2 Which of the following reactions to a traumatic event was required for the DSM-IV diagnosis of posttraumatic stress disorder (PTSD) but is not required for the DSM-5 diagnosis?

A. Intense fear, helplessness, or horror.
B. Insomnia or hypersomnia.
C. Avoidance.

D. A foreshortened sense of the future.

E. Flashbacks.

Correct Answer: A. Intense fear, helplessness, or horror.

Explanation: DSM-5 criteria for PTSD differ significantly from the DSM-IV criteria. The stressor criterion (Criterion A) is more explicit with regard to events that qualify as "traumatic" experiences. Also, DSM-IV Criterion A2 regarding the subjective reaction to the traumatic event (experiencing "intense fear, helplessness, or horror") has been eliminated in DSM-5.

7.2—Appendix / Highlights of Changes From DSM-IV to DSM-5 (p. 812)

7.3   Which of the following statements about reactive attachment disorder (RAD) is *true*?

A. RAD occurs only in children who lack healthy attachments.

B. RAD occurs only in children who have secure attachments.

C. RAD occurs only in children who have impaired communication.

D. RAD occurs in children without a history of severe social neglect.

E. RAD is a common condition, with a prevalence of 25% of children seen in clinical settings.

Correct Answer: A. RAD occurs only in children who lack attachments.

Explanation: Reactive attachment disorder of infancy or early childhood is characterized by a pattern of markedly disturbed and developmentally inappropriate attachment behaviors, in which a child rarely or minimally turns preferentially to an attachment figure for comfort, support, protection, and nurturance. The essential feature is absent or grossly underdeveloped attachment between the child and putative caregiving adults. Serious social neglect is a diagnostic requirement for reactive attachment disorder and is also the only known risk factor for the disorder. Children with reactive attachment disorder show social communicative functioning comparable to their overall level of intellectual functioning. The prevalence of RAD is unknown, but the disorder is seen relatively rarely in clinical settings. Even in populations of severely neglected children, the disorder is uncommon, occurring in less than 10% of such children.

7.3—Reactive Attachment Disorder / Diagnostic Features; Associated Features Supporting Diagnosis; Prevalence; Risk and Prognostic Factors (pp. 266–267)

7.4   A 4-year-old boy in day care often displays fear that does not seem to be related to any of his activities. Although frequently distressed, he does not seek contact with any of the staff and does not respond when a staff member tries to comfort him. What additional caregiver-obtained information about this child would be important in deciding whether his symptoms represent reactive attachment disorder (RAD) or autism spectrum disorder (ASD)?

A. Age at first appearance of the behavior.
B. Family history about his siblings.
C. History of language delay.
D. Indications that he has experienced severe social neglect.
E. Presence of selective attachment behaviors.

Correct Answer: D. Indications that he has experienced severe social neglect.

Explanation: Aberrant social behaviors manifest in young children with RAD, but they also are key features of ASD. Specifically, young children with either condition can manifest dampened expression of positive emotions, cognitive and language delays, and impairments in social reciprocity. As a result, RAD must be differentiated from ASD. These two disorders can be distinguished based on differential histories of neglect and on the presence of restricted interests or ritualized behaviors, specific deficit in social communication, and selective attachment behaviors. Children with RAD have experienced a history of severe social neglect, although it is not always possible to obtain detailed histories about the precise nature of their experiences, especially in initial evaluations. Children with ASD will only rarely have a history of social neglect. Children with ASD regularly show attachment behavior typical for their developmental level. In contrast, children with RAD do so only rarely or inconsistently, if at all.

> **7.4—Reactive Attachment Disorder / Differential Diagnosis (Autism spectrum disorder) (pp. 267–268)**

7.5 For a child diagnosed with reactive attachment disorder, which of the following situations would qualify for a disorder specifier of "severe"?

A. The child has been in five foster homes.
B. The child never expresses positive emotions when interacting with caregivers.
C. The disorder has been present for 18 months.
D. The child meets all symptoms of the disorder, with each symptom manifesting at relatively high levels.
E. There is a documented history of physical abuse of the child.

Correct Answer: D. The child meets all symptoms of the disorder, with each symptom manifesting at relatively high levels.

Explanation: Reactive attachment disorder is specified as severe when a child meets all symptoms of the disorder, with each symptom manifesting at relatively high levels.

> **7.5—Reactive Attachment Disorder / diagnostic criteria (p. 266)**

7.6   A 6-year-old girl has repeatedly approached strangers while in the park with her class. The teacher requests an evaluation of the behavior. The girl has a history of being placed in several different foster homes over the past 3 years. Which diagnosis is suggested from this history?

   A. Attention-deficit/hyperactivity disorder (ADHD).
   B. Disinhibited social engagement disorder (DSED).
   C. Autism spectrum disorder (ASD).
   D. Bipolar I disorder.
   E. Borderline personality disorder.

Correct Answer: B. Disinhibited social engagement disorder (DSED).

Explanation: The essential feature of DSED is a pattern of behavior that involves culturally inappropriate, overly familiar behavior with relative strangers (Criterion A). The behaviors must include socially disinhibited behavior, not just ADHD-like impulsivity (Criterion B), and the child must have experienced a pattern of extremes of insufficient care (Criterion C) as evidenced by at least one of the following:

1. Social neglect or deprivation in the form of persistent lack of having basic emotional needs for comfort, stimulation, and affection met by caregiving adults.
2. Repeated changes of primary caregivers that limit opportunities to form stable attachments (e.g., frequent changes in foster care).
3. Rearing in unusual settings that severely limit opportunities to form selective attachments (e.g., institutions with high child to caregiver ratios).

7.6—Disinhibited Social Engagement Disorder / diagnostic criteria (p. 268)

7.7   A 25-year-old woman, new to your practice, tells you that a little more than 3 months ago she was accosted on her way home. The attacker told her he had a gun, was going to rape her, and would shoot her if she resisted. He walked her toward an alley. She was sure he would kill her afterward no matter what she did, and therefore she pushed away from him, aware that she might be shot. She was able to escape unharmed. She describes not being able to fall asleep for the first 2 nights after the attack and of avoiding that particular street in her neighborhood for 2 days following the event. She thinks that the attacker might have touched her breasts but cannot remember for sure. She has recently started feeling anxious all of the time and is tearful, and she has stopped going to work. She fears that something about her makes her "look like a victim." What is the most likely diagnosis?

   A. Posttraumatic stress disorder.
   B. Acute stress disorder.
   C. Adjustment disorder.

D. Dissociative amnesia.

E. Personality disorder.

Correct Answer: C. Adjustment disorder.

Explanation: The patient developed emotional symptoms within 3 months of the stressor. The symptoms qualify as clinically significant, because although her distress is not out of proportion to the severity of the stressor precipitating the symptoms, she does demonstrate significant impairment in important areas of functioning. This symptom pattern is diagnostic for adjustment disorder. The essential feature of acute stress disorder is the development of acute posttraumatic symptoms within 1 month of exposure to extreme traumatic stressors. The full symptom picture of 9 or more (of a possible 12) symptoms must be present at least 3 days after the traumatic event and can be diagnosed up to 1 month after the event; symptoms that occur immediately after the event but resolve in less than 3 days would not qualify for a trauma- or stressor-related disorder diagnosis. The patient does not have dissociative experiences, flashbacks, dreams, or avoidance symptoms and does not meet the criteria for acute stress disorder or posttraumatic stress disorder. There is nothing to suggest that she has a personality disorder or that she has dissociative amnesia.

7.7—Posttraumatic Stress Disorder / Diagnostic Features; Differential Diagnosis (pp. 274–276, 279)

7.8   After a routine chest X ray, a 53-year-old man with a history of heavy cigarette use is told that he has a suspicious lesion in his lung. A bronchoscopy confirms the diagnosis of adenocarcinoma. The man delays scheduling a follow-up appointment with the oncologist for more than 2 weeks, describes feeling as if "all of this is not real," is having nightly dreams of seeing his own tombstone, and is experiencing intrusive flashbacks to the moment when he heard the physician saying, "The tests strongly suggest that you have cancer of the lung." He is tearful and is convinced he will die. He also feels intense guilt that his smoking caused the cancer and expresses the thought that he "deserves" to have cancer. What diagnosis best fits this clinical picture?

A. Acute stress disorder.

B. Posttraumatic stress disorder.

C. Adjustment disorder.

D. Major depressive disorder.

E. Generalized anxiety disorder.

Correct Answer: C. Adjustment disorder.

Explanation: The essential feature of acute stress disorder (ASD) is the development of characteristic symptoms lasting from 3 days to 1 month following exposure to one or more traumatic events. Traumatic events that are experienced directly include, but are not limited to, exposure to war as a combatant or civilian, threatened or actual violent personal assault (e.g., sexual assault, physical attack, active combat, mugging, childhood physical and/or sexual abuse, being kidnapped, being taken hostage, terrorist attack, or torture), natural or human-made disasters (e.g., earthquake, hurricane, airplane crash), and severe accidents (e.g., severe motor vehicle or industrial accident). A life-threatening illness or debilitating condition is not necessarily considered a traumatic event. Stressful events that do not meet Criterion A definitions for a diagnosis of ASD may nonetheless be sufficient to qualify for an adjustment disorder diagnosis.

7.8—Acute Stress Disorder / Diagnostic Features (pp. 281–282)

7.9   Criterion B for acute stress disorder requires the presence of nine (or more) symptoms from any of five categories of response. Which of the following is *not* one of these five categories?

   A. Intrusion.
   B. Dissociation.
   C. Confusion.
   D. Avoidance.
   E. Arousal.

Correct Answer: C. Confusion.

Explanation: Criterion B for acute stress disorder requires the presence of 9 (or more) of a total of 12 symptoms from any of the five categories of intrusion, negative mood, dissociation, avoidance, and arousal, beginning or worsening after the traumatic event(s) occurred.

7.9—Acute Stress Disorder / diagnostic criteria (pp. 280–281)

7.10   Which of the following stressful situations would meet Criterion A for the diagnosis of acute stress disorder (ASD)?

   A. Finding out that one's spouse has been fired.
   B. Failing an important final examination.
   C. Receiving a serious medical diagnosis.
   D. Being in the cross fire of a police shootout but not being harmed.
   E. Being in a subway train that gets stuck between stations.

Correct Answer: D. Being in the cross fire of a police shootout but not being harmed.

Explanation: The essential feature of ASD is the development of characteristic symptoms lasting from 3 days to 1 month following exposure to one or more traumatic events. Traumatic events that are experienced directly include, but are not limited to, exposure to war as a combatant or civilian, threatened or actual violent personal assault (e.g., sexual assault, physical attack, active combat, mugging, childhood physical and/or sexual abuse, being kidnapped, being taken hostage, terrorist attack, or torture), natural or human-made disasters (e.g., earthquake, hurricane, airplane crash), and severe accidents (e.g., severe motor vehicle or industrial accident).

Stressful events that do not meet Criterion A definitions for a diagnosis of ASD may nonetheless be sufficient to qualify for an adjustment disorder. In adjustment disorder, the stressor can be of any severity. The diagnosis of adjustment disorder is used when the response to an extreme stressor does not meet the full criteria for ASD (or another specific mental disorder) and for situations in which the stressor is not considered extreme (e.g., spouse leaving, being fired.)

7.10—Acute Stress Disorder / Diagnostic Features (pp. 281–282)

7.11   Following discharge from the hospital, a 22-year-old man describes vivid and intrusive memories of his stay in the intensive care unit (ICU), where he received treatment for smoke inhalation. Now at home, he states that he has memories of people being tortured and hearing their screams. He dreams of this every night, waking from sleep in a terror. He talks about not feeling like himself after the experience, finding little pleasure in life after what happened to him, and being easily angered by his family; in addition, he avoids his physician out of fear that he will be told he needs to return to the ICU. What is the most likely explanation for this patient's symptoms?

A. He has acute stress disorder because his life was in danger during the ICU stay.
B. He has posttraumatic stress disorder because his life was in danger during the ICU stay.
C. He has a delirium persisting from the ICU stay.
D. He had a delirium in the ICU and now has an adjustment disorder.
E. He has a psychotic disorder.

Correct Answer: D. He had a delirium in the ICU and now has an adjustment disorder.

Explanation: Flashbacks in acute stress disorder must be distinguished from illusions, hallucinations, and other perceptual disturbances that may occur in schizophrenia, other psychotic disorders, depressive or bipolar disorder with psychotic features, a delirium, substance/medication-induced disorders, and psychotic disorders due to another medical condition. Acute stress disorder flashbacks are distinguished from these other perceptual disturbances by being directly related to the traumatic experience and occurring in the absence of other psychotic or substance/medication-induced features.

7.11—Acute Stress Disorder / Differential Diagnosis (Psychotic disorders) (p. 286)

7.12   Which of the following experiences would *not* qualify as exposure to a traumatic event (Criterion A) in the diagnosis of acute stress disorder or posttraumatic stress disorder?

A. Hearing that one's brother was killed in combat.
B. Hearing that one's close childhood friend survived a motor vehicle accident
    but is paralyzed.
C. Hearing that one's child has been kidnapped.
D. Hearing that one's company had suddenly closed.
E. Hearing that one's spouse has been shot.

Correct Answer: D. Hearing that one's company had suddenly closed.

Explanation: The *directly experienced* traumatic events in Criterion A include,
but are not limited to, exposure to war as a combatant or civilian, threatened or
actual physical assault (e.g., physical attack, robbery, mugging, childhood
physical abuse), threatened or actual sexual violence (e.g., forced sexual penetration, alcohol/drug-facilitated sexual penetration, abusive sexual contact,
noncontact sexual abuse, sexual trafficking), being kidnapped, being taken
hostage, terrorist attack, torture, incarceration as a prisoner of war, natural or
human-made disasters, and severe motor vehicle accidents. A life-threatening
illness or debilitating medical condition is not necessarily considered a traumatic event. Medical incidents that qualify as traumatic events involve sudden, catastrophic events (e.g., waking during surgery, anaphylactic shock).
     Witnessed events include, but are not limited to, observing threatened or se-
rious injury, unnatural death, physical or sexual abuse of another person due
to violent assault, domestic violence, accident, war or disaster, or a medical catastrophe in one's child (e.g., a life-threatening hemorrhage).
     Indirect exposure through learning about an event is limited to experiences af-
fecting close relatives or friends and experiences that are violent or accidental
(e.g., death due to natural causes does not qualify). Such events include violent
personal assault, suicide, serious accident, and serious injury. The disorder
may be especially severe or long-lasting when the stressor is interpersonal and
intentional (e.g., torture, sexual violence).

7.12—Posttraumatic Stress Disorder / Diagnostic Features (p. 274)

7.13   A 31-year-old man narrowly escapes (without injury) from a house fire caused
when he dropped the lighter while trying to light his crack pipe. Six weeks
later, while smoking crack, he thinks he smells smoke and runs from the building in a panic, shouting, "It's on fire!" Which of the following symptoms or circumstances would rule out a diagnosis of posttraumatic stress disorder (PTSD)
for this patient?

A. Having difficulty falling asleep.
B. Being uninterested in going back to work.

C. Inappropriately getting angry at family members.

D. Experiencing symptoms only when smoking crack cocaine.

E. Concluding that "the world is completely dangerous."

Correct Answer: D. Experiencing symptoms only when smoking crack cocaine.

Explanation: Although the stressor and symptoms described would qualify this man for a diagnosis of PTSD, Criterion H states that "The disturbance is not attributable to the physiological effects of a substance (e.g., medication, alcohol) or another medical condition." If this man's symptoms occur only when he smokes crack cocaine, he would not meet criteria for PTSD.

7.13—Posttraumatic Stress Disorder / diagnostic criteria (pp. 271–272)

7.14 Criterion A4 of posttraumatic stress disorder requires "Experiencing repeated or extreme exposure to aversive details of the traumatic event." Which of the following would *not* qualify as an experiencing trauma under this criterion?

A. A police officer reviewing surveillance videotapes of homicides to identify perpetrators.

B. A social worker interviewing children who have been sexually abused and obtaining the details of the abuse.

C. A soldier sifting through the rubble of a collapsed building to retrieve remains of comrades.

D. A college student at a film festival watching a series of violent movies that contain graphic rape scenes.

E. A psychologist working with victims of torture who are seeking political asylum in the United States.

Correct Answer: D. A college student at a film festival watching a series of violent movies that contain graphic rape scenes.

Explanation: The examples given in Criterion A4 of posttraumatic stress disorder are first responders collecting human remains and police officers repeatedly exposed to details of child abuse. This criterion does not apply to exposure through electronic media, television, movies, or pictures, unless the exposure is work related.

7.14—Posttraumatic Stress Disorder / diagnostic criteria (pp. 271–272)

7.15 Which of the following statements about gender differences in the risk of developing posttraumatic stress disorder (PTSD) is *true?*

A. The risk is lower in females in preschool-age populations.

B. The risk is higher in females across the life span.

C. The risk is higher in males in elderly populations.

D. The risk is lower in middle-aged females than in middle-aged males.

E. The risk is higher in males across the life span.

Correct Answer: B. The risk is higher in females across the life span.

Explanation: PTSD is more prevalent among females than among males across the lifespan. Females in the general population experience PTSD for a longer duration than do males. At least some of the increased risk for PTSD in females appears to be attributable to a greater likelihood of exposure to traumatic events, such as rape, and other forms of interpersonal violence. Within populations exposed specifically to such stressors, gender differences in risk for PTSD are attenuated or nonsignificant.

7.15—Posttraumatic Stress Disorder / Gender-Related Diagnostic Issues (p. 278)

7.16 A 5-year-old child was present when her babysitter was sexually assaulted. Which of the following symptoms would be most suggestive of posttraumatic stress disorder (PTSD) in this child?

A. Playing normally with toys.

B. Having dreams about princesses and castles.

C. Taking the clothing off her dolls while playing.

D. Expressing no fear when talking about the event.

E. Talking about the event with her parents.

Correct Answer: C. Taking the clothing off her dolls while playing.

Explanation: The clinical expression of reexperiencing can vary across development. Young children may report new onset of frightening dreams without content specific to the traumatic event. Before age 6 years (see criteria for PTSD in children 6 years and younger), young children are more likely to express reexperiencing symptoms through play that refers directly or symbolically to the trauma. They may not manifest fearful reactions at the time of the exposure or during reexperiencing. Parents may report a wide range of emotional or behavioral changes in young children. Children may focus on imagined interventions in their play or storytelling. In addition to avoidance, children may become preoccupied with reminders. Because of young children's limitations in expressing thoughts or labeling emotions, negative alterations in mood or cognition tend to involve primarily mood changes.

7.16—Posttraumatic Stress Disorder / Development and Course (p. 277)

7.17 Which of the following statements about risk factors for developing posttraumatic stress disorder (PTSD) is *true?*

A. Sustaining personal injury does not affect the risk of developing PTSD.
B. Severity of the trauma influences the risk of developing PTSD.
C. Dissociation has no impact on the risk of developing PTSD.
D. Perceived life threat is the only risk factor for developing PTSD.
E. Prior mental disorders have little influence on the risk of developing PTSD.

Correct Answer: B. Severity of the trauma influences the risk of developing PTSD.

Explanation: Risk factors related to the traumatic event (i.e., peritraumatic factors) include severity (dose) of the trauma (the greater the magnitude of trauma, the greater the likelihood of PTSD), perceived life threat, personal injury, interpersonal violence (particularly trauma perpetrated by a caregiver or involving a witnessed threat to a caregiver in children), and, for military personnel, being a perpetrator, witnessing atrocities, or killing the enemy. Finally, dissociation that occurs during the trauma and persists afterward is a risk factor.

Risk factors related to temperament include childhood emotional problems by age 6 years (e.g., prior traumatic exposure, externalizing or anxiety problems) and prior mental disorders (e.g., panic disorder, depressive disorder, PTSD, or obsessive-compulsive disorder).

7.17—Posttraumatic Stress Disorder / Risk and Prognostic Factors / Pretraumatic factors / Temperamental; Peritraumatic factors / Environmental (pp. 277, 278)

7.18   How does the 12-month prevalence of posttraumatic stress disorder (PTSD) in the United States compare with that in European and Latin American countries?

A. It is much lower than that in other countries.
B. It is much higher than that in other countries.
C. It is equal to that in other countries.
D. It is somewhat higher than that in other countries.
E. It is somewhat lower than that in other countries.

Correct Answer: D. It is somewhat higher than that in other countries.

Explanation: The 12-month prevalence of PTSD among U.S. adults is about 3.5%. Lower estimates are seen in Europe and most Asian, African, and Latin American countries, clustering around 0.5%–1.0%. Although different groups have different levels of exposure to traumatic events, the conditional probability of developing PTSD following a similar level of exposure may also vary across cultural groups.

7.18—Posttraumatic Stress Disorder / Prevalence (p. 276)

7.19 A woman complains of sad mood and feeling hopeless 3 months after her husband files for divorce. She finds it difficult to take care of her home or make
meals for her family but has continued to fulfill her responsibilities. She denies
suicidal ideation, feels she was a good wife who "has nothing to feel guilty
about," and wishes she could "forget about the whole thing." She cannot stop
thinking about her situation. Which diagnosis best fits this symptom picture?

A. Adjustment disorder, with depressed mood.
B. Adjustment disorder, with disturbance of conduct.
C. Adjustment disorder, with anxiety.
D. Adjustment disorder, with mixed disturbance of emotions and conduct.
E. Adjustment disorder, unspecified.

Correct Answer: A. Adjustment disorder, with depressed mood.

Explanation: Among the various specifiers included in the adjustment disorder diagnostic criteria, "with depressed mood" best fits this patient's symptoms. The full set of specifiers is as follows:

> **With depressed mood:** Low mood, tearfulness, or feelings of hopelessness
> are predominant.
> **With anxiety:** Nervousness, worry, jitteriness, or separation anxiety is pre-
> dominant.
> **With mixed anxiety and depressed mood:** A combination of depression
> and anxiety is predominant.
> **With disturbance of conduct:** Disturbance of conduct is predominant.
> **With mixed disturbance of emotions and conduct:** Both emotional symp-
> toms (e.g., depression, anxiety) and a disturbance of conduct are predomi-
> nant.
> **Unspecified:** For maladaptive reactions that are not classifiable as one of
> the specific subtypes of adjustment disorder.

7.19—Adjustment Disorders / diagnostic criteria (p. 287)

7.20 Six months after the death of her husband, a 70-year-old woman is seen for
symptoms of overwhelming sadness, anger regarding her husband's unexpected death from a heart attack, intense yearning for him to come back, and
repeated unsuccessful attempts to begin moving out of her large home (which
she can no longer afford) due to inability to sort through and dispose of her
husband's belongings. What is the most appropriate diagnosis?

A. Major depressive disorder.
B. Posttraumatic stress disorder.
C. Adjustment disorder, with depressed mood.
D. Other specified trauma- and stressor-related disorder (persistent complex
bereavement disorder).
E. Normative stress reaction.

Correct Answer: C. Adjustment disorder, with depressed mood.

Explanation: The presence of emotional or behavioral symptoms in response to an identifiable stressor is the essential feature of adjustment disorders (Criterion A). The stressor may be a single event or there may be multiple stressors. There are several adjustment disorder specifiers, but "with depressed mood" best fits this patient's symptoms. Adjustment disorders may be diagnosed following the death of a loved one when the intensity, quality, or persistence of grief reactions exceeds what normally might be expected, when cultural, religious, or age-appropriate norms are taken into account. A more specific set of bereavement-related symptoms has been designated *persistent complex bereavement disorder* (see "Conditions for Further Study" in DSM-5 Section III). If this woman's symptoms persist for more than 12 months, a diagnosis of "other specified trauma- and stressor-related disorder (persistent complex bereavement disorder)" might be appropriate.

> 7.20—Adjustment Disorders / diagnostic criteria; Diagnostic Features (pp. 286–287); Other Specified Trauma- and Stressor-Related Disorder (p. 289); Conditions for Further Study / Persistent Complex Bereavement Disorder (pp. 789–790)

7.21 A 25-year-old woman with asthma becomes extremely anxious when she gets an upper respiratory infection. She presents to the emergency department with complaints of being unable to breathe. While there, she begins to hyperventilate and then reports feeling extremely dizzy. Her hyperventilation causes her to become fatigued, and when the medical evaluation indicates that she is retaining carbon dioxide (CO_2), it becomes necessary to admit her. The woman denies any other symptoms beyond anxiety. What is the most appropriate diagnosis?

A. Acute stress disorder.
B. Generalized anxiety disorder.
C. Adjustment disorder with anxiety.
D. Psychological factors affecting other medical conditions.
E. Factitious disorder.

Correct Answer: D. Psychological factors affecting other medical conditions.

Explanation: In psychological factors affecting other medical conditions, specific psychological entities (e.g., psychological symptoms, behaviors, other factors) exacerbate a medical condition. These psychological factors can precipitate, exacerbate, or put an individual at risk for medical illness, or they can worsen an existing condition. In contrast, an adjustment disorder is a reaction to the stressor (e.g., having a medical illness).

> 7.21—Adjustment Disorders / Differential Diagnosis (Psychological factors affecting other medical conditions) (p. 289)

7.22   How many Criterion B symptoms are required to be present for the diagnosis of acute stress disorder?

A. One.
B. Three.
C. Five.
D. Seven.
E. Nine.

Correct Answer: E. Nine.

Explanation: Criterion B for acute stress disorder requires the presence of 9 (or more) of a total of 12 symptoms from any of the five categories of intrusion, negative mood, dissociation, avoidance, and arousal, beginning or worsening after the traumatic event(s) occurred.

7.22—Acute Stress Disorder / diagnostic criteria (pp. 280–281)

7.23   How do the diagnostic criteria for posttraumatic stress disorder (PTSD) in preschool children differ from those for PTSD in individuals older than 6 years?

A. The preschool criteria incorporate simpler language that can be understood by children 6 years or younger.
B. The preschool criteria require one or more **intrusion** symptoms, one symptom representing *either* **avoidance** *or* **negative alterations in cognitions and mood,** and two or more **arousal/reactivity** symptoms, whereas the criteria for older individuals require symptoms in all four categories.
C. The criteria for individuals older than 6 years require one or more **intrusion** symptoms, one symptom representing *either* **avoidance** *or* **negative alterations in cognitions and mood,** and two or more **arousal/reactivity** symptoms, whereas the preschool criteria require symptoms in all four categories.
D. The preschool criteria require that the child directly experience the trauma, whereas the criteria for older individuals do not have this requirement.
E. The preschool criteria include only one type of traumatic exposure—witnessing of a traumatic event occurring to a parent or caregiving figure—as a qualifying traumatic event.

Correct Answer: B. The preschool criteria require one or more intrusion symptoms, one symptom representing *either* avoidance *or* negative alterations in cognitions and mood, and two or more arousal/reactivity symptoms, whereas the criteria for older individuals require symptoms in all four categories.

Explanation: The preschool criteria for PTSD include all of the types of traumatic exposure listed in the criteria for older individuals except for Criterion

A4 ("Experiencing repeated or extreme exposure to aversive details of the traumatic event"); in addition, Criterion A3 for preschool children specifies "parent or caregiving figure" instead of "a close family member or a close friend." The preschool criteria require one or more symptoms in Criterion B (intrusion), one or more symptoms in Criterion C (avoidance or negative alterations in cognitions or mood), and two or more symptoms in Criterion D (arousal and reactivity). By contrast, the criteria for individuals older than 6 years require one or more symptoms in Criterion B (intrusion), one or both symptoms in Criterion C (avoidance), two or more symptoms in Criterion D (negative alterations in cognitions or mood), and two or more symptoms in Criterion E (arousal and reactivity).

7.23—Posttraumatic Stress Disorder / diagnostic criteria (pp. 271–274)

7.25 Criterion B in the DSM-5 diagnostic criteria for acute stress disorder (ASD) requires the presence of symptoms from **five** different categories: *Intrusion, Negative Mood, Dissociative, Avoidance,* and *Arousal.* Match each of the following symptoms to the appropriate category (each symptom may be placed into only one category).

    a. Recurrent, involuntary, and intrusive distressing memories of the traumatic event(s).
    b. Problems with concentration.
    c. Persistent inability to experience positive emotions (e.g., inability to experience happiness, satisfaction, or loving feelings).
    d. An altered sense of the reality of one's surroundings or oneself (e.g., seeing oneself from another's perspective, being in a daze, time slowing).
    e. Efforts to avoid external reminders (people, places, conversations, activities, objects, situations) that arouse distressing memories, thoughts, or feelings about or closely associated with the traumatic event(s).
    f. Irritable behavior and angry outbursts (with little or no provocation), typically expressed as verbal or physical aggression toward people or objects.
    g. Inability to remember an important aspect of the traumatic event(s) (typically due to dissociative amnesia and not to other factors such as head injury, alcohol, or drugs).
    h. Recurrent distressing dreams in which the content and/or affect of the dream is related to the event(s).
    i. Hypervigilance.
    j. Dissociative reactions (e.g., flashbacks) in which the individual feels or acts as if the traumatic event(s) were recurring.
    k. Exaggerated startle response.
    l. Efforts to avoid distressing memories, thoughts, or feelings about or closely associated with the traumatic event(s).
    m. Sleep disturbance (e.g., difficulty falling or staying asleep, restless sleep).

n.　Intense or prolonged psychological distress or marked physiological reactions in response to internal or external cues that symbolize or resemble an aspect of the traumatic event(s).

Correct Matches:
Intrusion: a, h, j, n;
Negative Mood: c;
Dissociative: d, g;
Avoidance: e, l;
Arousal: b, f, i, k, m.

Explanation: Psychological distress following exposure to a traumatic or stressful event is quite variable. In some cases, symptoms can be well understood within an anxiety- or fear-based context. It is clear, however, that many individuals who have been exposed to a traumatic or stressful event exhibit a phenotype in which, rather than anxiety- or fear-based symptoms, the most prominent clinical characteristics are anhedonic and dysphoric symptoms, externalizing angry and aggressive symptoms, or dissociative symptoms. Furthermore, it is not uncommon for the clinical picture to include some combination of the above symptoms (with or without anxiety- or fear-based symptoms).

7.24—chapter intro (p. 265); Acute Stress Disorder / diagnostic criteria (pp. 271–272)

7.25　The DSM-5 diagnostic criteria for posttraumatic stress disorder (PTSD) require the presence of symptoms from **four** different categories: *Intrusion* (Criterion B), *Avoidance* (Criterion C), *Negative Alterations in Cognitions and Mood* (Criterion D), and *Arousal* (Criterion E). Match each of the following symptoms to the appropriate category (each symptom may be placed into only one category).

　　a.　Irritable behavior and angry outbursts (with little or no provocation), typically expressed as verbal or physical aggression toward people or objects.
　　b.　Avoidance of or efforts to avoid distressing memories, thoughts, or feelings about or closely associated with the traumatic event(s).
　　c.　Recurrent, involuntary, and intrusive distressing memories of the traumatic event(s).
　　d.　Inability to remember an important aspect of the traumatic event(s) (typically due to dissociative amnesia and not to other factors such as head injury, alcohol, or drugs).
　　e.　Avoidance of or efforts to avoid external reminders (people, places, conversations, activities, objects, situations) that arouse distressing memories, thoughts, or feelings about or closely associated with the traumatic event(s).
　　f.　Reckless or self-destructive behavior.
　　g.　Recurrent distressing dreams in which the content and/or affect of the dream is related to the event(s).

h. Persistent and exaggerated negative beliefs or expectations about oneself, others, or the world (e.g., "I am bad," "No one can be trusted," "The world is completely dangerous," "My whole nervous system is permanently ruined").

i. Hypervigilance.

j. Dissociative reactions (e.g., flashbacks) in which the individual feels or acts as if the traumatic event(s) were recurring.

k. Persistent, distorted cognitions about the cause or consequences of the traumatic event(s) that lead the individual to blame himself/herself or others.

l. Exaggerated startle response.

m. Persistent negative emotional state (e.g., fear, horror, anger, guilt, or shame).

n. Problems with concentration.

o. Markedly diminished interest or participation in significant activities.

p. Intense or prolonged psychological distress at exposure to internal or external cues that symbolize or resemble an aspect of the traumatic event(s).

q. Sleep disturbance (e.g., difficulty falling or staying asleep, restless sleep).

r. Feelings of detachment or estrangement from others.

s. Marked physiological reactions to internal or external cues that symbolize or resemble an aspect of the traumatic event(s).

t. Persistent inability to experience positive emotions (e.g., inability to experience happiness, satisfaction, or loving feelings).

Correct Matches:
Intrusion: c, g, j, p, s;
Avoidance: b, e;
Negative Alterations in Cognitions and Mood: d, h, k, m, o, r, t;
Arousal: a, f, i, l, n, q.

Explanation: DSM-5 criteria for PTSD differ significantly from the DSM-IV criteria. Whereas there were three major symptom clusters in DSM-IV—reexperiencing, avoidance/numbing, and arousal—there are now four symptom clusters in DSM-5, because the avoidance/numbing cluster is divided into two distinct clusters: avoidance and persistent negative alterations in cognitions and mood. This latter category, which retains most of the DSM-IV numbing symptoms, also includes new or reconceptualized symptoms, such as persistent negative emotional states. The final cluster—alterations in arousal and reactivity—retains most of the DSM-IV arousal symptoms. It also includes irritable behavior or angry outbursts and reckless or self-destructive behavior.

7.25—Posttraumatic Stress Disorder / diagnostic criteria (pp. 271–272); Appendix / Highlights of Changes From DSM-IV to DSM-5 (p. 812)

7.26   Eighteen months following the death of her son, a 49-year-old woman consults you for psychotherapy. She reports that her son died following a skiing accident on a trip that she gave him as a gift for his 17th birthday. She is preoccupied with the death and blames herself for providing the gift of the trip.

Although she denies any overt suicidal plans, she describes longing for her son and an intense wish to be with him. She has not entered her son's room since his death, has difficulty relating to her husband and feels anger toward him for agreeing to allow their son to go on the ski trip, and reports arguments between them regarding her social isolation and her lack of interest in maintaining their home and preparing meals for their other children. She was treated with a selective serotonin reuptake inhibitor at full dose for 6 months after her son's death but reports that the medication had no impact on her symptoms. What is the most appropriate diagnosis?

A. Major depressive disorder.
B. Posttraumatic stress disorder.
C. Other specified trauma- and stressor-related disorder.
D. Normal grief.
E. Adjustment disorder.

Correct Answer: C. Other specified trauma- and stressor-related disorder.

Explanation: The severe and persistent grief and mourning reactions that characterize this woman's symptom presentation meet criteria for the proposed diagnosis *persistent complex bereavement disorder,* which appears in Section III ("Conditions for Further Study") of DSM-5. However, because the proposed criteria sets in Section III are not intended for clinical use, the appropriate diagnosis in this case would be *other specified trauma- and stressor-related disorder (persistent complex bereavement disorder).* This woman's symptoms do not meet criteria for major depressive disorder, posttraumatic stress disorder, or an adjustment disorder. The "other specified trauma- and stressor-related disorder" category applies to presentations in which symptoms characteristic of a trauma- and stressor-related disorder that cause clinically significant distress or impairment in social, occupational, or other important areas of functioning predominate but do not meet the full criteria for any of the disorders in the trauma- and stressor-related disorders diagnostic class.

7.26—Other Specified Trauma- and Stressor-Related Disorder (p. 289); Conditions for Further Study (Section III) / Persistent Complex Bereavement Disorder (pp. 789–792)

CHAPTER 8

Dissociative Disorders

8.1   Which of the following is *not* a way in which DSM-5 classification of dissociative disorders differs from DSM-IV?

A. In DSM-IV, derealization occurring without depersonalization was classified under dissociative disorder not otherwise specified (NOS), whereas in DSM-5 it is classified as depersonalization/derealization disorder.
B. In DSM-IV, dissociative fugue was a separate diagnosis, whereas in DSM-5, it is a subtype of dissociative amnesia.
C. In DSM-IV, experiences of possession could not be part of the diagnosis of dissociative identity disorder (DID); in DSM-5, they can be.
D. In keeping with the empirical basis of DSM-5, DID can be diagnosed only if the clinician or a reliable family member witnesses the claimed disruption of identity; in DSM-IV, this restriction did not apply.
E. The criteria for DID have been changed to indicate that gaps in the recall of events may occur for everyday events and not just traumatic events.

Correct Answer: D. In keeping with the empirical basis of DSM-5, DID can be diagnosed only if the clinician or a reliable family member witnesses the claimed disruption of identity; in DSM-IV, this restriction did not apply.

Explanation: In DSM-5, self-reports of identity disruptions are sufficient to make the diagnosis, whereas in DSM-IV, these disruptions (e.g., change of personality to an alter) had to be observed in order to make the diagnosis. This is now also true for possession-form experiences; that is, a self-report of experiencing possession (without a frank psychotic delusion) can also be used to diagnose DID. In DSM-5, derealization occurring without depersonalization is classified as depersonalization/derealization disorder; in other words, derealization symptoms and depersonalization symptoms are given equal weight, and one can make the diagnosis of depersonalization/derealization disorder with either derealization or depersonalization symptoms alone or a combination of them. In DSM-IV, dissociative fugue was a separate diagnosis, but in DSM-5, it is a subtype of dissociative amnesia. Finally, in DSM-5, the amnesia symptoms in DID include amnesia for everyday events, not just traumatic events.

8.1—Dissociative Identity Disorder / diagnostic criteria (p. 292); Appendix / Highlights of Changes From DSM-IV to DSM-5 (p. 812)

8.2   Dissociative disorders involve disruptions or discontinuities in the operation and integration of many areas of psychological functioning. Which of the following is *not* a functional area affected in dissociative disorders?

A. Memory.
B. Consciousness.
C. Perception.
D. Delusional beliefs.
E. Emotional responses.

Correct Answer: D. Delusional beliefs.

Explanation: Dissociative disorders encompass disruptions and discontinuities in many areas of psychological functioning, including normal integration of consciousness, memory, identity, emotion, perception, body representation, motor control, and behavior. If frank psychotic symptoms such as delusional beliefs are present, one must consider a diagnosis outside the dissociative disorders arena to account for the symptoms.

8.2—chapter intro (p. 291)

8.3   Which of the following statements correctly describes the meanings of the adjectives *positive* and *negative* when applied to dissociative symptoms?

A. When applied to dissociative disorder symptoms, the adjectives *positive* and *negative* have the same meanings as they do in schizophrenia.
B. "Positive" dissociative symptoms refer to those accompanied by euphoric moods.
C. "Negative" dissociative symptoms refer to inability to access mental content or to control mental functions in a normal fashion.
D. "Negative" dissociative symptoms refer to the belief that one has ceased to exist.
E. The adjectives *positive* and *negative* are not appropriately applied to dissociative symptoms because these symptoms are value neutral.

Correct Answer: C. "Negative" dissociative symptoms refer to inability to access mental content or to control mental functions in a normal fashion.

Explanation: Dissociative symptoms are experienced as 1) unbidden intrusions into awareness and behavior, with accompanying losses of continuity in subjective experience (i.e., "positive" dissociative symptoms such as fragmentation of identity, depersonalization, and derealization) and/or 2) inability to access information or to control mental functions that normally are readily amenable to access or control (i.e., "negative" dissociative symptoms such as amnesia).

8.3—chapter intro (p. 291)

8.4   Which of the following statements about depersonalization/derealization disorder is *true*?

A. Although transient symptoms of depersonalization/derealization are common in the general population, symptomatology that meets full criteria for depersonalization/derealization disorder is markedly less common.
B. Women are 1.5 times more likely than men to develop depersonalization/derealization disorder.
C. Age at onset of the disorder is most commonly between 25 and 35 years.
D. During episodes of depersonalization/derealization, individuals may feel that they are "going crazy" and typically lose reality testing.
E. The most common childhood traumatic experience in persons with depersonalization/derealization disorder is sexual abuse.

Correct Answer: A. Although transient symptoms of depersonalization/derealization are common in the general population, symptomatology that meets full criteria for depersonalization/derealization disorder is markedly less common.

Explanation: Transient depersonalization/derealization symptoms lasting hours to days are common in the general population; approximately one-half of all adults have experienced at least one lifetime episode of depersonalization/derealization. However, symptomatology that meets full criteria for depersonalization/derealization disorder is markedly less common than transient symptoms. Women and men have the disorder with equal frequency (gender ratio of 1:1). The mean age at onset of the disorder is 16 years; only 5% of individuals experience onset after age 25. Individuals with depersonalization/derealization disorder may have difficulty describing their symptoms and may think they are "crazy" or "going crazy"; however, Criterion B specifies that reality testing remains intact during these experiences. There is a clear association between depersonalization/derealization disorder and childhood interpersonal traumas in a substantial portion of individuals, although this association is not as prevalent or as extreme in the nature of the traumas as in other dissociative disorders, such as dissociative identity disorder. In particular, emotional abuse and emotional neglect have been most strongly and consistently associated with the disorder. Other stressors can include physical abuse; witnessing domestic violence; growing up with a seriously impaired, mentally ill parent; or unexpected death or suicide of a family member or close friend. Sexual abuse is a much less common antecedent but can be encountered.

8.4—Depersonalization/Derealization Disorder / Associated Features Supporting Diagnosis (p. 303); Prevalence (p. 303); Development and Course (pp. 303–304); Risk and Prognostic Factors (p. 304)

8.5   Criterion A for the diagnosis of dissociative identity disorder (DID) requires
       the presence of two or more distinct personality states or an experience of pos-
       session. Which of the following symptom presentations would *not* qualify as a
       manifestation of an alternate identity?

       A. An intrusive but nonhallucinatory voice that is not recognized as being part
          of one's own normal thought flow.
       B. Suddenly emergent strong impulses or emotions.
       C. Acute changes in personal preferences in areas such as food, clothing, or
          even political convictions.
       D. An acute sense of being in a different body, such as an adult feeling like he
          or she is in a child's body.
       E. A religious experience of being reborn into a new spiritual state that affects
          multiple domains of the individual's behavior.

       **Correct Answer: E. A religious experience of being reborn into a new spiri-
       tual state that affects multiple domains of the individual's behavior.**

       Explanation: Personality changes do not qualify as part of Criterion A symp-
       toms if they are a normal part of a broadly accepted cultural or religious prac-
       tice. Personality changes that *do* count toward Criterion A are related to
       discontinuities of experience that can affect any aspect of an individual's func-
       tioning. Individuals with dissociative identity disorder may report the feeling
       that they have suddenly become depersonalized observers of their "own"
       speech and actions, which they may feel powerless to stop (sense of self). Such
       individuals may also report perceptions of voices (e.g., a child's voice; crying;
       the voice of a spiritual being). In some cases, voices are experienced as multi-
       ple, perplexing, independent thought streams over which the individual expe-
       riences no control. Strong emotions, impulses, and even speech or other actions
       may suddenly emerge, without a sense of personal ownership or control (sense
       of agency). These emotions and impulses are frequently reported as ego-dys-
       tonic and puzzling. Attitudes, outlooks, and personal preferences (e.g., about
       food, activities, dress) may suddenly shift and then shift back. Individuals may
       report that their bodies feel different (e.g., like a small child, like the opposite
       gender, huge and muscular). Alterations in sense of self and loss of personal
       agency may be accompanied by a feeling that these attitudes, emotions, and
       behaviors—even one's body—are "not mine" and/or are "not under my con-
       trol."

       **8.5—Dissociative Identity Disorder / diagnostic criteria; Diagnostic Features (pp. 292–
       293)**

8.6   Criterion B for the diagnosis of dissociative identity disorder (DID) requires re-
       current gaps in the recall of everyday events, important personal information,
       and/or traumatic events that are inconsistent with ordinary forgetting. Which
       of the following statements about Criterion B–qualifying amnesia is *false?*

A. Gaps in recall of remote life events do not meet Criterion B definitions for amnesia.
B. It is common for individuals with DID to minimize their amnesia symptoms.
C. Individuals with DID may discover evidence of their past actions or experiences, such as finding clothing in the closet they do not recall buying, or seeing a photo of a trip they don't recall taking.
D. Forgetting of skills such as those involved in playing a musical instrument would count as amnesia for the purposes of Criterion B.
E. Dissociative fugues in which an individual finds him- or herself in a location with no memory of having traveled there are common in DID and represent a form of amnesia.

Correct Answer: A. Gaps in recall of remote life events do not meet Criterion B definitions for amnesia.

Explanation: The dissociative amnesia of individuals with DID manifests in three primary ways: as 1) gaps in remote memory of personal life events (e.g., periods of childhood or adolescence; some important life events, such as the death of a grandparent, getting married, giving birth); 2) lapses in dependable memory (e.g., of what happened today, of well-learned skills such as how to do their job, use a computer, read, drive); and 3) discovery of evidence of their everyday actions and tasks that they do not recollect doing (e.g., finding unexplained objects in their shopping bags or among their possessions; finding perplexing writings or drawings that they must have created; discovering injuries; "coming to" in the midst of doing something). Dissociative fugues, wherein the person discovers dissociated travel, are common. Thus, individuals with DID may report that they have suddenly found themselves at the beach, at work, in a nightclub, or somewhere at home (e.g., in the closet, on a bed or sofa, in the corner) with no memory of how they came to be there. Amnesia in individuals with DID is not limited to stressful or traumatic events; these individuals often cannot recall everyday events as well.

8.6—Dissociative Identity Disorder / Diagnostic Features (pp. 292–293)

8.7   Dissociative amnesia most often involves which of the following types of amnesia?

A. Continuous amnesia.
B. Permanent, irreversible amnesia.
C. Localized or selective amnesia for specific events.
D. Generalized amnesia similar to that seen in neurological toxicity.
E. Systematized amnesia.

Correct Answer: C. Localized or selective amnesia for specific events.

Explanation: The defining characteristic of dissociative amnesia is an inability to recall important autobiographical information that 1) should be successfully stored in memory and 2) ordinarily would be readily remembered (Criterion A). Dissociative amnesia differs from the permanent amnesias due to neurobiological damage or toxicity that prevent memory storage or retrieval in that it is always potentially reversible because the memory has been successfully stored.

Criterion A notes that dissociative amnesia most often consists of localized or selective amnesia for a specific event or events; or generalized amnesia for identity and life history. *Localized amnesia,* a failure to recall events during a circumscribed period of time, is the most common form of dissociative amnesia. In *selective amnesia,* the individual can recall some, but not all, of the events during a circumscribed period of time. Thus, the individual may remember part of a traumatic event but not other parts. Some individuals report both localized and selective amnesias.

Generalized amnesia, a complete loss of memory for one's life history, is rare. Individuals with generalized amnesia may forget personal identity. Some lose previous knowledge about the world (i.e., semantic knowledge) and can no longer access well-learned skills (i.e., procedural knowledge). Generalized amnesia may be more common among combat veterans, sexual assault victims, and individuals experiencing extreme emotional stress or conflict.

Individuals with dissociative amnesia are frequently unaware (or only partially aware) of their memory problems. Many, especially those with localized amnesia, minimize the importance of their memory loss and may become uncomfortable when prompted to address it. In *systematized amnesia,* the individual loses memory for a specific category of information (e.g., all memories relating to one's family, a particular person, or childhood sexual abuse). In *continuous amnesia,* an individual forgets each new event as it occurs.

8.7—Dissociative Amnesia / Diagnostic Features (pp. 298–299)

8.8 How does DSM-5 differ from DSM-IV in its classification of dissociative fugue?

A. Unlike DSM-IV, DSM-5 allows a fugue event to be diagnosed as dissociative identity disorder (DID) if it takes place in conjunction with the symptoms of DID.

B. Unlike DSM-IV, DSM-5 allows a fugue event secondary to temporal lobe epilepsy to be diagnosed as dissociative fugue.

C. Whereas dissociative fugue was a separate diagnosis in DSM-IV, it is a specifier of dissociative amnesia in DSM-5 (i.e., dissociative amnesia with dissociative fugue).

D. Unlike DSM-IV, DSM-5 recognizes that fugue states are more common in dissociative amnesia than in dissociative identity disorder.

E. Whereas DSM-IV treated dissociative fugue as an independent diagnostic entity, DSM-5 recognizes that fugue states most commonly present in the context of identity pathology.

Correct Answer: C. Whereas dissociative fugue was a separate diagnosis in DSM-IV, it is a specifier of dissociative amnesia in DSM-5 (i.e., dissociative amnesia with dissociative fugue).

Explanation: In DSM-5 the emphasis is on the amnestic aspect of fugue rather than on the identity discontinuity. Thus, the specifier "with dissociative fugue"—defined as "apparently purposeful travel or bewildered wandering that is associated with amnesia for identity or for other important autobiographical information"—is provided in the DSM-5 diagnostic criteria for dissociative amnesia, not in the criteria for dissociative identity disorder. A patient who presents with fugue would receive the diagnosis *dissociative amnesia, with dissociative fugue*. Like DSM-IV, DSM-5 recognizes that fugue events actually present more commonly as part of a more global disorder—namely, dissociative identity disorder. A fugue event secondary to temporal lobe epilepsy was excluded from receiving a DSM-IV diagnosis of dissociative fugue and is also excluded from receiving a DSM-5 diagnosis of dissociative amnesia with dissociative fugue.

8.8—Appendix / Highlights of Changes From DSM-IV to DSM-5 (p. 812)

CHAPTER 9

Somatic Symptom and Related Disorders

9.1   Somatoform Disorders in DSM-IV are referred to as Somatic Symptom and Related Disorders in DSM-5. Which of the following features characterizes the major diagnosis in this class, somatic symptom disorder?

A. Medically unexplained somatic symptoms.
B. Underlying psychic conflict.
C. Masochism.
D. Distressing somatic symptoms and abnormal thoughts, feelings, and behaviors in response to these symptoms.
E. Comorbidity with anxiety and depressive disorders.

Correct Answer: D. Distressing somatic symptoms and abnormal thoughts, feelings, and behaviors in response to these symptoms.

Explanation: Somatic symptom disorder emphasizes diagnosis made on the basis of positive symptoms and signs (distressing somatic symptoms plus abnormal thoughts, feelings, and behaviors in response to these symptoms) rather than the absence of a medical explanation for somatic symptoms. A distinctive characteristic of many individuals with somatic symptom disorder is not the somatic symptoms per se, but instead the way they present and interpret them. Incorporating affective, cognitive, and behavioral components into the criteria for somatic symptom disorder provides a more comprehensive and accurate reflection of the true clinical picture than can be achieved by assessing the somatic complaints alone.

9.1—chapter intro (p. 309)

9.2   In DSM-IV, a patient with a high level of anxiety about having a disease and many associated somatic symptoms would have been given the diagnosis of hypochondriasis. What DSM-5 diagnosis would apply to this patient?

A. Hypochondriasis.
B. Illness anxiety disorder.
C. Somatic symptom disorder.
D. Generalized anxiety disorder.
E. Unspecified somatic symptom and related disorder.

Correct Answer: C. Somatic symptom disorder.

Explanation: All of these disorders are characterized by the prominent focus on somatic concerns and their initial presentation mainly in medical rather than mental health care settings. Somatic symptom disorder offers a more clinically useful method of characterizing individuals who may have been considered in the past for a diagnosis of somatization disorder. Furthermore, approximately 75% of individuals previously diagnosed with hypochondriasis are subsumed under the diagnosis of somatic symptom disorder. However, about 25% of individuals with hypochondriasis have high health anxiety in the absence of somatic symptoms, and many such individuals' symptoms would not qualify for an anxiety disorder diagnosis. The DSM-5 diagnosis of illness anxiety disorder is for this latter group of individuals. Illness anxiety disorder can be considered either in this diagnostic section or as an anxiety disorder. Because of the strong focus on somatic concerns, and because illness anxiety disorder is most often encountered in medical settings, for utility it is listed with the somatic symptom and related disorders. Hypochondriasis has been eliminated as a diagnostic label. Individuals with a high level of anxiety about having an illness but without prominent somatic symptoms are now included in illness anxiety disorder.

9.2—Somatic Symptom Disorder / chapter intro (p. 310)

9.3   In DSM-III and DSM-IV, a large number of somatic symptoms were needed to qualify for the diagnosis of somatization disorder. How many somatic symptoms are needed to meet symptom criteria for the DSM-5 diagnosis of somatic symptom disorder?

　　A. Four: at least one pseudoneurological, one pain, one sexual, and one gastrointestinal symptom.
　　B. Fifteen, distributed across several organ systems.
　　C. One.
　　D. At least one that is medically unexplained.
　　E. None.

Correct Answer: C. One.

Explanation: The diagnosis of somatic symptom disorder requires one or more somatic symptoms that are distressing or result in disruption of daily life (Criterion A). The individual must also manifest "excessive thoughts, feelings, or behaviors related to the somatic symptoms or associated health concerns" (Criterion B). with persistence of the symptomatic state (typically for more than 6 months) (Criterion C). The excessive symptoms in Criterion B may manifest in one of the following ways: 1) disproportionate and persistent thoughts about the seriousness of one's symptoms; 2) persistently high level of anxiety about health or symptoms; 3) excessive time and energy devoted to these symptoms or health concerns. A symptom need not be medically unexplained—it is the presence of the symptom along with the "excessive" cognitive-affective-behavioral response that defines the disorder.

9.3—Somatic Symptom Disorder / diagnostic criteria; Diagnostic Features (pp. 311–312)

9.4   After an airplane flight, a 60-year-old woman with a history of chronic anxiety develops deep vein thrombophlebitis and a subsequent pulmonary embolism. Over the next year, she focuses relentlessly on sensations of pleuritic chest pain and repeatedly seeks medical attention for this symptom, which she worries is due to recurrent pulmonary emboli, despite negative test results. Review of systems reveals that she also has chronic back pain and that she has consulted many physicians for symptoms of culture-negative cystitis. What diagnosis best fits this clinical picture?

A. Post–pulmonary embolism syndrome.
B. Chest pain syndrome.
C. Hypochondriasis.
D. Pain disorder.
E. Somatic symptom disorder.

Correct Answer: E. Somatic symptom disorder.

Explanation: This patient's pain preoccupations, anxiety about her symptoms, and medical care–seeking behaviors in the aftermath of her pulmonary embolism are the basis for making the diagnosis of somatic symptom disorder. The issue of whether her pleuritic pain symptoms can be explained as caused by her previous pulmonary embolism is not relevant to this determination; what matters is her abnormal appraisal of, focus on, and behavioral response to the pain. In the DSM-IV classification, she might have received a dual diagnosis of hypochondriasis and pain disorder; in DSM-5 her anxiety about the significance of her somatic symptoms and her ongoing pain complaints point to a diagnosis of somatic symptom disorder.

9.4—Somatic Symptom Disorder / Diagnostic Features (p. 311)

9.5   Which of the following is a descriptive specifier included in the diagnostic criteria for somatic symptom disorder?

A. With predominant pain.
B. With hypochondriasis.
C. With psychological comorbidity.
D. Psychotic type.
E. Undifferentiated.

Correct Answer: A. With predominant pain.

Explanation: The "with predominant pain" specifier is used for individuals whose somatic symptoms predominantly involve pain.

9.5—Somatic Symptom Disorder / diagnostic criteria (p. 311)

9.6 A 60-year-old man has prostate cancer with bony metastases that cause persistent pain. He is treated with antiandrogen medications that result in hot flashes. He is unable to work because of his symptoms, but he is stoical, hopeful, and not anxious. What is the appropriate diagnosis?

A. Pain disorder.
B. Illness anxiety disorder.
C. Somatic symptom disorder.
D. Psychological factors affecting other medical conditions.
E. No diagnosis.

Correct Answer: E. No diagnosis.

Explanation: This patient has "medically explained" symptoms, but they are still somatic symptoms that result in disruption of important daily life functions. He therefore meets Criterion A for somatic symptom disorder; however, he does *not* meet Criterion B, which requires excessive thoughts, feelings, or behaviors related to the symptoms. Pain disorder is not a DSM-5 diagnostic category. The patient has a somatic symptom but is not anxious, so he does not have illness anxiety disorder. The diagnosis psychological factors affecting other medical conditions refers to emotional, cognitive, or behavioral issues that worsen prognosis or interfere with management of a physical condition; that diagnosis would not apply to the patient in this vignette.

9.6—Somatic Symptom Disorder / diagnostic criteria (p. 311)

9.7 Illness anxiety disorder involves a preoccupation with having or acquiring a serious illness. How severe must the accompanying somatic symptoms be to meet criteria for the diagnosis of illness anxiety disorder?

A. Mild to moderate severity.
B. Moderate to high severity.
C. Any level of severity.
D. Mild severity at most, but there need not be any somatic symptoms.
E. None of the above; the presence of *any* somatic symptoms rules out the diagnosis of illness anxiety disorder.

Correct Answer: D. Mild severity at most, but there need not be any somatic symptoms.

Explanation: Criterion B for illness anxiety disorder states, "Somatic symptoms are not present or, if present, are only mild in intensity." The hallmark of the disorder is chronic, excessive, and disproportionate preoccupation and worry about having or acquiring a serious medical illness, rather than a somatic complaint. If somatic symptoms are present, it is likely that a diagnosis of somatic symptom disorder is more appropriate.

9.7—Illness Anxiety Disorder / diagnostic criteria (p. 315)

9.8   Over a period of several years, a 50-year-old woman visits her dermatologist's office every few weeks to be evaluated for skin cancer, showing the dermatologist various freckles, nevi, and patches of dry skin about which she has become concerned. None of the skin findings have ever been abnormal, and the dermatologist has repeatedly reassured her. The woman does not have pain, itching, bleeding, or other somatic symptoms. She does have a history of occasional panic attacks. What is the most likely diagnosis?

A. Unspecified anxiety disorder.
B. Illness anxiety disorder.
C. Hypochondriasis.
D. Somatic symptom disorder.
E. Factitious disorder.

Correct Answer: B. Illness anxiety disorder.

Explanation: One should consider the possibility that the presenting problem is better accounted for by another psychiatric disorder that would preclude a diagnosis of illness anxiety disorder, but the mere presence of another anxiety symptom (panic attacks) is not sufficient to conclude that another anxiety disorder diagnosis better explains the patient's problem. Illness anxiety disorder is the appropriate diagnosis because the patient has no somatic symptom but does have a persistent worry that she has a serious illness (skin cancer), is easily alarmed by minor somatic changes (patches of dry skin), and repeatedly and excessively seeks reassurance through medical checkups, with persistence of the problem for more than 6 months. The term *hypochondriasis* as a synonym for illness anxiety is no longer used as a diagnostic label. The absence of a somatic symptom rules out somatic symptom disorder. Factitious disorder entails willful falsification of signs or symptoms.

9.8—Illness Anxiety Disorder / diagnostic criteria (p. 315)

9.9   A 45-year-old man with a family history of early-onset coronary artery disease avoids climbing stairs, eschews exercise, and abstains from sexual activity for fear of provoking a heart attack. He frequently checks his pulse, reads extensively about preventive cardiology, and tries many health food supplements alleged to be good for the heart. When he experiences an occasional twinge of chest discomfort, he rests in bed for 24 hours; however, he does not go to doctors because he fears hearing bad news about his heart from them. What diagnosis best fits this clinical picture?

A. Persistent complex bereavement disorder.
B. Adjustment disorder.
C. Illness anxiety disorder.
D. Unspecified somatic symptom and related disorder.
E. Somatic symptom disorder.

Correct Answer: C. Illness anxiety disorder.

Explanation: This man has the anxiety and preoccupation about somatic illness and the reassurance seeking without relief that are characteristic of illness anxiety disorder. The fact that he does not go to doctors does not preclude the diagnosis. (He would fit the "care-avoidant" type.) One might surmise that his family history fuels his anxiety, and perhaps bereavement after the early death of a loved one from coronary disease plays a role in his illness, but we are provided with no data to support this conjecture. Major life stress, including the death of a loved one, is considered a risk factor for illness anxiety disorder. Somatic symptoms are not a prominent part of the clinical presentation; rather, worry and preoccupation with having a disease are the main feature, so a somatic symptom disorder diagnosis would be inappropriate.

9.9—Illness Anxiety Disorder / diagnostic criteria (p. 315)

9.10   A 25-year-old woman is hospitalized for evaluation of episodes in which she appears to lose consciousness, rocks her head from side to side, and moves her arms and legs in a nonsynchronous, bicycling pattern. The episodes occur a few times per day and last for 2–5 minutes. Electroencephalography during the episodes does not reveal any ictal activity. Immediately after a fit, her sensorium appears clear. What is the most likely diagnosis?

A. Epilepsy.
B. Malingering.
C. Somatic symptom disorder.
D. Conversion disorder (functional neurological symptom disorder), with attacks or seizures.
E. Factitious disorder.

Correct Answer: D. Conversion disorder (functional neurological symptom disorder), with attacks or seizures.

Explanation: The essential feature of conversion disorder (functional neurological symptom disorder) is the presence of one or more symptoms that cause clinically significant distress or impairment in social, occupational, or other important areas of functioning (or warrant medical attention); are incompatible with recognized neurological or medical conditions; and cannot be better explained by another mental disorder. This patient's pattern of movement, duration of attack, and return to clear consciousness at the end of the attack are incompatible with a diagnosis of epilepsy (as is underscored by the electroencephalogram) and lack resemblance to any other medical or neurological disorder that would account for them. Although factitious disorder, with conscious feigning of symptoms, has not been absolutely ruled out, the diagnosis of conversion disorder does *not* require certainty that symptoms are not consciously feigned, in recognition of the fact that reliability in ascertaining conscious feigning is poor. Positive evidence of feigning would rule out conversion disorder; in that case, the diagnosis would be factitious disorder.

> **9.10—Conversion Disorder (Functional Neurological Symptom Disorder) / diagnostic criteria (pp. 318–319)**

9.11 Which of the following symptoms is incompatible with a diagnosis of conversion disorder (functional neurological symptom disorder)?

A. Light-headedness upon standing up.
B. Dystonic movements.
C. Tunnel vision.
D. Touch and temperature anesthesia with intact pinprick sensation over the left forearm.
E. Transient leg weakness in a patient with known multiple sclerosis.

Correct Answer: A. Light-headedness upon standing up.

Explanation: The diagnosis of conversion disorder requires the presence of a voluntary motor or sensory symptom; "autonomic" symptoms such as orthostatic light-headedness would not be included in this category and would be better accommodated by a diagnosis of somatic symptom disorder. Tunnel vision ("tubular visual field") and localized anesthesia for some but not all sensory modalities that are carried in the same nerve distribution are classic examples of sensory deficit symptoms that would be considered functional or psychogenic neurological symptoms. In a patient with a medical/neurological diagnosis such as multiple sclerosis that might account for a new neurological symptom, great caution should be exercised before labeling a symptom as psychogenic or functional, but it is possible even for patients with such illnesses to have functional symptoms.

> **9.11—Conversion Disorder (Functional Neurological Symptom Disorder) / diagnostic criteria / Diagnostic Features (pp. 318–319)**

9.12 Why is *la belle indifférence* (apparent lack of concern about the symptom) not included as a diagnostic criterion for conversion disorder (functional neurological symptom disorder)?

A. It has poor interrater reliability.
B. It has poor specificity.
C. It has poor sensitivity.
D. It pathologizes stoicism.
E. It has poor test-retest reliability.

Correct Answer: C. It has poor sensitivity.

Explanation: Although classically described as a feature of conversion disorder, *la belle indifférence* (i.e., apparent lack of concern about the nature or implications of the symptom) is not specific for conversion disorder and should not be used to make the diagnosis.

> **9.12—Conversion Disorder (Functional Neurological Symptom Disorder) / Associated Features Supporting Diagnosis (p. 320)**

9.13 A 20-year-old man presents with the complaint of acute onset of decreased visual acuity in his left eye. Physical, neurological, and laboratory examinations are entirely normal, including stereopsis testing, fogging test, and brain magnetic resonance imaging. The remainder of the history is negative except for the patient's report that since his midteens he has felt that his left cheekbone and eyebrow are too big. He spends a lot of time comparing the right and left sides of his face in the mirror. He is planning to have plastic surgery as soon as he graduates from college. Which of the following diagnoses are suggested?

A. Somatic symptom disorder and delusional disorder, somatic subtype.
B. Somatic symptom disorder and illness anxiety disorder.
C. Body dysmorphic disorder and conversion disorder (functional neurological symptom disorder).
D. Somatic symptom disorder, illness anxiety disorder, and body dysmorphic disorder.
E. Delusional disorder, somatic subtype.

Correct Answer: C. Body dysmorphic disorder and conversion disorder (functional neurological symptom disorder).

Explanation: The vision complaint and normal examinations are consistent with a diagnosis of a functional neurological symptom disorder, specifically a functional visual acuity problem ("special sensory" subtype of conversion disorder). The long-standing concern about the appearance of the left side of his face is consistent with a diagnosis of body dysmorphic disorder, as is the plan for plastic surgery in the absence of any visible cosmetic defect. An individual can have both of these diagnoses. One might speculate about the relationship, in this case, of preoccupation with the appearance of the left side of the face in particular and the development of functional symptoms in the left eye, but these speculations are beyond the scope of DSM-5 diagnosis.

9.13—Conversion Disorder (Functional Neurological Symptom Disorder) / Differential Diagnosis (p. 321)

9.14   A 50-year-old man with hard-to-control hypertension acknowledges to his physician that he regularly "takes breaks" from his medication regimen because he was brought up with the belief that pills are bad and natural remedies are better. He is well aware that his blood pressure becomes dangerously high when he does not follow the regimen. Which diagnosis best fits this case?

   A. Nonadherence to medical treatment.
   B. Unspecified anxiety disorder.
   C. Denial of medical illness.
   D. Adjustment disorder.
   E. Psychological factors affecting other medical conditions.

Correct Answer: E. Psychological factors affecting other medical conditions.

Explanation: DSM-5 includes nonadherence to medical treatment as a matter that may be the subject of clinical attention but not as a diagnosis per se. It receives a V code. If noncompliance becomes the major focus of clinical attention, then the V code would apply. We do not have evidence to support a diagnosis of an anxiety disorder. Denial of illness is not a diagnosis, although it may certainly command clinical attention, and the use of denial as a coping mechanism, if it interferes with obtaining treatment in a timely way, would be an example of a psychological factor affecting another medical condition; however, this patient does not deny his hypertension or the potential consequences. An adjustment disorder diagnosis applies to a clinically significant psychological response to a stressor, such as mood or anxiety symptoms. The diagnosis of psychological factors affecting another medical condition applies when a medical symptom or condition is present AND psychological or behavioral factors adversely affect the medical condition in one of the following ways: 1) close temporal association of the psychological factor and the onset or exacerbation or delay in recovery of the medical condition; 2) the factors interfere with treatment; 3) the factors add to the individual's health risk; 4) the factors influence the pathophysiology to precipitate or exacerbate symptoms. In this vignette, the patient's long-standing belief that pills are "bad" interferes with treatment adherence for his acknowledged hypertension, adding to his health risk.

9.14—Psychological Factors Affecting Other Medical Conditions / diagnostic criteria (pp. 322–323)

9.15   A 60-year-old man has prostate cancer with bony metastases that cause persistent pain. He is being treated with antiandrogen medications that result in hot flashes. Although (by his own assessment) his pain is well controlled with analgesics, he states that he is unable to work because of his symptoms. Despite reassurance that his medications are controlling his metastatic disease, every instance of pain leads him to worry that he has new bony lesions and is about to die, and he continually expresses fears about his impending death to his wife and children. Which diagnosis best fits this patient's presentation?

A. Panic disorder.
B. Illness anxiety disorder.
C. Somatic symptom disorder.
D. Psychological factors affecting other medical conditions.
E. Adjustment disorder with anxious mood.

Correct Answer: C. Somatic symptom disorder.

Explanation: In this vignette the patient's somatic symptoms are "medically explained" by the metastatic disease and antiandrogen therapy; however, their presence in conjunction with an excessively high level of anxiety, anticipatory fearfulness, and behavioral reactivity point to a diagnosis of somatic symptom disorder. It is not the experience of uncontrolled pain that is the patient's problem, it is his conviction that pain signifies progression of his cancer.

The diagnosis of psychological factors affecting another medical condition applies when a medical symptom or condition is present *AND* psychological or behavioral factors adversely affect the medical condition in one of the following ways: 1) close temporal association of the psychological factor and the onset or exacerbation or delay in recovery of the medical condition; 2) the factors interfere with treatment; 3) the factors add to the individual's health risk; 4) the factors influence the pathophysiology to precipitate or exacerbate symptoms.

When dysfunctional illness anxiety accompanies a prominent somatic symptom, somatic symptom disorder is a more appropriate diagnosis than illness anxiety disorder. If the patient had no somatic symptoms but had recently been told that his illness had taken a turn for the worse, and then transiently experienced worry, jitteriness, and sleeplessness, one might label his condition an adjustment disorder with anxious mood.

9.15—Somatic Symptom Disorder / diagnostic criteria (p. 311)

9.16   A 60-year-old man with a history of coronary disease and emphysema continues to smoke one pack of cigarettes daily despite his doctor's clear advice that abstinence is important for his survival. He says he's tried to quit a dozen times but has always relapsed due to withdrawal symptoms or feelings of tension relieved by smoking. What is the most likely diagnosis?

A. Psychological factors affecting other medical conditions.
B. Tobacco use disorder.
C. Denial of illness.
D. Nonadherence to medical treatment.
E. Adjustment disorder.

Correct Answer: B. Tobacco use disorder.

Explanation: When a substance use disorder adversely affects a physical condition, the substance use disorder diagnosis is "usually sufficient" and the diagnosis of psychological factor affecting a physical condition would be superfluous. If subthreshold substance use affects the course of the medical condition, the "psychological factors" diagnosis would be applied. In this vignette, the patient does not manifest denial of illness, nonadherence to medical treatment (neither of which is a DSM diagnosis), or a maladaptive psychological response to a stressor (the *sine qua non* for an adjustment disorder.)

9.16—Psychological Factors Affecting Other Medical Conditions / Diagnostic Features (pp. 322–323)

9.17   What is the essential diagnostic feature of factitious disorder?

   A. Somatic symptoms.
   B. Conscious misrepresentation and deception.
   C. External gain associated with illness.
   D. Absence of another medical disorder that may cause the symptoms.
   E. Normal physical examination and laboratory tests.

Correct Answer: B. Conscious misrepresentation and deception.

Explanation: The essential feature of factitious disorder is the falsification of medical or psychological signs and symptoms in oneself or others that are associated with the identified deception. Individuals with factitious disorder can also seek treatment for themselves or another following induction of injury or disease. The diagnosis requires demonstrating that the individual is taking surreptitious actions to misrepresent, simulate, or cause signs or symptoms of illness or injury in the absence of obvious external rewards. Methods of illness falsification can include exaggeration, fabrication, simulation, and induction. While a preexisting medical condition may be present, the deceptive behavior or induction of injury associated with deception causes others to view such individuals (or another) as more ill or impaired, and this can lead to excessive clinical intervention.

9.17—Factitious Disorder / Diagnostic Features (p. 325)

9.18   A 19-year-old man is brought to the emergency department by his family with acute onset of hemoptysis. Although he denies any role in the genesis of the symptom, he is observed in the waiting area to be surreptitiously inhaling a solution that provokes violent coughing. On confrontation he eventually acknowledges his action but explains that he heard an angel's voice instructing him to purify himself for a divine mission for which he will receive a heavenly reward. He was therefore trying to expunge all "evil vapors" from his lungs but felt obliged to keep this a secret. Why would this patient *not* be considered to have factitious disorder?

A. Consequences of religious or culturally normative practices are exempt from consideration as fabricated illnesses.
B. Factitious disorder occurs almost exclusively in women.
C. Repeated instances of illness fabrication are necessary for a diagnosis of factitious disorder.
D. The patient expects to receive an external reward and therefore should be considered to be malingering.
E. The presence of a psychotic illness that better accounts for the symptoms precludes the diagnosis of factitious disorder.

Correct Answer: E. The presence of a psychotic illness that better accounts for the symptoms precludes the diagnosis of factitious disorder.

Explanation: The presence of bizarre delusions and command auditory hallucinations strongly suggests a psychotic disorder. When another mental illness better accounts for the presentation, a diagnosis of factitious disorder should not be made (Criterion D). DSM-5 seeks to be respectful of variations in experience and modes of self-expression that are aspects of an individual's cultural and religious background, but it is unlikely that such factors would result in fabrication of illness presentation, and "rewards from heaven" would not generally be considered to be "obvious external rewards." Factitious disorder is more common in women, but it also occurs in men. Both single and recurrent episodes of fabrication qualify for diagnosis and should be specified.

9.18—Factitious Disorder / diagnostic criteria (p. 324)

9.19 When a mother knowingly and deceptively reports signs and symptoms of illness in her preschool-aged child, resulting in the child's hospitalization and subjection to numerous tests and procedures, what diagnosis would be recorded for the child?

A. Munchausen syndrome by proxy.
B. Factitious disorder by proxy.
C. No diagnosis.
D. Munchausen syndrome imposed on another.
E. Factitious disorder imposed on another.

Correct Answer: C. No diagnosis.

Explanation: Situations in which an individual falsifies illness in another in the absence of obvious external rewards and presents that person to others as ill, impaired, or injured qualify for a diagnosis of factitious disorder imposed on another. This diagnosis pertains to the perpetrator of the falsification, not the victim. In addition to other people, animals (e.g., pets) may be victims of such falsification. The diagnosis of factitious disorder is not made when the behavior is better explained by another mental disorder. The victim of this kind of falsification is not coded as having a mental disorder diagnosis (unless another diagnosis is present). The term *Munchausen syndrome* is not used in DSM-5, and the DSM-IV term *by proxy* has been replaced with *imposed on another*. DSM-5 states that the victim "may" be given an abuse diagnosis (if warranted).

9.19—Factitious Disorder / Recording Procedures (p. 325)

9.20 A 25-year-old woman with a history of intravenous heroin abuse is admitted to the hospital with infective endocarditis. Blood cultures are positive for several fungal species. Search of the patient's belongings discloses hidden syringes and needles and a small bag of dirt, which, when cultured, yields the same fungal species. Which of the following diagnoses are likely to apply?

A. Infective endocarditis, opioid use disorder, malingering, factitious disorder, and antisocial personality disorder.
B. Opioid use disorder and malingering.
C. Infective endocarditis, opioid use disorder, and factitious disorder.
D. Malingering and antisocial personality disorder.
E. Malingering and factitious disorder.

Correct Answer: C. Infective endocarditis, opioid use disorder, and factitious disorder.

Explanation: Although intravenous drug use is often the route of infection in infective endocarditis, in this vignette the infection is due to soil flora, suggesting that the patient injected dirt from the sample hidden in her belongings to cause the infection. Factitious illness includes some instances in which the patient actually surreptitiously causes a medical condition, not just cases in which the patient deceives others about factitious signs and symptoms. We have no evidence of external reward to justify considering a diagnosis of malingering, and, apart from deception about her illness, nothing to suggest antisocial personality disorder.

9.20—Factitious Disorder / Diagnostic Features (p. 325)

9.21 After finding a breast lump, a 50-year-old woman with a family history of breast cancer is overwhelmed by feelings of anxiety. Consultation with a breast surgeon, mammogram, and biopsy show the lump to be benign. The surgeon tells her that she requires no treatment; however, she continues to ruminate about the possibility of cancer and surgery that will result in disfigurement. Her sleep is restless, and she is having trouble concentrating at work. After 6 weeks of these symptoms, her primary physician refers her for psychiatric consultation. Her medical and psychiatric history is otherwise negative. Which diagnosis best fits this presentation?

A. Somatic symptom disorder.
B. Illness anxiety disorder.
C. Unspecified somatic symptom and related disorder.
D. Other specified somatic symptom and related disorder.
E. Adjustment disorder with anxious mood.

Correct Answer: D. Other specified somatic symptom and related disorder.

Explanation: This patient does not have somatic symptom disorder but does have the cardinal feature of illness anxiety disorder: excessive, intrusive anxiety about having a serious medical illness. However, the course of her illness has been too brief (6 weeks) to qualify for a diagnosis of illness anxiety disorder. A "brief illness anxiety disorder" with duration of less than 6 months is best classified as an "other specified somatic symptom and related disorder." If the mammogram was equivocal and the patient was anxious while awaiting further consultation and workup, clinical judgment might not label her anxiety "excessive," and a diagnosis of adjustment disorder with anxious mood might better apply. When a diagnosis of "other specified somatic symptom and related disorder" is made, the clinician should specify the reason that criteria for a specific disorder are not met; in this example, the specifier might be "illness anxiety of less than 6 months' duration."

9.21—Other Specified Somatic Symptom and Related Disorder (p. 327)

9.22   After finding a breast lump, a 53-year-old woman with a family history of breast cancer is overwhelmed by feelings of anxiety. Consultation with a breast surgeon, mammogram, and biopsy show the lump to be benign. The surgeon indicates that she requires no treatment; however, she continues to ruminate about the possibility of cancer and surgery that will result in disfigurement. Her sleep is restless and she is having trouble concentrating at work. After 6 weeks in this state, her primary physician requests that she consult a psychiatrist. On initial evaluation the patient weeps throughout the interview, and is so distraught that the evaluator is unable to elicit details of her medical and psychiatric history beyond reviewing the current "crisis." Which diagnosis best fits this presentation?

A. Somatic symptom disorder.
B. Illness anxiety disorder.
C. Unspecified somatic symptom and related disorder.
D. Other specified somatic symptom and related disorder.
E. Adjustment disorder with anxious mood.

Correct Answer: C. Unspecified somatic symptom and related disorder.

Explanation: This vignette can be contrasted with the one presented in question 9.21 above. The patient has the cardinal feature of illness anxiety disorder:

excessive, intrusive anxiety about having a serious medical illness; however, in this case, because the patient's emotional state has precluded sufficient history-gathering, the psychiatric evaluation does not provide sufficient data to determine whether she meets the full criteria for illness anxiety disorder or better fulfills criteria for another diagnosis. In contrast to the "other specified somatic symptom and related disorder" category, the "unspecified" category should be used when insufficient data are available or when the clinician chooses not to specify why the criteria for a specific diagnosis are not met.

9.22—Unspecified Somatic Symptom and Related Disorder (p. 327)

CHAPTER 10

Feeding and Eating Disorders

10.1   Which DSM-5 diagnosis replaced the DSM-IV diagnosis of feeding disorder of infancy or early childhood?

A. Anorexia nervosa.
B. Unspecified feeding or eating disorder.
C. Anorexia nervosa of early childhood.
D. Avoidant/restrictive food intake disorder.
E. Pica.

Correct Answer: D. Avoidant/restrictive food intake disorder.

Explanation: Because of the elimination of the DSM-IV chapter "Disorders Usually First Diagnosed During Infancy, Childhood, or Adolescence," the DSM-5 Feeding and Eating Disorders chapter describes several disorders found in the DSM-IV section "Feeding and Eating Disorders of Infancy or Early Childhood," such as *pica* and *rumination disorder.* The DSM-IV category *feeding disorder of infancy or early childhood* has been renamed *avoidant/restrictive food intake disorder,* and the criteria are significantly expanded.

10.1—Appendix / Highlights of Changes From DSM-IV to DSM-5 (p. 813)

10.2   Which of the following statements about DSM-5 changes in the diagnostic criteria for anorexia nervosa is *true?*

A. The requirement for menorrhagia has been eliminated.
B. The requirement for amenorrhea has been eliminated.
C. The requirements for amenorrhea and menorrhagia have been eliminated.
D. Low body weight is no longer required.
E. Developmental stage is no longer a significant issue.

Correct Answer: B. The requirement for amenorrhea has been eliminated.

Explanation: The core diagnostic criteria for anorexia nervosa are conceptually unchanged from DSM-IV with one exception: the requirement for amenorrhea is eliminated. As in DSM-IV, individuals with this disorder are required by Criterion A to be at a significantly low body weight for their developmental stage.

The wording of the criterion is changed for clarification, and guidance regarding how to judge whether an individual is at or below a significantly low weight is provided in the text. In DSM-5, Criterion B is expanded to include not only overtly expressed fear of weight gain but also persistent behavior that interferes with weight gain.

10.2—Appendix / Highlights of Changes From DSM-IV to DSM-5 (p. 813)

10.3 Which of the following statements about DSM-5 changes in the diagnostic criteria for bulimia nervosa is *true?*

    A. There is an increase in the required numbers of binge-eating episodes and inappropriate compensatory behaviors per week, from twice to three times weekly.
    B. There is an increase in the numbers of episodes of using ipecac or vomiting per week, from three to four.
    C. There is a reduction in the required minimum frequency of binge eating and inappropriate compensatory behavior frequency, from twice to once weekly.
    D. There is a requirement for an episode of pica, at least once in the last year.
    E. There is a requirement for electrolyte imbalances to be demonstrated at least twice in the past 2 years.

Correct Answer: C. There is a reduction in the required minimum frequency of binge eating and inappropriate compensatory behavior frequency, from twice to once weekly.

Explanation: The only change in the DSM-IV criteria for bulimia nervosa is a reduction in the required minimum average frequency of binge eating and inappropriate compensatory behavior frequency from twice to once weekly.

10.3—Appendix / Highlights of Changes From DSM-IV to DSM-5 (p. 813)

10.4 What is the minimum average frequency of binge eating required for a diagnosis of DSM-5 binge-eating disorder?

    A. Once weekly for the last 3 months.
    B. Once weekly for the last 4 months.
    C. Every other week for the last 3 months.
    D. Every other week for the last 4 months.
    E. Once a month for the last 3 months.

Correct Answer: A. Once weekly for the last 3 months.

Explanation: Binge eating is reliably associated with obesity and overweight status in individuals who seek treatment. The extensive research that followed the promulgation of preliminary criteria for binge-eating disorder in Appendix

B of DSM-IV documented the clinical utility and validity of binge-eating disorder. The only significant difference from the preliminary criteria is that the minimum average frequency of binge eating required for diagnosis is once weekly over the last 3 months, which is identical to the frequency criterion for bulimia nervosa (rather than at least 2 days a week for 6 months in DSM-IV).

10.4—Appendix / Highlights of Changes From DSM-IV to DSM-5 (p. 813)

10.5 In avoidant/restrictive food intake disorder, the eating or feeding disturbance is manifested by persistent failure to meet appropriate nutritional and/or energy needs associated with one or more of four specified features. Which of the following options correctly lists these four features?

   A. Manic or hypomanic symptoms; ruminative behaviors; compulsive thoughts; marked interference with psychosocial functioning.
   B. Significant weight loss; significant nutritional deficiency; dependence on enteral feeding or oral nutritional supplements; marked interference with psychosocial functioning.
   C. Significant weight loss; ruminative behaviors; delusions or hallucinations; manic or hypomanic symptoms.
   D. Significant nutritional deficiency; increased use of alcohol or other substances; manic or hypomanic symptoms; delusions or hallucinations.
   E. Dependence on enteral feeding or oral nutritional supplements; ruminative behaviors; delusions or hallucinations; manic or hypomanic symptoms.

Correct Answer: B. Significant weight loss; significant nutritional deficiency; dependence on enteral feeding or oral nutritional supplements; marked interference with psychosocial functioning.

Explanation: Avoidant/restrictive food intake disorder replaces and extends the DSM-IV diagnosis of feeding disorder of infancy or early childhood. The main diagnostic feature of avoidant/restrictive food intake disorder is avoidance or restriction of food intake (Criterion A) manifested by clinically significant failure to meet requirements for nutrition or insufficient energy intake through oral intake of food. One or more of the following key features must be present: significant weight loss, significant nutritional deficiency (or related health impact), dependence on enteral feeding or oral nutritional supplements, or marked interference with psychosocial functioning. The determination of whether weight loss is significant (Criterion A1) is a clinical judgment; instead of losing weight, children and adolescents who have not completed growth may not maintain weight or height increases along their developmental trajectory.

Determination of significant nutritional deficiency (Criterion A2) is also based on clinical assessment (e.g., assessment of dietary intake, physical examination, and laboratory testing). In severe cases, particularly in infants, malnutrition can be life threatening. "Dependence" on enteral feeding or oral nutritional supplements (Criterion A3) means that supplementary feeding is required to sustain adequate intake. Examples of individuals requiring supplementary feeding include infants with failure to thrive who require nasogastric tube feeding, children with neurodevelopmental disorders who are dependent on nutritionally complete supplements, and individuals who rely on gastrostomy tube feeding or complete oral nutrition supplements in the absence of an underlying medical condition.

10.5—Avoidant/Restrictive Food Intake Disorder / Diagnostic Features (pp. 234–235)

10.6   Which of the following statements about onset and prevalence of avoidant/restrictive food intake disorder is *true*?

A. The disorder occurs mostly in females, with onset typically in older adolescence.
B. The disorder occurs mostly in males, with onset typically in early childhood.
C. The disorder is more common in childhood and more common in females than in males.
D. The disorder is more common in childhood and equally common in males and females.
E. The disorder is extremely common in elderly adults, who often manifest an age-related reduction in intake.

Correct Answer: D. The disorder is more common in childhood and equally common in males and females.

Explanation: Avoidant/restrictive food intake disorder is equally common in males and females in infancy and early childhood. The disorder manifests more commonly in children than in adults, and there may be a long delay between onset and clinical presentation. Avoidant/restrictive food intake disorder does not include avoidance or restriction of food intake related to lack of availability of food or to cultural practices (e.g., religious fasting or normal dieting) (Criterion B), nor does it include developmentally normal behaviors (e.g., picky eating in toddlers, reduced intake in older adults).

10.6—Avoidant/Restrictive Food Intake Disorder / Diagnostic Features (pp. 334–335)

10.7   A 45-year-old woman had a choking episode 3 years ago after eating salad. Since that time she has been afraid to eat a wide range of foods, fearing that she will choke. This fear has affected her functionality and her ability to eat out with friends and has contributed to weight loss. Which diagnosis best fits this clinical picture?

A. Bulimia nervosa.
B. Schizophrenia.
C. Avoidant/restrictive food intake disorder.

D. Binge-eating disorder.

E. Adjustment disorder.

Correct Answer: C. Avoidant/restrictive food intake disorder.

Explanation: Food avoidance or restriction may also represent a conditioned negative response associated with food intake following, or in anticipation of, an aversive experience, such as choking; a traumatic investigation, usually involving the gastrointestinal tract (e.g., esophagoscopy); or repeated vomiting. The terms *functional dysphagia* and *globus hystericus* have also been used for such conditions.

10.7—Avoidant/Restrictive Food Intake Disorder / Diagnostic Features (p. 335)

10.8 What are the two subtypes of anorexia nervosa?

A. Restricting type and binge-eating/purging type.

B. Energy-sparing type and binge-eating/purging type.

C. Low-calorie/low-carbohydrate type and restricting type.

D. Low-carbohydrate/low-fat type and restricting type.

E. Restricting type and low-weight type.

Correct Answer: A. Restricting type and binge-eating/purging type.

Explanation: The subtype specifiers describe the primary mode of weight loss used for the past 3 months. In the restricting subtype of anorexia nervosa, weight loss is accomplished primarily through dieting, fasting, and/or excessive exercise; in the binge-eating/purging subtype, it is accomplished through recurrent episodes of binge eating or purging behavior (i.e., self-induced vomiting or the misuse of laxatives, diuretics, or enemas).

Most individuals with the binge-eating/purging type of anorexia nervosa who binge eat also purge through self-induced vomiting or the misuse of laxatives, diuretics, or enemas. Some individuals with this subtype of anorexia nervosa do not binge eat but do regularly purge after the consumption of small amounts of food. Crossover between the subtypes over the course of the disorder is not uncommon; therefore, subtype description should be used to describe current symptoms rather than longitudinal course.

10.8—Anorexia Nervosa / diagnostic criteria; Subtypes (p. 339)

10.9 What are the three essential diagnostic features of anorexia nervosa?

A. Persistently low self-confidence, intense fear of becoming fat, and disturbance in motivation.

B. Low self-esteem, disturbance in self-perceived weight or shape, and persistent energy restriction.

C. Restricted affect, disturbance in motivation, and low calorie intake.

D. Persistent restriction of energy intake, intense fear of becoming fat, and disturbance in self-perceived weight or shape.

E. Persistent lack of weight gain, disturbance in motivation, and restricted affect.

Correct Answer: D. Persistent restriction of energy intake, intense fear of becoming fat, and disturbance in self-perceived weight or shape.

Explanation: There are three essential features of anorexia nervosa: persistent energy intake restriction; intense fear of gaining weight or of becoming fat, or persistent behavior that interferes with weight gain; and a disturbance in self-perceived weight or shape.

10.9—Anorexia Nervosa / Diagnostic Features (p. 239)

10.10 What laboratory abnormalities are commonly found in individuals with anorexia nervosa?

A. Elevated blood urea nitrogen (BUN); low triiodothyronine (T_3); hyperadrenocorticism; low serum estrogen (females) or testosterone (males); bradycardia; low bone mineral density.

B. Low BUN; hypercholesterolemia; high thyroxine (T_4); hypoadrenocorticism; short QTc; low bone mineral density.

C. Blast cells; thrombocytosis; hyperphosphatemia; hypoamylasemia; high serum estrogen (females) or testosterone (males).

D. Hyperzincemia; hypermagnesemia; hyperchloremia; hyperkalemia.

E. C and D.

Correct Answer: A. Elevated blood urea nitrogen (BUN); low triiodothyronine (T_3); hyperadrenocorticism; low serum estrogen (females) or testosterone (males); bradycardia; low bone mineral density.

Explanation: Individuals with anorexia nervosa may have dehydration, reflected by elevated BUN levels. They may be cachectic and semistarved, reflected in other abnormal laboratory indices such as hypozincemia and hypophosphatemia. Purging, vomiting, and use of laxatives may lead to metabolic alkalosis, hypochloremia, and hypokalemia.

10.10—Anorexia Nervosa / Diagnostic Markers (pp. 342–343)

10.11 A 27-year-old graduate student has a 10-year history of anorexia nervosa. Her boyfriend is quite concerned because she has extreme fears related to cleanliness. She washes her hands more than 12 times a day and is excessively worried about contamination. What would be the best decision by the mental health professional at this point regarding these symptoms?

A. Assume that the patient's obsessive-compulsive symptoms are related to her anorexia nervosa.
B. Further evaluate the obsessive-compulsive features, because if they are not related to anorexia nervosa, a new diagnosis of obsessive-compulsive disorder might be warranted.
C. Ask the patient to wait 1 year and see how this evolves.
D. Make a diagnosis of body dysmorphic disorder.
E. Refer the patient for a colonoscopy.

Correct Answer: B. Further evaluate the obsessive-compulsive features, because if they are not related to anorexia nervosa, a new diagnosis of obsessive-compulsive disorder might be warranted.

Explanation: Obsessive-compulsive features, both related and unrelated to food, are often prominent in anorexia nervosa. Most individuals with anorexia nervosa are preoccupied with thoughts of food. Some collect recipes or hoard food. Observations of behaviors associated with other forms of starvation suggest that obsessions and compulsions related to food may be exacerbated by undernutrition. When individuals with anorexia nervosa exhibit obsessions and compulsions that are not related to food, body shape, or weight, an additional diagnosis of obsessive-compulsive disorder may be warranted

10.11—Anorexia Nervosa / Associated Features Supporting Diagnosis (p. 341)

10.12 What are the three essential diagnostic features of bulimia nervosa?

A. Recurrent episodes of binge eating; recurrent inappropriate compensatory behaviors to prevent weight gain; self-evaluation that is unduly influenced by body shape and weight.
B. Recurrent restriction of food; self-evaluation that is unduly influenced by body shape and weight; mood instability.
C. Delusions regarding body habitus; obsessional focus on food; recurrent purging.
D. Hypomanic symptoms for 1 month; mood instability; self-evaluation that is unduly influenced by body shape and weight.
E. Self-evaluation that is unduly influenced by body shape and weight; history of anorexia nervosa; recurrent inappropriate compensatory behaviors to gain weight.

Correct Answer: A. Recurrent episodes of binge eating; recurrent inappropriate compensatory behaviors to prevent weight gain; self-evaluation that is unduly influenced by body shape and weight.

Explanation: There are three essential features of bulimia nervosa: recurrent episodes of binge eating, recurrent inappropriate compensatory behaviors to prevent weight gain, and self-evaluation that is unduly influenced by body shape and weight. To qualify for the diagnosis, the binge eating and inappropriate compensatory behaviors must occur, on average, at least once per week for 3 months. An "episode of binge eating" is defined as eating, in a discrete period of time, an amount of food that is definitely larger than most individuals would eat in a similar period of time under similar circumstances.

10.12—Bulimia Nervosa / Diagnostic Features (p. 345)

10.13 What are the subtypes of bulimia nervosa?

A. Restrictive.
B. Purging.
C. Restrictive and purging.
D. None.
E. With normal weight/abnormal weight.

Correct Answer: D. None.

Explanation: There are no subtypes for bulimia nervosa in DSM-5.

10.13—Bulimia Nervosa / diagnostic criteria (p. 345)

10.14 What minimum average frequency of binge eating is required to qualify for a diagnosis of binge-eating disorder?

A. At least once a week for 3 months.
B. At least twice a week for 3 months.
C. At least once a week for 6 months.
D. At least twice a week for 6 months.
E. None of the above.

Correct Answer: A. At least once a week for 3 months.

Explanation: The essential feature of binge-eating disorder is recurrent episodes of binge eating that must occur, on average, at least once per week for 3 months. An "episode of binge eating" is defined as eating, in a discrete period of time, an amount of food that is definitely larger than most people would eat in a similar period of time under similar circumstances.

10.14—Binge-Eating Disorder / Diagnostic Features (pp. 350–351)

CHAPTER 1 1

Elimination Disorders

11.1   A 7-year-old boy with mild to moderate developmental delay presents with a chronic history of wetting his clothes during the day about once weekly, even during school. He is now refusing to go to school for fear of wetting his pants and being ridiculed by his classmates. Which of the following statements accurately describes the diagnostic options regarding enuresis in this case?

   A. He should not be diagnosed with enuresis because the frequency is less than twice per week.
   B. He should be diagnosed with enuresis because the incontinence is resulting in impairment of age-appropriate role functioning.
   C. He should not be diagnosed with enuresis because his mental age is likely less than 5 years old.
   D. He should be diagnosed with enuresis, diurnal only subtype.
   E. He should not be diagnosed with enuresis because the events are restricted to the daytime.

   Correct Answer: C. He should not be diagnosed with enuresis because his mental age is likely less than 5 years old.

   Explanation: Criterion C requires than an individual be of an age in which consistent continence can be reasonably expected. While this is ordinarily at age 5, in the case of developmental delay one goes by the child's mental age. In this vignette it is likely that the child has not yet attained a mental age of 5 and is ineligible for the diagnosis even though he has clinically significant distress. Criterion B requires that the incontinence be clinically significant, and this condition can be met by the frequency/duration requirement of twice weekly for 3 months, or by the fact that it causes clinically significant distress. In this vignette the latter condition is fulfilled (because the child has clinically significant distress) and so Criterion B is met, and would not be a reason to withhold the diagnosis. Although the general public may think of nighttime incontinence as a central aspect, enuresis can present as, and can be specified as, nocturnal only, diurnal only, or nocturnal and diurnal (i.e., combined presentation).

   11.1—Enuresis / diagnostic criteria (p. 355)

11.2   Which of the following statements about enuresis is *true?*

A. Over 60% of children diagnosed with enuresis have a comorbid DSM-5 disorder.
B. Developmental delays are no more common in children with enuresis than in other children.
C. Urinary tract infections are more common in children with enuresis.
D. While embarrassing, enuresis has no effect on children's self-esteem.
E. Prevalence rates for enuresis at age 10 are similar to those at age 5.

Correct Answer: C. Urinary tract infections are more common in children with enuresis.

Explanation: Urinary tract infections are more common in children with enuresis. Although most children with enuresis do not have a comorbid DSM-5 diagnosis, those with enuresis do have higher rates of behavioral problems such as developmental delays. Children with enuresis often present with significant self-esteem issues. The prevalence of enuresis declines with older age.

11.2—Enuresis / Prevalence; Functional Consequences of Enuresis; Comorbidity (pp. 356–357)

11.3 Which of the following statements about the diurnal-only subtype of enuresis is *true?*

A. This subtype is more common in males.
B. This subtype is more common after age 9 years.
C. This subtype is sometimes referred to as *monosymptomatic enuresis.*
D. This subtype is more common than the nocturnal-only subtype.
E. This subtype includes a subgroup of individuals with "voiding postponement," in which micturition is consciously deferred because of a social reluctance to use the bathroom or to interrupt a play activity.

Correct Answer: E. This subtype includes a subgroup of individuals with "voiding postponement," in which micturition is consciously deferred because of a social reluctance to use the bathroom or to interrupt a play activity.

Explanation: The diurnal-only subtype of enuresis involves incontinence only during the day and is also referred to as *urinary incontinence.* It is more common in females and is uncommon after age 9. In daytime (diurnal) enuresis, the child defers voiding until incontinence occurs, sometimes because of a reluctance to use the toilet as a result of social anxiety or a preoccupation with school or play activity. The enuretic event most commonly occurs in the early afternoon on school days and may be associated with symptoms of disruptive behavior.

11.3—Enuresis / Subtypes; Development and Course; Gender-Related Diagnostic Issues (pp. 355–357)

11.4   Which of the following statements correctly identifies a distinction between primary enuresis and secondary enuresis?

A. Secondary enuresis is due to an identified medical condition; primary enuresis has no known etiology.
B. Children with secondary enuresis have higher rates of psychiatric comorbidity than do children with primary enuresis.
C. Primary enuresis has a typical onset at age 10, much later than the onset of secondary enuresis.
D. Primary enuresis is never preceded by a period of continence, whereas secondary enuresis is always preceded by a period of continence.
E. Unlike primary enuresis, secondary enuresis tends to persist into late adolescence.

Correct Answer: D. Primary enuresis is never preceded by a period of continence, whereas secondary enuresis is always preceded by a period of continence.

Explanation: In primary enuresis, the individual has never established urinary continence; in secondary enuresis, incontinence develops after a period of established continence. By definition, primary incontinence begins when a child reaches the mental age of 5. Prior to this there is no expectation of consistent continence, and incontinence of urine is not considered pathological. After age 5, a child has either established continence and lost it or never developed continence, in which case the onset should be considered to be at age 5, regardless of age at presentation. Urinary incontinence secondary to another medical condition is not diagnosed as enuresis because Criterion D rules this out. Secondary enuresis is not associated with higher rates of psychiatric comorbidity, and both forms tend to disappear by late adolescence (when prevalence rates approach 1%).

11.4—Enuresis / Development and Course (p. 356)

11.5   Which of the following statements correctly describes factors related to the etiology and/or onset of enuresis?

A. Enuresis has been shown to be heritable, with a child being twice as likely to have the diagnosis if either parent has had it.
B. Mode of toilet training or its neglect can affect rates of enuresis, as shown by high rates seen in orphanages.
C. In girls with enuresis, nocturnal enuresis is the more common form.
D. Rates of enuresis are much higher in European countries than in developing countries.
E. The development of modern diapers is believed to speed toilet training and reduce enuresis.

Correct Answer: B. Mode of toilet training or its neglect can affect rates of enuresis, as shown by high rates seen in orphanages.

Explanation: Enuresis has etiological sources in both genetics and learned behaviors. There are very high rates of enuresis in orphanages and other residential institutions, likely related to the mode and environment in which toilet training occurs. Heritability has been shown in family, twin, and segregation analyses. The relative risk of having a child who develops enuresis is greater for previously enuretic fathers (odds ratio of 10.1) than for previously enuretic mothers (odds ratio of 3.6). Nocturnal enuresis is more common in males; diurnal incontinence is more common in females. Enuresis has been reported in a variety of European, African, and Asian countries as well as in the United States. At a national level, prevalence rates are remarkably similar, and there is great similarity in the developmental trajectories found in different countries.

11.5—Enuresis / Risk and Prognostic Factors; Culture-Related Diagnostic Issues; Gender-Related Diagnostic Issues (pp. 356–357)

11.6   A 6-year-old boy with mild to moderate developmental delay presents with a history of passing feces into his underwear during the day about once every 2 weeks, even during school. He is now refusing to go to school for fear of soiling his pants and being ridiculed by his classmates. Which of the following statements accurately describes the diagnostic options regarding encopresis in this case?

A. He should not be diagnosed with encopresis because the frequency is less than twice per week.
B. He should be diagnosed with encopresis because the incontinence is resulting in impairment of age-appropriate role functioning.
C. He should not be diagnosed with encopresis because his mental age is likely less than 4 years old.
D. He should be diagnosed with encopresis.
E. He should not be diagnosed with encopresis because the events are restricted to the daytime.

Correct Answer: C. He should not be diagnosed with encopresis because his mental age is likely less than 4 years old.

Explanation: Criterion C requires than an individual be of an age in which consistent continence can be reasonably expected. Although this is ordinarily at age 4 years, in the case of developmental delay, one goes by the child's mental age. In this case it is likely that the child has not yet attained a mental age of 4 and is ineligible for the diagnoses even though he has clinically significant distress. Criterion B requires that the incontinence be clinically significant, and this condition can be met by the frequency/duration requirement of once monthly for 3 months. In this case, the child has sufficient frequency, and so

Criterion B is met, and would not be a reason to withhold the diagnosis. Unlike enuresis, encopresis has no specification regarding time of day.

11.6—Encopresis / diagnostic criteria (pp. 357–358)

11.7   Which of the following statements about encopresis is *true?*

A. When oppositional defiant disorder or conduct disorder is present, one cannot diagnose encopresis.
B. When constipation is present, one cannot diagnose encopresis.
C. Urinary tract infections can be comorbid with encopresis and are more common in girls.
D. Although it is embarrassing, encopresis has no effect on children's self-esteem.
E. Prevalence rates for encopresis at age 5 are estimated to be 5%.

Correct Answer: C. Urinary tract infections can be comorbid with encopresis and are more common in girls.

Explanation: Urinary tract infections are more common in children with encopresis. Although most children with encopresis do not have a comorbid DSM-5 diagnosis, those with encopresis do have higher rates of behavioral problems such as developmental delays. Children with encopresis often present with significant self-esteem issues. The prevalence of encopresis declines with older age. When the passage of feces is involuntary rather than intentional, it is often related to constipation, impaction, and retention with subsequent overflow. Smearing feces may be deliberate or accidental, resulting from the child's attempt to clean or hide feces that were passed involuntarily. When the incontinence is clearly deliberate, features of oppositional defiant disorder or conduct disorder may also be present.

11.7—Encopresis / Prevalence; Comorbidity (p. 359)

11.8   Which of the following statements correctly describes clinical aspects of the diagnosis of encopresis?

A. Encopresis with constipation and overflow incontinence is often involuntary.
B. Encopresis with constipation and overflow incontinence always involves well-formed stool.
C. Encopresis with constipation and overflow incontinence cannot be diagnosed if the behavior results from avoidance of defecation that develops for psychological reasons.
D. In encopresis with constipation and overflow incontinence, leakage usually occurs during sleep.

E. Encopresis with constipation and overflow incontinence rarely resolves after treatment of the constipation.

Correct Answer: A. Encopresis with constipation and overflow incontinence is often involuntary.

Explanation: When the passage of feces is involuntary rather than intentional, it is often related to constipation, impaction, and retention with subsequent overflow. The constipation may develop for psychological reasons (e.g., anxiety about defecating in a particular place, a more general pattern of anxious or oppositional behavior), leading to avoidance of defecation.

Feces in the *with constipation and overflow incontinence subtype* are characteristically (but not invariably) poorly formed, and leakage can be infrequent to continuous, occurring mostly during the day and rarely during sleep. Only part of the feces is passed during toileting, and the incontinence resolves after treatment of the constipation. In the *without constipation and overflow incontinence subtype*, feces are likely to be of normal form and consistency, and soiling is intermittent. Feces may be deposited in a prominent location. This is usually associated with the presence of oppositional defiant disorder or conduct disorder or may be the consequence of anal masturbation. Soiling without constipation appears to be less common than soiling with constipation.

Smearing feces may be deliberate or accidental, resulting from the child's attempt to clean or hide feces that were passed involuntarily. When the incontinence is clearly deliberate, features of oppositional defiant disorder or conduct disorder may also be present.

11.8—Encopresis / Subtypes; Diagnostic Features; Associated Features Supporting Diagnosis (pp. 358–359)

CHAPTER 12

Sleep-Wake Disorders

12.1   Which of the following is a core feature of insomnia disorder?

A. Depressed mood.
B. Dissatisfaction with sleep quantity or quality.
C. Cognitive impairment.
D. Abnormal behaviors during sleep.
E. Daytime fatigue.

Correct Answer: B. Dissatisfaction with sleep quantity or quality.

Explanation: Individuals with insomnia disorder typically present with sleep-wake complaints of dissatisfaction regarding the quality, timing, or amount of sleep. Resulting distress and impairment are core features.

12.1—Insomnia Disorder / diagnostic criteria (p. 362)

12.2   Which of the following is necessary to make a diagnosis of insomnia disorder?

A. Difficulty being fully awake after awakening.
B. Difficulty with sleep initiation or sleep maintenance, or early-morning awakening with inability to return to sleep.
C. Absence of a coexisting mental disorder.
D. Documented insufficient opportunity for sleep.
E. Persistence of sleep difficulties despite use of sedative-hypnotic agents.

Correct Answer: B. Difficulty with sleep initiation or sleep maintenance, or early-morning awakening with inability to return to sleep.

Explanation: The key features of insomnia disorder in DSM-5 are dissatisfaction with sleep quality, trouble initiating or maintaining sleep, or early-morning awakening or, in children, resistance to going to bed, and distress or impairment in daytime functioning, despite adequate opportunity to sleep, with the problem occurring frequently and persisting for at least 3 months. An important change from DSM-IV is the possibility of making an independent diagnosis of insomnia disorder even when another disorder such as major depressive disorder might include sleep disturbance as a diagnostic feature. In such a case, both diagnoses would be appropriate, and the comorbid psychiatric disorder listed as a clinical comorbid condition specifier (i.e., "With non–sleep disorder mental comorbidity").

12.2—Insomnia Disorder / diagnostic criteria (pp. 362–363)

12.3   An 80-year-old man has a history of myocardial infarction and had coronary artery bypass graft surgery 8 years ago. He plays tennis three times a week, takes care of his grandchildren 2 afternoons each week, generally enjoys life, and manages all of his activities of daily living independently; however, he complains of excessively early morning awakening. He goes to sleep at 9:00 P.M. and sleeps well, with nocturia once nightly, but wakes at 3:30 A.M. although he would like to rise at 5:00 A.M. He does not endorse daytime sleepiness as a problem. His physical examination, mental status, and cognitive function are normal. What is the most likely sleep-wake disorder diagnosis?

A. Insomnia disorder.
B. Rapid eye movement (REM) sleep behavior disorder.
C. Restless legs syndrome.
D. Obstructive sleep apnea hypopnea.
E. The man is a short sleeper, which is not a DSM-5 diagnosis.

Correct Answer: E. The man is a short sleeper, which is not a DSM-5 diagnosis.

Explanation: Although he complains about his sleep timing and endorses early awakening as a complaint, this man has no other features of impairment to justify a diagnosis of insomnia disorder. Many older adults are short sleepers. This man has no evidence of functional impairment such as excessive daytime sleepiness interfering with activities.

12.3—Insomnia Disorder / Differential Diagnosis (p. 367)

12.4   Which of the following symptoms is most likely to indicate the presence of hypersomnolence disorder?

A. Sleep inertia.
B. Nonrefreshing sleep in main sleep episode.
C. Automatic behavior.
D. Frequent napping.
E. Headache.

Correct Answer: A. Sleep inertia.

Explanation: Sleep inertia is a period of impaired performance and reduced vigilance, following waking from the main episode of sleep or from a nap that persists for several minutes or more. Although some patients with hypersomnolence disorder have one or more of the other symptoms listed, these symptoms are not as specific to hypersomnolence disorder as is sleep inertia.

12.4—Hypersomnolence Disorder / diagnostic criteria; Diagnostic Features (pp. 368–369)

12.5 An obese 52-year-old man complains of daytime sleepiness, and his partner confirms that he snores, snorts, and gasps during nighttime sleep. What polysomnographic finding is needed to confirm the diagnosis of obstructive sleep apnea hypopnea?

A. No polysomnography is necessary.
B. Polysomnographic evidence of at least 5 apnea or hypopnea episodes per hour of sleep.
C. Polysomnographic evidence of at least 10 apnea or hypopnea episodes per hour of sleep.
D. Polysomnographic evidence of at least 15 apnea or hypopnea episodes per hour of sleep.
E. Polysomnographic evidence of resolution of apneas/hypopneas with application of continuous positive airway pressure.

Correct Answer: B. Polysomnographic evidence of at least 5 apnea or hypopnea episodes per hour of sleep.

Explanation: The diagnostic criteria for obstructive sleep apnea hypopnea are as follows:

A. Either (1) or (2):

1. Evidence by polysomnography of at least five obstructive apneas or hypopneas per hour of sleep and either of the following sleep symptoms:
   a. Nocturnal breathing disturbances: snoring, snorting/gasping, or breathing pauses during sleep.
   b. Daytime sleepiness, fatigue, or unrefreshing sleep despite sufficient opportunities to sleep that is not better explained by another mental disorder (including a sleep disorder) and is not attributable to another medical condition.

2. Evidence by polysomnography of 15 or more obstructive apneas and/or hypopneas per hour of sleep regardless of accompanying symptoms.

12.5—Obstructive Sleep Apnea Hypopnea / diagnostic criteria (p. 378)

12.6 In addition to requiring recurrent sleep attacks, the diagnostic criteria for narcolepsy require the presence of cataplexy, hypocretin deficiency, *or* characteristic abnormalities on sleep polysomnography or multiple sleep latency testing. Which of the following is a defining characteristic of cataplexy?

A. It is sudden.
B. It is induced by suggestion.
C. It occurs unilaterally.
D. It persists for hours.
E. It is accompanied by hypertonia.

Correct Answer: A. It is sudden.

Explanation: The definition of cataplexy differs according to patient characteristics. In individuals with long-standing narcolepsy, cataplexy is defined as brief (seconds to minutes) episodes of sudden bilateral loss of muscle tone with maintained consciousness that are precipitated by laughter or joking. In children or in individuals within 6 months of onset, cataplexy takes the form of spontaneous grimaces or jaw-opening episodes with tongue thrusting or a global hypotonia, without any obvious emotional triggers.

12.6—Narcolepsy / diagnostic criteria (pp. 372–373)

12.7 In DSM-IV, the diagnosis of breathing-related sleep disorder would be given to an individual complaining of excessive daytime sleepiness, with nocturnal polysomnography demonstrating episodic loss of ventilatory effort and resulting apneic episodes occurring 10–20 times per hour, whose symptoms cannot be attributed to another mental disorder, a medication or substance, or another medical condition. What is the appropriate DSM-5 diagnosis for the same individual?

A. Insomnia disorder.
B. Narcolepsy.
C. Obstructive sleep apnea hypopnea.
D. Central sleep apnea.
E. Other specified hypersomnolence disorder.

Correct Answer: D. Central sleep apnea.

Explanation: The diagnosis of central sleep apnea is made on the basis of five or more central apneic episodes per hour on polysomnography and absence of another sleep disorder. Unlike DSM-IV, DSM-5 codes central and obstructive sleep apnea syndromes as different diagnoses within a larger group of breathing-related sleep disorders that also includes sleep-related hypoventilation. Central apneas are characterized by a loss of respiratory drive rather than by mechanical obstruction.

12.7—Central Sleep Apnea / Diagnostic Features (pp. 383–384)

12.8 Which of the following metabolic changes is the cardinal feature of sleep-related hypoventilation?

A. Insulin resistance.
B. Hypoxia.
C. Hypercapnia.
D. Low arterial hemoglobin oxygen saturation.
E. Elevated vasopressin.

Correct Answer: C. Hypercapnia.

Explanation: Sleep-related hypoventilation is diagnosed using polysomnography showing sleep-related hypoxemia and hypercapnia that is not better explained by another breathing-related sleep disorder. The documentation of increased arterial pCO_2 levels to greater than 55 mmHg during sleep or a 10 mmHg or greater increase in pCO_2 levels (to a level that also exceeds 50 mmHg) during sleep in comparison to awake supine values, for 10 minutes or longer, is the gold standard for diagnosis. However, obtaining arterial blood gas determinations during sleep is impractical, and noninvasive measures of pCO_2 have not been adequately validated during sleep and are not widely used during polysomnography in adults. Prolonged and sustained decreases in oxygen saturation (oxygen saturation of less than 90% for more than 5 minutes with a nadir of at least 85%, or oxygen saturation of less than 90% for at least 30% of sleep time) in the absence of evidence of upper airway obstruction are often used as an indication of sleep-related hypoventilation; however, this finding is not specific, as there are other potential causes of hypoxemia, such as that due to lung disease.

12.8—Sleep-Related Hypoventilation / Diagnostic Markers (p. 389)

12.9   A 51-year-old man presents with symptoms of chronic fatigue and excessive worrying about current life stressors. He has a strong family history of depression and a past history of a major depressive episode, with some improvement while maintained on antidepressants. On weekday nights, it takes him several hours to fall asleep, and he then has difficulty getting up to go to work in the morning, experiencing sleepiness for the first few hours of awake time. On weekends, he awakens later in the morning and feels less fatigue and sleepiness. Which of the following diagnoses apply?

A. Major depressive disorder, in partial remission.
B. Generalized anxiety disorder.
C. Insomnia disorder.
D. Major depressive disorder in partial remission and circadian rhythm sleep-wake disorder, delayed sleep phase type.
E. Major depressive disorder in partial remission; generalized anxiety disorder; circadian rhythm sleep-wake disorder, delayed sleep phase type; and insomnia disorder.

Correct Answer: D. Major depressive disorder in partial remission and circadian rhythm sleep-wake disorder, delayed sleep phase type.

Explanation: In this case, both diagnoses should be coded, even though insomnia can be considered as a symptom of major depressive disorder. Circadian rhythm sleep-wake disorder, delayed sleep phase type, is characterized by delayed onset (usually more than 2 hours) of the major sleep period in relation to the desired sleep and wake times appropriate to the individual's personal and occupational obligations, with resulting symptoms of tiredness and insomnia complaints. When allowed to set their own schedule, individuals with this condition have normal (for age) quality and quantity of sleep.

12.9—Circadian Rhythm Sleep-Wake Disorders / diagnostic criteria (pp. 390–391)

12.10 A 67-year-old woman complains of insomnia. She does not have trouble falling asleep between 10 and 11 P.M., but after 1–2 hours she awakens for several hours in the middle of the night, sleeps again for 2–4 hours in the early morning, and then naps three or four times during the day for 1–3 hours at a time. She has a family history of dementia. On exam she appears fatigued and has deficits in short-term memory, calculation, and abstraction. What is the most likely diagnosis?

A. Major neurocognitive disorder (NCD).
B. Circadian rhythm sleep-wake disorder, irregular sleep-wake type, and unspecified NCD.
C. Narcolepsy.
D. Insomnia disorder.
E. Major depressive disorder.

Correct Answer: B. Circadian rhythm sleep-wake disorder, irregular sleep-wake type, and unspecified NCD.

Explanation: The DSM-5 circadian rhythm sleep-wake disorders retained three of the DSM-IV subtypes—delayed sleep phase type, shift work type, and unspecified type—and expanded to include advanced sleep phase type and irregular sleep-wake type, whereas the jet lag type was removed. In this patient's presentation, there is no major sleep period and no discernible circadian rhythm to the sleep-wake cycle; her sleep is fragmented into five or six periods across the 24-hour day. *Irregular sleep-wake type* is commonly associated with NCDs, including major NCDs such as Alzheimer's disease, Parkinson's disease, and Huntington's disease, as well as NCDs in children. Insufficient data are provided to justify a diagnosis of major NCD or depression. This woman does not have narcolepsy, which is characterized by frequent irresistible urges to sleep, but also requires the presence of at least one of the following: 1) cataplexy, 2) hypocretin deficiency, or 3) characteristic abnormalities on nocturnal polysomnography or multiple sleep latency testing.

12.10—Circadian Rhythm Sleep-Wake Disorders / Irregular Sleep-Wake Type (pp. 394–395); Narcolepsy / diagnostic criteria (pp. 372–373)

12.11 Following a traumatic brain injury resulting in blindness, a 50-year-old man develops waxing and waning daytime sleepiness interfering with daytime activity. Serial actigraphy (a method of measuring human activity/rest cycles) demonstrates that the time of onset of the major sleep period occurs progressively later day after day, with a normal duration of the major sleep period. What is the most likely diagnosis?

A. Circadian rhythm sleep-wake disorder, unspecified type.
B. Circadian rhythm sleep-wake disorder, delayed sleep phase type.
C. Circadian rhythm sleep-wake disorder, non-24-hour sleep-wake type.
D. Pineal gland injury.
E. Malingering.

Correct Answer: C. Circadian rhythm sleep-wake disorder, non-24-hour sleep-wake type.

Explanation: Non-24-hour sleep-wake type circadian rhythm sleep disorder is common in individuals with blindness. The endogenous sleep-wake cycle is longer than 24 hours and is not entrained by light cues, resulting in onset of sleepiness at later and later times of day. When the onset of sleepiness occurs at night, there is low interference with normal daytime activities; however, as the onset of sleepiness cycles toward the daytime hours there is greater impairment in social-occupational function. In DSM-IV, this disorder was included in the "unspecified" type of circadian rhythm sleep disorder.

12.11—Circadian Rhythm Sleep-Wake Disorders / Diagnostic Features (p. 396)

12.12 A 50-year-old emergency department nurse complains of sleepiness at work interfering with her ability to function. She recently switched from the 7 A.M.– 4 P.M. day shift to the 11 P.M.–8 A.M. night shift in order to have her afternoons free. Even with this schedule change, she finds it difficult to sleep in the mornings at home, has little energy for recreational activities or household chores in the afternoon, and feels exhausted by the middle of her overnight shift. What is the most likely diagnosis?

A. Normal variation in sleep secondary to shift work.
B. Circadian rhythm sleep-wake disorder, shift work type.
C. Bipolar disorder.
D. Insomnia disorder.
E. Hypersomnolence disorder.

Correct Answer: B. Circadian rhythm sleep-wake disorder, shift work type.

Explanation: The criteria for circadian rhythm sleep-wake disorder, shift work type, are a gradual reversion from conventional daylight hours as the main period of occupational engagement, difficulty sleeping in the day, and sleepiness at night during the work shift. The daylight sleeping problem might be mistaken for insomnia and the work shift sleepiness problem for hypersomnolence, but the presence of both symptoms in this context clarifies the diagnosis. The daytime and nighttime symptoms must be clinically significant in terms of distress or impairment in function, which is largely a clinical judgment, and the boundary between normal variation in sleep and sleepiness due to shift work versus the shift work type of circadian rhythm sleep-wake disorder is not sharply demarcated. Bipolar disorder may be destabilized by shift work that interferes with stable circadian rhythms and adequate sleep at nighttime, but mania resulting from such destabilization does not generally manifest as complaints of sleepiness or insomnia.

12.12—Circadian Rhythm Sleep-Wake Disorders / Shift Work Type (pp. 397–398)

12.13 A 14-year-old girl frequently wakes in the morning with clear recollection of very frightening dreams. Once she awakens, she is normally alert and oriented, but the dreams are a persistent source of distress. Her mother reports that the girl sometimes murmurs or groans but does not talk or move during the period before waking. Her history is otherwise notable for having been homeless and living with her mother in a series of temporary shelter accommodations for 1 year when she was 10 years old. What is the most likely diagnosis?

A. Unspecified anxiety disorder.
B. Rapid eye movement (REM) sleep behavior disorder.
C. Non–rapid eye movement sleep arousal disorders.
D. Posttraumatic stress disorder.
E. Nightmare disorder.

Correct Answer: E. Nightmare disorder.

Explanation: Nightmare disorder is characterized by repeated nightmares, which are extended, dysphoric, and well-remembered dreams occurring mostly in the second half of the major sleep episode and which usually involve threats to one's survival, security, or physical integrity. On awakening, the affected individual returns quickly to a normal level of consciousness with normal orientation, but the dreams cause persistent distress and/or impairment in function. Coexisting medical and mental disorders do not adequately explain the predominant complaint of dysphoric dreams. In children, nightmare disorder occurs most often after exposure to severe psychosocial stressors. Nightmares occur during REM sleep, when skeletal muscle tone decreases, so vocalization and body movement does not occur, except possibly at the very end of the REM sleep period. Nightmare disorder is common in childhood, and may continue to occur in women into adulthood, but is less common in men in adulthood. In contrast to nightmares, sleep terrors are associated with non-REM deep-stage sleep, generally occur earlier in the major sleep period, and are characterized by poor recall, only partial arousal, and confusion and disorientation at the end of the terror event. Amnesia for the event is common after the end of the sleep period. REM sleep behavior disorder is characterized by violent dream enactment or other complex motor behavior during sleep, and it is most common in middle-aged or older, male patients. Nightmares can occur in posttraumatic stress disorder (PTSD) as part of the "reexperiencing" phenomena but are insufficient alone to make a diagnosis of PTSD.

12.13—Non–Rapid Eye Movement Sleep Arousal Disorders / diagnostic criteria (p. 399); Nightmare Disorder / diagnostic criteria (p. 404); Rapid Eye Movement Sleep Behavior Disorder / diagnostic criteria (pp. 407–408)

12.14 Which of the following is a type of non–rapid eye movement (REM) sleep arousal disorder in DSM-5?

A. REM sleep behavior disorder.
B. Sleep terrors.
C. Nightmare disorder.
D. Fugue.
E. Obstructive sleep apnea hypopnea.

Correct Answer: B. Sleep terrors.

Explanation: DSM-5 includes sleep terrors and sleepwalking in the diagnostic category of non-REM sleep arousal disorders. *Sleep terrors* are associated with a sense of terror and distress, but with incomplete awakening and poor recall, and they tend to occur early in the major sleep period, when non-REM sleep predominates. *REM sleep behavior disorder* episodes occur in REM sleep, which is predominantly in the later part of the sleep episode, with complex behaviors that are often recalled as "acting out" of a dream, sometimes violently. Nightmares are also a REM sleep phenomenon. Patients with *nightmare disorder* awaken and rapidly reorient and achieve full alertness, in contrast to those with sleep terrors. *Fugue* states are not sleep disorders.

12.14—Non–Rapid Eye Movement Sleep Arousal Disorders / diagnostic criteria (p. 399)

12.15 Which of the following is a specific subtype of non–rapid eye movement sleep arousal disorder, sleepwalking type?

A. Rapid eye movement (REM) sleep behavior disorder.
B. Sleep-related seizure disorder.
C. Sleep-related sexual behavior (sexsomnia).
D. Complex motor behavior during alcoholic blackout.
E. Nocturnal panic attack.

Correct Answer: C. Sleep-related sexual behavior (sexsomnia).

Explanation: The essential feature of sleepwalking is repeated episodes of complex motor behavior initiated during sleep, including rising from bed and walking about. Sleep-related sexual behavior and sleep-related eating are recognized as specific subtypes. Sleepwalking arises in non-REM sleep, not during REM sleep. Sleepwalking episodes can begin with a confusional arousal but progress to more complex motor behaviors and ambulation. Alcoholic blackouts do not occur during sleep or unconsciousness but involve loss of memory for events during the drinking episode. Sleep-related seizures are in the differential diagnosis of non-REM sleep arousal disorders but tend to be more stereotypic rather than complex motor behaviors.

12.15—Non–Rapid Eye Movement Sleep Arousal Disorders / diagnostic criteria; Diagnostic Features (pp. 399–400)

12.16 What is the difference between sleep terrors and nightmare disorder?

A. In nightmare disorder, arousal or awakening from the nightmare is incomplete, whereas sleep terrors result in complete awakening.
B. In sleep terrors, episodes are concentrated in the final hours of the sleep period, whereas nightmares occur mostly early in the sleep period.
C. Sleep terrors are characterized by clear recall of vivid dreams with frightening content, whereas nightmares are not recalled.
D. Sleep terrors occur during rapid eye movement (REM) sleep, whereas nightmares occur in non-REM sleep.
E. Sleep terrors are precipitous but incomplete awakenings from sleep beginning with a panicky scream or cry, with little recall, whereas nightmares are characterized by full arousal and vivid recall.

Correct Answer: E. Sleep terrors are precipitous but incomplete awakenings from sleep beginning with a panicky scream or cry, with little recall, whereas nightmares are characterized by full arousal and vivid recall.

Explanation: Sleep terrors are a non-REM sleep phenomenon and therefore tend to occur in the early period of sleep when non-REM sleep predominates; autonomic arousal, fearful crying out, incomplete awakening, and little recall or total amnesia characterize the episodes. Nightmares are REM sleep phenomena and therefore tend to be more prominent in the later part of the sleep period, and may be vividly recalled. Arousal after a nightmare tends to be to full consciousness.

12.16—Nightmare Disorder / diagnostic criteria (p. 404)

12.17 What is the key abnormality in sleep physiology in rapid eye movement (REM) sleep behavior disorder?

A. REM starts earlier than normal in the sleep cycle.
B. There is more REM sleep than normal.
C. Delta wave activity is increased.
D. Skeletal muscle tone is preserved during REM sleep.
E. Total sleep time is greater than normal.

Correct Answer: D. Skeletal muscle tone is preserved during REM sleep.

Explanation: REM sleep without atonia is a sine qua non for the diagnosis of REM sleep behavior disorder. Normally there is loss of muscle tone during REM sleep, so no voluntary motor activity occurs, but when muscle atonia is not present, the dreaming individual "enacts" his or her actions in the ongoing dream. In an individual with an established synucleinopathy diagnosis, a history suggestive of REM sleep behavior disorder, even in the absence of polysomnographic evidence of REM sleep without atonia, is adequate to make the diagnosis of REM sleep behavior disorder.

12.17—Rapid Eye Movement Sleep Behavior Disorder / Diagnostic Features (p. 408)

12.18 Which of the following conditions is commonly associated with rapid eye movement (REM) sleep behavior disorder?

A. Attention-deficit/hyperactivity disorder.
B. Synucleinopathies.
C. Tourette's syndrome.
D. Sleep terrors.
E. Epilepsy.

Correct Answer: B. Synucleinopathies.

Explanation: Based on findings from individuals presenting to sleep clinics, most individuals (>50%) with initially "idiopathic" REM sleep behavior disorder will eventually develop a neurodegenerative disease—most notably, one of the synucleinopathies (Parkinson's disease, multiple system atrophy, or major or mild neurocognitive disorder with Lewy bodies). REM sleep behavior disorder often predates any other sign of these disorders by many years (often more than a decade). Nocturnal seizures may perfectly mimic REM sleep behavior disorder, but the behaviors are generally more stereotyped. Polysomnographic monitoring employing a full electroencephalographic seizure montage may differentiate the two. REM sleep without atonia is not present on polysomnographic monitoring.

12.18—Rapid Eye Movement Sleep Behavior Disorder / Development and Course (p. 408–409)

12.19 Which of the following classes of psychotropic drugs may result in rapid eye movement (REM) sleep without atonia and REM sleep behavior disorder?

A. Selective serotonin reuptake inhibitors.
B. Benzodiazepines.
C. Phenothiazines.
D. Second-generation antipsychotics.
E. Monoamine oxidase inhibitors.

Correct Answer: A. Selective serotonin reuptake inhibitors.

Explanation: Many widely prescribed medications, including tricyclic antidepressants, selective serotonin reuptake inhibitors, serotonin-norepinephrine reuptake inhibitors, and beta-blockers, may result in polysomnographic evidence of REM sleep without atonia and in frank REM sleep behavior disorder. It is not known whether the medications per se result in REM sleep behavior disorder or they unmask an underlying predisposition

12.19—Rapid Eye Movement Sleep Behavior Disorder / Risk and Prognostic Factors (p. 409)

12.20 A 10-year-old boy is referred by his teacher for evaluation of his difficulty sitting still in school, which is interfering with his academic performance. The boy complains of an unpleasant "creepy-crawly" sensation in his legs and an urge to move them when sitting still that is relieved by movement. This symptom bothers him most of the day, but less when playing sports after school or watching television in the evening, and it generally does not bother him in bed at night. What aspect of his clinical presentation rules out a diagnosis of restless legs syndrome (RLS)?

A. He is too young for a diagnosis of RLS.
B. He does not have a sleep complaint.
C. He does not complain of daytime fatigue or sleepiness.
D. His symptoms occur in the daytime as much as or more than in the evening or at night.
E. He does not have impaired social functioning.

Correct Answer: D. His symptoms occur in the daytime as much as or more than in the evening or at night.

Explanation: The diagnostic criteria for RLS specify that symptoms are worse in the evening or night, and in some individuals occur only in the evening or night. The symptoms can delay sleep onset and awaken the individual from sleep, resulting in significant sleep fragmentation and daytime sleepiness. RLS symptoms are accompanied by significant distress or impairment in social, occupational, educational, academic, behavioral, or other important areas of functioning. Although it is more common in adults, RLS can be diagnosed in children.

12.20—Restless Legs Syndrome / diagnostic criteria (p. 410); Diagnostic Features; Development and Course (p. 411)

12.21 A 28-year-old woman who is in her thirty-fourth week of pregnancy reports that for the past few weeks she has experienced restlessness and difficulty falling asleep at the onset of the sleep period, as well as daytime fatigue. She works during the day and has not changed her schedule. She states that as she becomes increasingly tired, she feels more irritable and depressed. What sleep disorder is suggested by the onset of these symptoms in the third trimester of pregnancy?

A. Circadian rhythm sleep-wake disorder, delayed sleep phase type.
B. Insomnia disorder.
C. Rapid eye movement (REM) sleep behavior disorder.
D. Restless legs syndrome.
E. Hypersomnolence disorder.

Correct Answer: D. Restless legs syndrome.

Explanation: The onset of symptoms late in pregnancy is a common feature of restless legs syndrome; the prevalence of restless legs syndrome in pregnant women is two to three times higher than that in the general population. In this case, one would want to know more about the patient's sense of restlessness in order to determine whether she has the unpleasant sensations and urge to move her legs, with relief of the unpleasant sensations after moving, that are the hallmark of the disorder.

12.21—Restless Legs Syndrome / Gender-Related Diagnostic Issues (p. 412)

12.22 Which of the following sleep disturbances or disorders occurs during rapid eye movement (REM) sleep?

A. Nightmare disorder.
B. Confusional arousals.
C. Sleep terrors.
D. Obstructive sleep apnea hypopnea.
E. Central sleep apnea.

Correct Answer: A. Nightmare disorder.

Explanation: Nightmares occur during REM sleep, which makes up a larger part of the sleep cycle later in the sleep period. Confusional arousals and sleep terrors are non-REM sleep phenomena. Obstructive sleep apneas and especially central sleep apneas tend to occur in deeper stages of sleep but can occur in lighter sleep as well, and they are not REM related.

12.22—Nightmare Disorder / Diagnostic Features (pp. 404–405)

12.23 Which of the following sleep disturbances is associated with chronic opiate use?

A. Excessive daytime sleepiness.
B. Insomnia.
C. Periodic limb movements in sleep.

D. Obstructive sleep apnea hypopnea.
E. Parasomnias.

Correct Answer: B. Insomnia.

Explanation: Although acute opiate intoxication tends to lead to sedation, habituation may result in eventual complaints of insomnia. Opiates may also decrease respiratory drive, resulting in central sleep apneas.

12.23—Substance/Medication-Induced Sleep Disorder / Associated Features Supporting Diagnosis (p. 417)

12.24 Which of the following substances is associated with parasomnias?

A. Cannabis.
B. Zolpidem.
C. Methadone.
D. Cocaine.
E. Mescaline.

Correct Answer: B. Zolpidem.

Explanation: Benzodiazepine receptor agonists, especially at high doses, may cause parasomnias. These would be classified as a zolpidem-induced sleep disorder, with onset during intoxication, parasomnia type.

12.24—Substance/Medication-Induced Sleep Disorder / Associated Features Supporting Diagnosis (p. 417)

12.25 A psychiatric consultation is requested for evaluation and help with management of severe insomnia in a 65-year-old man, beginning the day after elective hip replacement surgery and continuing for 2 days. On evaluation the patient acknowledges heavy drinking until the day before surgery, and he appears to be in alcohol withdrawal, with autonomic instability, confusion, and tremor. Why would a diagnosis of substance/medication-induced sleep disorder be inappropriate in this situation?

A. The insomnia is an understandable emotional reaction to the anxiety provoked by having surgery.
B. The insomnia is not causing functional impairment.
C. The insomnia has not been documented with polysomnography or actigraphy.
D. The insomnia is occurring during acute alcohol withdrawal.
E. The insomnia might be related to postoperative pain.

Correct Answer: D. The insomnia is occurring during acute alcohol withdrawal.

Explanation: A substance/medication-induced sleep disorder diagnosis should be made instead of a diagnosis of substance withdrawal only when the sleep disturbance symptoms "predominate in the clinical picture" and are "sufficiently severe to warrant clinical attention." Otherwise, a diagnosis of substance withdrawal is more appropriate. Pain and emotional stress may result in insomnia and should certainly be considered in the differential diagnosis of this patient's problems. Functional impairment may be hard to judge in a medically hospitalized patient, but it can sometimes be understood in terms of the patient's ability to participate appropriately with care. Polysomnography and actigraphy are useful tools in sleep disorder diagnosis in general, but they are not required to make this particular diagnosis.

12.25—Substance/Medication-Induced Sleep Disorder / diagnostic criteria (pp. 413–414)

12.26 A 56-year-old college professor complains of having difficulty sleeping for more than 5 hours per night over the past few weeks, leaving her feeling tired in the daytime. She awakens an hour or two before her intended waking time in the morning, experiencing restless sleep with frequent awakenings until it is time to get up. She does not have initial insomnia and is not depressed. The patient attributes the sleep trouble to intrusive thoughts that arise, after she initially awakens momentarily, about the need to complete an overdue academic project. What is the most appropriate diagnosis?

A. Adjustment disorder with anxious mood.
B. Obsessive-compulsive personality disorder.
C. Insomnia disorder.
D. Other specified insomnia disorder (brief insomnia disorder).
E. Unspecified insomnia disorder.

Correct Answer: D. Other specified insomnia disorder (brief insomnia disorder).

Explanation: According to DSM-5, "The other specified insomnia disorder category is used in situations in which the clinician chooses to communicate the specific reason that the presentation does not meet the criteria for insomnia disorder or any specific sleep-wake disorder. This is done by recording 'other specified insomnia disorder' followed by the specific reason (e.g., brief insomnia disorder)." In this case we do not have sufficient evidence to justify a diagnosis of adjustment disorder or obsessive-compulsive personality disorder. The patient has an insomnia problem but does not meet the duration criterion for insomnia disorder. She can be given the diagnosis of other specified insomnia disorder because the clinician can specify the way in which her disorder differs from one of the DSM-5 insomnia diagnoses. If the clinician lacked specifying information or had reason to choose not to provide specification, the diagnosis would be unspecified insomnia disorder.

12.26—Other Specified Insomnia Disorder (p. 420)

12.27 A 74-year-old woman has a history of daytime sleepiness interfering with her ability to carry out her daily routine. She reports that it has become progressively worse over the past year. Polysomnography reveals sleep apnea without evidence of airway obstruction with two or three apneic episodes per hour. What is the most appropriate diagnosis?

A. Central sleep apnea.
B. Other specified sleep-wake disorder (atypical central sleep apnea).
C. Unspecified sleep-wake disorder.
D. Rapid eye movement (REM) sleep behavior disorder.
E. Circadian rhythm sleep-wake disorder.

Correct Answer: B. Other specified sleep-wake disorder (atypical central sleep apnea).

Explanation: The patient does not meet full criteria for central sleep apnea because her apneic episodes occur at a frequency of fewer than five per hour. This deviation from diagnostic criteria can be specified. Therefore, "other specified" rather than "unspecified" sleep-wake disorder is the appropriate diagnosis.

12.27—Other Specified Hypersomnolence Disorder (p. 421)

CHAPTER 13

Sexual Dysfunctions

13.1 According to "Highlights of Changes From DSM-IV to DSM-5" in the DSM-5 Appendix, which of the following DSM-IV sexual dysfunction diagnoses is still included in DSM-5?

A. Sexual aversion disorder.
B. Female orgasmic disorder.
C. Dyspareunia.
D. Vaginismus.
E. None of the above.

Correct Answer: B. Female orgasmic disorder.

Explanation: An updated definition of female orgasmic disorder is included in DSM-5. Sexual aversion disorder was removed from DSM-5 because it was infrequently used and there was little research justifying this disorder. Vaginismus and dyspareunia, which had high comorbidity and poor diagnostic reliability as independent diagnoses, have now been combined into genito-pelvic pain/penetration disorder.

13.1—Appendix / Highlights of Changes From DSM-IV to DSM-5 (p. 814)

13.2 Female sexual interest/arousal disorder requires a lack of, or significantly reduced, sexual interest/arousal, as manifested by at least three of six possible indicators. Which of the following is *not* one of these six indicators?

A. No/reduced initiation of sexual activity, and typically unreceptive to a partner's attempts to initiate.
B. Absent/reduced sexual excitement/pleasure during sexual activity with the opposite sex.
C. Absent/reduced genital or nongenital sensations during sexual activity in almost all or all sexual encounters.
D. Absent/reduced interest in sexual activity.
E. Absent/reduced sexual/erotic thoughts or fantasies.

Correct Answer: B. Absent/reduced sexual excitement/pleasure during sexual activity with the opposite sex.

Explanation: There are no sexual dysfunction criteria that specify the sex or gender of the individual's choice of sexual partner. Therefore, the diagnosis can be given without regard to sexual orientation. All of the other options are indicators that can be used to fulfill Criterion A.

13.2—Female Sexual Interest/Arousal Disorder / diagnostic criteria (p. 433)

13.3 Several of the sexual dysfunctions have criteria that contain the phrase "almost all or all"; for example, "Absent/reduced sexual excitement/pleasure during sexual activity in almost all or all sexual encounters." How is "almost all or all" defined?

    A. At least 75%.
    B. At least 90%.
    C. Approximately 75%–100%.
    D. Approximately 90%–100%.
    E. In the clinician's best estimate.

Correct Answer: C. Approximately 75%–100%.

Explanation: For all of the sexual dysfunctions, whenever the term *almost all or all* is used in regard to a symptom, it is defined as "approximately 75%–100%."

13.3—diagnostic criteria for various sexual dysfunctions

13.4 Which of the following is a subtype of sexual dysfunction in DSM-5?

    A. Lifelong.
    B. Secondary to a medical condition.
    C. Due to relationship factors.
    D. Due to psychological factors.
    E. None of the above.

Correct Answer: A. Lifelong.

Explanation: Whereas DSM-IV included three possible subtypes for sexual dysfunction, DSM-5 includes only two—lifelong/acquired and generalized/situational. The DSM-IV specifiers "due to psychological factors" and "due to combined factors" were eliminated in DSM-5 because most clinical presentations have both psychological and biological contributors.

    Lifelong refers to a sexual problem that has been present from first sexual experiences, and *acquired* applies to sexual disorders that develop after a period of relatively normal sexual function. *Generalized* refers to sexual difficulties that are not limited to certain types of stimulation, situations, or partners, and *situational* refers to sexual difficulties that only occur with certain types of stimulation, situations, or partners. In addition to these subtypes, a number of factors must be considered during the assessment of sexual dysfunction, given that they may be relevant to etiology and/or treatment, and that may contribute, to varying degrees, across individuals: 1) partner factors (e.g., partner's sexual problems; partner's health status); 2) relationship factors (e.g., poor communication; discrepancies in desire for sexual activity); 3) individual vulnerability factors (e.g., poor body image; history of sexual or emotional abuse), psychiatric comorbidity (e.g., depression, anxiety), or stressors (e.g., job loss, bereavement); 4) cultural or religious factors (e.g., inhibitions related to prohibitions against sexual activity or pleasure; attitudes toward sexuality); and 5) medical factors relevant to prognosis, course, or treatment.

13.4—chapter intro (p. 423)

13.5   In all of the sexual dysfunctions except substance/medication-induced sexual dysfunction, symptoms must be present for what minimum duration to qualify for the diagnosis?

A. Approximately 1 month.
B. Approximately 3 months.
C. Approximately 6 months.
D. Approximately 1 year.
E. Approximately 2 years.

Correct Answer: C. Approximately 6 months.

Explanation: Substance/medication-induced sexual dysfunction has no minimum duration. In all of the other sexual dysfunctions, symptoms must have been present for a minimum duration of approximately 6 months. The use of "approximately" allows for clinician judgment in cases where the symptoms have not lasted a full 6 months.

13.5—diagnostic criteria for various sexual dysfunctions (pp. 423–450); Appendix / Highlights of Changes From DSM-IV to DSM-5 (p. 814)

13.6   A 65-year-old man who presented with difficulty in obtaining an erection due to diabetes and severe vascular disease had received a DSM-IV diagnosis of Sexual Dysfunction Due to…[Indicate the General Medical Condition] (coded as *607.84 male erectile disorder due to diabetes mellitus*). What DSM-5 diagnosis would be given to a person with this presentation?

A. Sexual dysfunction due to a general medical condition.
B. Erectile disorder.
C. Somatic symptom disorder.
D. A dual diagnosis of erectile disorder and somatic symptom disorder.
E. No diagnosis.

Correct Answer: E. No diagnosis.

Explanation: The DSM-IV diagnosis of *Sexual Dysfunction Due to…[Indicate the General Medical Condition]* no longer exists. In DSM-5, a sexual dysfunction that is fully explained by medical factors would not receive a diagnosis.

The diagnosis of somatic symptom disorder requires the presence of distressing somatic symptoms *and* abnormal thoughts, feelings, and behaviors in response to these symptoms. An individual who presents with erectile dysfunction but shows no disproportionate anxiety or distress would not be given this diagnosis.

> 13.6—Erectile Disorder / diagnostic criteria (p. 426); Diagnostic Features (p. 427); Somatic Symptom and Related Disorders chapter / Somatic Symptom Disorder / diagnostic criteria (p. 311)

13.7   A 35-year-old man with new-onset diabetes presents with a 6-month history of inability to maintain an erection. His erectile dysfunction had a sudden onset: he was fired from his job a month before the symptoms began. His serum glucose is well controlled with oral hypoglycemic medication. What is the appropriate DSM-5 diagnosis?

A. Sexual dysfunction due to a general medical condition.
B. Erectile disorder.
C. Adjustment disorder.
D. Unspecified sexual dysfunction.
E. No diagnosis.

Correct Answer: B. Erectile disorder.

Explanation: The DSM-IV diagnosis of *Sexual Dysfunction Due to…[Indicate the General Medical Condition]* no longer exists. In DSM-5, erectile problems that are fully explained by the effects of a medical condition would not receive a diagnosis of a erectile dysfunction. The distinction between erectile disorder as a mental disorder and erectile dysfunction as the result of another medical condition is usually unclear, and many cases will have complex, interactive biological and psychiatric etiologies. If the individual is older than 40–50 years and/or has concomitant medical problems, the differential diagnosis should include medical etiologies, especially vascular disease. The presence of an organic disease known to cause erectile problems does not confirm a causal relationship. For example, a man with diabetes mellitus can develop erectile disorder in response to psychological stress. In general, erectile dysfunction due to organic factors is generalized and gradual in onset. An exception would be erectile problems after traumatic injury to the nervous innervation of the genital organs (e.g., spinal cord injury). Erectile problems that are situational and inconsistent and that have an acute onset after a stressful life event are most often due to psychological events. An age of less than 40 years is also suggestive of a psychological etiology to the difficulty.

> 13.7—Erectile Disorder / diagnostic criteria (p. 426); Differential Diagnosis (p. 429)

13.8   Which of the following factors should be considered during assessment and diagnosis of a sexual dysfunction?

A. Partner factors.
B. Relationship factors.
C. Cultural or religious factors.
D. Individual vulnerability factors, psychiatric comorbidity, or stressors.
E. All of the above.

Correct Answer: E. All of the above.

Explanation: In addition to the subtypes "lifelong/acquired" and "general-
ized/situational," the following five factors must be considered during assessment and diagnosis of a sexual dysfunction, given that they may be relevant to
etiology and/or treatment: 1) *partner factors* (e.g., partner's sexual problems,
partner's health status); 2) *relationship factors* (e.g., poor communication, discrepancies in desire for sexual activity); 3) *individual vulnerability factors* (e.g.,
poor body image; history of sexual or emotional abuse), *psychiatric comorbidity*
(e.g., depression, anxiety), or *stressors* (e.g., job loss, bereavement); 4) *cultural/
religious factors* (e.g., inhibitions related to prohibitions against sexual activity;
attitudes toward sexuality); and 5) *medical factors relevant to prognosis, course, or
treatment.* Each of these factors may contribute differently to the presenting
symptoms of different individuals with this disorder.

13.8—chapter introduction (p. 423)

13.9   A 30-year-old woman comes to your office and reports that she is there only
because her mother pleaded with her to see you. She tells you that although
she has a good social network with friends of both sexes, she has never had any
feelings of sexual arousal in response to men or women, does not have any
erotic fantasies, and has little interest in sexual activity. She has found other
like-minded individuals, and she and her friends accept themselves as asexual.
What is the appropriate diagnosis, if any?

A. Female sexual interest/arousal disorder, lifelong, mild.
B. Female sexual interest/arousal disorder, lifelong, severe.
C. Hypoactive sexual desire disorder.
D. No diagnosis, because she does not have the minimum number of symp-
toms required (Criterion A) for female sexual interest/arousal disorder.
E. No diagnosis, because she does not have clinically significant distress or
impairment.

**Correct Answer: E. No diagnosis, because she does not have clinically signif-
icant distress or impairment.**

Explanation: At first glance, this woman appears to meet criteria for female
sexual interest/arousal disorder, severe. She has three of the six possible indi-

cators in Criterion A, which is the minimum number needed; however, Criterion C requires "clinically significant distress." Therefore, no diagnosis would be made in an individual who self-identifies as asexual. In DSM-IV a diagnosis of hypoactive sexual desire disorder could apply to men or women. In DSM-5 the disorder applies exclusively to men, a change reflected in the new name *male hypoactive sexual desire disorder*. A woman with hypoactive sexual desire and clinical distress who does not meet criteria for female sexual interest/arousal disorder would now be given the diagnosis *other specified sexual dysfunction (hypoactive sexual desire)*.

> **13.9—Female Sexual Interest/Arousal Disorder / diagnostic criteria (p. 433) / Other Specified Sexual Dysfunction (p. 450)**

13.10 Which of the following symptoms or conditions would rule out a diagnosis of erectile disorder?

A. Presence of diabetes mellitus.
B. Marked decrease in erectile rigidity.
C. Age over 60 years.
D. Presence of alcohol use disorder.
E. Presence of symptom for less than 3 months.

Correct Answer: E. Presence of symptoms for less than 3 months.

Explanation: A marked decrease in erectile rigidity is one of the three options from Criterion A, any one of which is sufficient to meet the criterion. The symptoms must have persisted for a minimum duration of approximately 6 months; a duration of less than 3 months would not meet this criterion. The presence of diabetes mellitus does not *in itself* rule out erectile disorder, as long as the diabetes is not the cause of the erectile dysfunction. Similarly, the mere presence of alcohol use disorder does not rule out the possibility of a separate, concurrent erectile disorder. However, if the erectile dysfunction developed during or soon after alcohol intoxication or withdrawal, and there was no evidence to suggest that the dysfunction was unrelated to this exposure, the correct diagnosis would be substance/medication-induced sexual dysfunction rather than erectile disorder. Finally, although the prevalence of problems with erection is greater for older men (approximately 40%–50% of men older than 60–70 years vs. only 2% of men younger than 40 years), there is no age limit for the diagnosis of erectile disorder.

> **13.10—Erectile Disorder / diagnostic criteria (p. 426); Substance/Medication-Induced Sexual Dysfunction / diagnostic criteria (p. 446)**

13.11 Which of the following statements about the diagnoses of premature (early) ejaculation and delayed ejaculation is *true?*

A. Criterion A for both diagnoses includes a specific time period following penetration during which ejaculation must or must not have occurred.

B. Criterion A for both diagnoses specifies "partnered sexual activity."

C. Early ejaculation, but not delayed ejaculation, may be diagnosed even when there is no clinically significant distress.

D. Estimated and measured intravaginal ejaculatory latencies are poorly correlated.

E. For both diagnoses, the severity is based on the level of distress experienced by the individual.

Correct Answer: B. Criterion A for both diagnoses specifies "partnered sexual activity."

Explanation: Although both premature ejaculation and delayed ejaculation may be diagnosed without regard to the gender of the man's sexual partner, the criteria for both disorders specify that symptoms must be experienced in the context of partnered sexual activity. For early ejaculation, an ejaculatory latency of approximately 1 minute following vaginal penetration is the duration defined by Criterion A of the diagnosis; for delayed ejaculation, no specific duration is defined. Both diagnoses require the presence of clinically significant distress. Estimated and recorded intravaginal ejaculatory latencies are well correlated, so a self-report is sufficient to make the diagnosis. For delayed ejaculation, current severity is based on the level of distress over the symptoms. For early ejaculation, current severity is based on how quickly the person ejaculates following initiation of sexual activity: mild is approximately 30–60 seconds, moderate is approximately 15–30 seconds, and severe is prior to or at initiation, or within approximately 15 seconds.

13.11—Delayed Ejaculation / diagnostic criteria (p. 424); Premature Ejaculation / diagnostic criteria (p. 443)

13.12 Which of the following statements about sexual dysfunction occurring in the context of substance or medication use is *true*?

A. It is more frequently caused by buprenorphine than by methadone.

B. It occurs more commonly in 3,4-methylenedioxymethamphetamine (MDMA) abusers than in heroin abusers.

C. It occurs in approximately 50% of patients taking antipsychotics.

D. Less than 10% of individuals with orgasm delay from antidepressants will experience spontaneous remission of the dysfunction within 6 months.

E. The overall incidence and prevalence of medication-induced sexual dysfunction are well delineated, based on extensive research.

Correct Answer: C. It occurs in approximately 50% of patients taking antipsychotics.

Explanation: Approximately 50% of individuals taking antipsychotic medications will experience adverse sexual side effects, including problems with sexual desire, erection, lubrication, ejaculation, or orgasm. These sexual problems have occurred with typical as well as atypical agents. Although the incidence of these side effects among different antipsychotic agents is unclear, problems are less common with prolactin-sparing antipsychotics.

The prevalence and the incidence of substance/medication-induced sexual dysfunction are unclear, likely because of underreporting of treatment-emergent sexual side effects. The most commonly reported side effect of antidepressant drugs is difficulty with orgasm or ejaculation. Approximately 30% of individuals with mild to moderate orgasm delay will experience spontaneous remission of the dysfunction within 6 months.

Individuals who use illicit substances have elevated rates of sexual dysfunction. The prevalence of sexual problems appears related to chronic drug abuse and appears higher in individuals who abuse heroin (approximately 60%–70%) than in individuals who abuse amphetamines or MDMA. Elevated rates of sexual dysfunction are also seen in individuals receiving methadone but are seldom reported by patients receiving buprenorphine.

13.12—Substance/Medication-Induced Sexual Dysfunction / Associated Features Supporting Diagnosis; Prevalence (pp. 448–449)

13.13 Which of the following conditions would be appropriately diagnosed as "other specified sexual dysfunction"?

A. Substance/medication-induced sexual dysfunction.
B. Sexual aversion.
C. Erectile dysfunction.
D. Female sexual interest/arousal disorder.
E. Delayed ejaculation.

Correct Answer: B. Sexual aversion.

Explanation: All of the options except sexual aversion are diagnosable disorders in the sexual dysfunctions category, each with its own specific set of criteria. The DSM-IV diagnosis of sexual aversion disorder, defined as "persistent or recurrent extreme aversion to, and avoidance of, all or almost all genital sexual contact with a sexual partner," is no longer a recognized disorder and is not included among the DSM-5 sexual dysfunctions. However, if this condition causes clinically significant distress to the individual, it can be diagnosed as "other specified sexual dysfunction (sexual aversion)."

13.13—Other Specified Sexual Dysfunction (p. 450)

CHAPTER 14

Gender Dysphoria

14.1 In order for a child to meet criteria for a diagnosis of gender dysphoria, which of the following *must* be present?

A. A co-occurring disorder of sex development.
B. A strong desire to be of the other gender or an insistence that one *is* the other gender.
C. A strong dislike of one's sexual anatomy.
D. A stated wish to change gender.
E. A strong desire for the primary and/or secondary sex characteristics that match one's experienced gender.

Correct Answer: B. A strong desire to be the other gender or an insistence that one *is* the other gender.

Explanation: For a child to meet criteria for a gender dysphoria diagnosis, there must be a strong desire to be the other gender or an insistence that one *is* the other gender (Criterion A1). The inclusion of this criterion in DSM-5 makes the diagnosis more conservative. The strong desire need not be stated aloud, because DSM-5 recognizes that social and/or cultural factors may inhibit this expression. There may be a strong dislike of one's sexual anatomy, or a strong desire for sex characteristics that match one's experienced gender, but these are not necessary for the diagnosis. There may be a co-occurring disorder of sex development, but this is not necessary for the diagnosis.

14.1—Gender Dysphoria in Children / diagnostic criteria (pp. 542–453)

14.2 Which of the following statements about the diagnosis of gender dysphoria in adolescents and adults is *true?*

A. The "posttransition" specifier is used to indicate that the individual has undergone or is pursuing treatment procedures to support the new gender assignment.
B. To qualify for the diagnosis, the individual must be pursuing some kind of sex reassignment treatment.
C. To qualify for the diagnosis, the individual must have a strong desire to be the other gender or must insist that he or she *is* the other gender.
D. To qualify for the diagnosis, the individual must have an associated disorder of sex development.

E. To qualify for the diagnosis, the individual must engage in cross-dressing behavior.

Correct Answer: A. The "posttransition" specifier is used to indicate that the individual has undergone or is pursuing treatment procedures to support the new gender assignment.

Explanation: In the diagnostic criteria for adolescents and adults, the "post-transition" specifier is used to identify individuals who have undergone at least one medical procedure or treatment to support the new gender assignment (e.g., cross-sex hormone treatment). Although the concept of posttransition is modeled on the concept of full or partial remission, the term *remission* has implications in terms of symptom reduction that do not apply directly to gender dysphoria.

Unlike the case for a child, an adolescent or adult need not have a strong desire to be the other gender or insist that he or she *is* the other gender to qualify for the diagnosis of gender dysphoria.

> 14.2—Gender Dysphoria in Adolescents and Adults / diagnostic criteria; Specifiers (pp. 542–453)

14.3   Match each of the following terms (A–E) to its correct definition (i–v).

A. Transgender.
B. Gender.
C. Sex.
D. Transsexual.
E. Gender dysphoria.

  i.   The biological indicators of male or female seen in an individual.
 ii.   The distress that may accompany the incongruence between one's experienced or expressed gender and one's assigned gender.
iii.   An individual's lived role in society as boy or girl, man or woman.
 iv.   An individual who transiently or persistently identifies with a gender different from his or her natal gender.
  v.   An individual who seeks, or has undergone, a social transition from male to female or female to male.

Correct Answer: A: iv, B: iii, C: i, D: v, E. ii.

Explanation: The area of sex and gender is highly controversial and has led to a proliferation of terms whose meanings vary over time and within and between disciplines. The words *sex, gender, transgender,* and *transsexual* should be used properly. In general, *sex* refers to the biological indicators of male and female (understood in the context of reproductive capacity), such as in sex chromosomes, gonads, sex hormones, and nonambiguous internal and external genitalia; *gender* is used to denote the public (and usually legally recognized) lived role as boy or girl, man or woman. *Transgender* refers to the broad spectrum of individuals who transiently or persistently identify with a gender different from their natal gender. *Transsexual* denotes an individual who seeks, or has undergone, a social transition from male to female or female to male, which in many, but not all, cases also involves a somatic transition by cross-sex hormone treatment and genital surgery (sex reassignment surgery). *Gender dysphoria* refers to the distress that may accompany the incongruence between one's experienced or expressed gender and one's assigned gender.

14.3—chapter intro (p. 451)

14.4 Which of the following statements about gender is *true?*

A. An individual's gender cannot always be predicted from his or her biological indicators.
B. An individual's gender is determined by cultural factors.
C. An individual's gender is determined by assignment at birth (natal gender).
D. An individual's gender is determined by psychological factors.
E. An individual's gender cannot be determined when there is a concurrent disorder of sexual development.

Correct Answer: A. An individual's gender cannot always be predicted from his or her biological indicators.

Explanation: Gender is a complexly determined outcome that includes biological, social, cultural, and psychological factors.

Disorders of sex development denote conditions of inborn somatic deviations of the reproductive tract from the norm and/or discrepancies among the biological indicators of male and female. The need to introduce the term *gender* arose with the realization that for individuals with conflicting or ambiguous biological indicators of sex (i.e., "intersex"), the lived role in society and/or the identification as male or female could not be uniformly associated with or predicted from the biological indicators and, later, that some individuals develop an identity as female or male at variance with their uniform set of classical biological indicators. Thus, *gender* is used to denote the public (and usually legally recognized) lived role as boy or girl, man or woman, but, in contrast to certain social constructionist theories, biological factors are seen as contributing, in interaction with social and psychological factors, to gender development. *Gender assignment* refers to the initial assignment as male or female. This occurs usually at birth and, thereby, yields the "natal gender."

14.4—chapter intro (p. 451)

14.5   What new DSM-5 diagnosis has re placed the former DSM-IV diagnosis of gender identity disorder?

A. Gender aversion disorder.
B. Gender dysmorphic disorder.
C. Gender dysphoria.
D. Cross-gender identity disorder.
E. Gender incongruence.

Correct Answer: C. Gender dysphoria.

Explanation: Gender dysphoria is a new diagnostic class in DSM-5 and reflects a change in conceptualization of the disorder's defining features by emphasizing the phenomenon of "gender incongruence" rather than cross-gender identification per se, as was the case in DSM-IV gender identity disorder. Gender dysphoria includes separate sets of criteria: for children and for adults and adolescents. For the adolescents and adults criteria, the previous Criterion A (cross-gender identification) and Criterion B (aversion toward one's gender) are merged. In the wording of the criteria, "the other sex" is replaced by "the other gender" (or "some alternative gender")." *Gender* instead of *sex* is used systematically because the concept "sex" is inadequate when referring to individuals with a disorder of sex development. In the child criteria, "strong desire to be of the other gender" replaces the previous "repeatedly stated desire to be...the other sex" to capture the situation of some children who, in a coercive environment, may not verbalize the desire to be of another gender. For children, Criterion A1 ("a strong desire to be of the other gender or an insistence that he or she is the other gender") is now necessary (but not sufficient), which makes the diagnosis more restrictive and conservative. The subtyping on the basis of sexual orientation is removed because the distinction is no longer considered clinically useful.

14.5—Appendix / Highlights of Changes From DSM-IV to DSM-5 (p. 814)

CHAPTER 15

Disruptive, Impulse-Control, and Conduct Disorders

15.1 An 11-year-old boy has shown extreme stubbornness and defiance since early childhood. This behavior is seen primarily at home and does not typically involve significant mood instability or anger, although he occasionally can be spiteful and vindictive. These symptoms have affected his sibling relationships in an extremely negative fashion, and more recently this behavior has been seen with peers and has begun to affect his friendships. His parents demonstrate a somewhat hostile parenting style. Which of the following statements correctly summarizes the appropriateness of a diagnosis of oppositional defiant disorder (ODD) for this patient?

A. The boy does not qualify for a diagnosis of ODD because his symptoms lack a significant mood component and seem to be confined primarily to the home setting.
B. Although the boy does not have a persistently negative mood, he may nevertheless qualify for a diagnosis of ODD if he meets the other symptom criteria.
C. If as a preschooler the boy had demonstrated temper outbursts that occurred on a weekly basis on most days during a 6-week period, he might have received a diagnosis of ODD at that point, as long as he had four or more of the required symptoms for 6 months.
D. The boy does not qualify for a diagnosis of ODD; the hostile parenting style is probably the cause of his oppositional behavior.
E. If the boy meets criteria for ODD, then he probably has begun to acknowledge his own role in overreacting to reasonable demands.

Correct Answer: B. Although the boy does not have a persistently negative mood, he may nevertheless qualify for a diagnosis of ODD if he meets the other symptom criteria.

Explanation: According to DSM-5, some individuals with ODD may not have the negative mood often associated with the disorder, and they may exhibit the symptoms primarily at home. There is a requirement that symptoms be observed with others besides the child's siblings. DSM-5 emphasizes the need for multiple informants that have observed the child or adolescent in different settings. The hostile parenting style sometimes seen with these individuals is often part of a dynamic process, or in response to the child's behavior, not necessarily the cause of the behavior. Individuals with ODD generally do not acknowledge their own role in what precipitates their defiance or anger, and typically externalize blame on unreasonable demands or situations as the rationale for their anger or misbehavior.

15.1—Oppositional Defiant Disorder / diagnostic criteria (pp. 462–463)

15.2   A 3-year-old boy has rather severe temper tantrums that have occurred at least weekly for a 6-week period. Although the tantrums can sometimes be associated with defiant behavior, they often result from a change in routine, fatigue, or hunger, and he only rarely does anything destructive. He is generally well behaved in nursery school and during periods between his tantrums. Which of the following conclusions best fits this child's presentation?

A. The boy does not meet criteria for oppositional defiant disorder (ODD).
B. The boy meets criteria for ODD because of the presence of tantrums and defiant behavior.
C. The boy could be diagnosed with ODD as long as it does not appear that his home environment is harsh, neglectful, or inconsistent.
D. The boy's symptoms more likely represent intermittent explosive disorder than ODD.
E. The boy's symptoms more likely represent disruptive mood dysregulation disorder than ODD.

Correct Answer: A. The boy does not meet criteria for oppositional defiant disorder (ODD).

Explanation: Criterion A for ODD requires a pattern of angry/irritable mood, argumentative/defiant behavior, or vindictiveness lasting at least 6 months as evidenced by at least four symptoms from any of the following categories, and exhibited during interaction with at least one individual who is not a sibling:

Angry/Irritable Mood
1. Loses temper.
2. Is touchy or easily annoyed by others.
3. Is angry and resentful.
Defiant/Headstrong Behavior
4. Argues with adults.
5. Actively defies or refuses to comply with adults' request or rules.
6. Deliberately annoys people.
7. Blames others for his or her mistakes or misbehavior.
Vindictiveness
8. Has been spiteful or vindictive at least twice within the past 6 months.

In this vignette, the child's tantrums are the sole symptom; therefore, he would not meet Criterion A. In addition, whereas his tantrums have occurred at least weekly for a 6-week period, DSM-5 specifically notes that for a child younger than 5 years, behavior meeting Criterion A can be considered a symptom of ODD only if it occurs *on most days* for the preceding 6 months. Finally, the tantrums do not appear to cause significant distress or impairment in functioning (Criterion B) and could be developmental in nature.

15.2—Oppositional Defiant Disorder / diagnostic criteria (p. 462)

15.3 The diagnostic criteria for oppositional defiant disorder (ODD) include specifiers for indicating severity of the disorder as manifested by pervasiveness of symptoms across settings and relationships. Which of the following specifiers would be appropriate for an 11-year-old boy who meets Criterion A symptoms in two settings?

A. Mild.
B. Moderate.
C. Severe.
D. Extreme.
E. There is not enough information to code the specifier.

Correct Answer: B. Moderate.

Explanation: The "mild" specifier requires symptoms to be confined to one setting, the "moderate" specifier requires symptoms to be present in at least two settings, and the "severe" specifier requires symptoms to be present in at least three settings. There is no "extreme" specifier.

15.3—Oppositional Defiant Disorder / diagnostic criteria; Specifiers (pp. 462–463)

15.4 A previously well-behaved 13-year-old girl begins to display extremely defiant and oppositional behavior, with vindictiveness. She is angry, argumentative, and refuses to accept responsibility for her behavior, which is affecting both her home life and school life in a significant way. What is the *least likely* diagnosis?

A. Major depressive disorder.
B. Bipolar disorder.
C. Oppositional defiant disorder.
D. Adjustment disorder.
E. Substance use disorder.

Correct Answer: C. Oppositional defiant disorder.

Explanation: Oppositional defiant disorder is an unlikely diagnosis if the onset is in adolescence after a childhood marked by compliant behavior. In this case, the relatively acute onset suggests a mood disorder (major depressive disorder or bipolar disorder), an adjustment disorder (to a stressor not described in the vignette), or a substance use disorder.

15.4—Oppositional Defiant Disorder / Development and Course (p. 464)

15.5 Which of the following statements about prevalence/course of and risk factors for oppositional defiant disorder (ODD) is *false?*

A. ODD is more prevalent in boys than in girls by a ratio of 1.4:1.
B. Harsh, inconsistent, or neglectful child-rearing practices are common in the families of individuals with ODD.
C. ODD tends to be moderately stable across childhood and adolescence.
D. Individuals with ODD as children or adolescents are at higher risk as adults for difficulties with antisocial behavior, impulse-control problems, anxiety, substance abuse, and depression.
E. Biological factors such as lower heart rate and skin conductance reactivity, reduced basal cortisol reactivity, and abnormalities in the prefrontal cortex and the amygdala have been associated with ODD and can be used diagnostically.

Correct Answer: E. Biological factors such as lower heart rate and skin conductance reactivity, reduced basal cortisol reactivity, and abnormalities in the prefrontal cortex and the amygdala have been associated with ODD and can be used diagnostically.

Explanation: Although a number of neurobiological markers (e.g., lower heart rate and skin conductance reactivity; reduced basal cortisol reactivity; abnormalities in the prefrontal cortex and amygdala) have been identified in association with ODD, they cannot be used diagnostically because the vast majority of studies have not separated children with ODD from those with conduct disorder. Thus, it is unclear whether there are markers specific to ODD.

15.5—Oppositional Defiant Disorder / Development and Course; Risk and Prognostic Factors (pp. 467–468)

15.6 A 16-year-old boy with a long history of defiant behavior toward authority figures also has a history of aggression toward peers (gets into fights at school), toward his parents, and toward objects (punching holes in walls, breaking doors). He frequently lies, and he has recently begun to steal merchandise from stores and money and jewelry from his parents. He does not seem pervasively irritable or depressed, and he has no sleep disturbance or psychotic symptoms. What is the most likely diagnosis?

A. Oppositional defiant disorder (ODD).
B. Conduct disorder.
C. Attention-deficit/hyperactivity disorder (ADHD).
D. Major depressive disorder.
E. Disruptive mood dysregulation disorder.

Correct Answer: B. Conduct disorder.

Explanation: This boy displays aggression toward people, destruction of property, and deceitfulness or theft—all part of Criterion A for conduct disorder in DSM-5. Individuals with ODD are not typically aggressive toward people or animals, and they do not generally destroy property or exhibit patterns of behavior involving theft or deceit. In addition, individuals with ODD have problems with emotional dysregulation as a more prominent and pervasive feature of their presentation. There is not enough information from the vignette to establish a diagnosis of ADHD. The lack of a pervasive mood disturbance argues against a diagnosis of major depressive disorder or disruptive mood dysregulation disorder.

15.6—Conduct Disorder / diagnostic criteria (pp. 469–471)

15.7   A 15-year-old boy has a history of episodic violent behavior that is out of proportion to the precipitant. During a typical episode, which will escalate rapidly, he will become extremely angry, punching holes in walls or destroying furniture in the home. There seems to be no specific purpose or gain associated with the outbursts, and within 30 minutes he is calm and "back to himself," a state that is not associated with any predominant mood disturbance. What diagnosis best fits this clinical picture?

A. Bipolar disorder.
B. Disruptive mood dysregulation disorder (DMDD).
C. Intermittent explosive disorder (IED).
D. Conduct disorder.
E. Attention-deficit/hyperactivity disorder (ADHD).

Correct Answer: C. Intermittent explosive disorder (IED).

Explanation: This boy's presentation is characteristic of IED. The fact that there is no mood disturbance between episodes argues against bipolar disorder or DMDD. Although individuals with conduct disorder can exhibit aggressive behavior, the behavior of this patient lacks a proactive and predatory component. The aggression in IED is impulsive and is not associated with an overall disregard for rules and social or societal norms. ADHD can be comorbid with IED, but ADHD symptoms other than impulsivity (inattention and restlessness) are not described in this vignette.

15.7—Intermittent Explosive Disorder / diagnostic criteria (p. 466)

15.8   Which of the following statements about the risk and prognostic factors in intermittent explosive disorder (IED) is *true?*

A. First-degree relatives of individuals with IED show no increased risk of having IED themselves.

B. The etiology for the disorder is thought to be predominantly environmentally determined, and twin studies have not demonstrated a significant genetic influence for the impulsive aggression.

C. Individuals with antisocial personality disorder or borderline personality disorder and those who have a history of disorders with disruptive behaviors (e.g., attention-deficit/hyperactivity disorder [ADHD], conduct disorder, oppositional defiant disorder) are at greater risk of comorbid IED.

D. The course of IED is usually not chronic and persistent.

E. The prevalence in males versus females across cultures and studies is consistently about 4:1.

Correct Answer: C. Individuals with antisocial personality disorder or borderline personality disorder and those who have a history of disorders with disruptive behaviors (e.g., attention-deficit/hyperactivity disorder [ADHD], conduct disorder, oppositional defiant disorder) are at greater risk of comorbid IED.

Explanation: According to DSM-5, first-degree relatives of individuals with IED are at higher risk of also having the disorder, which has a strong genetic component to the impulsive aggression. The course typically is chronic and persistent, and the prevalence is greater in males than in females across some studies (odds ratios range from 1.4 to 2.3), although in other studies there is no gender difference. (In some cultures, the overall prevalence is lower.) Individuals with antisocial personality disorder or borderline personality disorder and those who have a history of disorders with disruptive behaviors (e.g., ADHD, conduct disorder, oppositional defiant disorder) are at greater risk of comorbid IED.

15.8—Intermittent Explosive Disorder / Risk and Prognostic Factors; Comorbidity (pp. 467–468, 469)

15.9   Which of the following biological markers is associated with intermittent explosive disorder (IED)?

A. Serotonergic abnormalities globally and in the limbic system and orbitofrontal cortex.

B. Reduced amygdala responses to anger stimuli during functional magnetic resonance imaging (fMRI) scanning.

C. Atrophy of the cerebral cortex.

D. Abnormalities in adrenal function.

E. Increased urinary catecholamines.

Correct Answer: A. Serotonergic abnormalities globally and in the limbic system and orbitofrontal cortex.

Explanation: Research provides neurobiological support for the presence of serotonergic abnormalities, globally and in the brain, specifically in areas of the limbic system (anterior cingulate) and orbitofrontal cortex in individuals with IED. Amygdala responses to anger stimuli during fMRI scanning are *greater* in individuals with IED compared with healthy individuals. There is no evidence for the abnormalities described in options C, D, and E.

15.9—Intermittent Explosive Disorder / Risk and Prognostic Factors (p. 468)

15.10 Which of the following statements about the differential diagnosis of intermittent explosive disorder (IED) is *false?*

A. The diagnosis of IED can be made even if the impulsive aggressive outbursts occur in the context of an adjustment disorder.
B. In contrast to IED, disruptive mood dysregulation disorder is characterized by a persistently negative mood state (i.e., irritability, anger) most of the day, nearly every day, between impulsive aggressive outbursts.
C. The level of impulsive aggression in individuals with antisocial personality disorder or borderline personality disorder is lower than that in individuals with IED.
D. A diagnosis of IED should not be made when aggressive outbursts are judged to result from the physiological effects of another diagnosable medical condition.
E. Aggression in oppositional defiant disorder is typically characterized by temper tantrums and verbal arguments with authority figures, whereas impulsive aggressive outbursts in IED are in response to a broader array of provocation and include physical assault.

Correct Answer: A. The diagnosis of IED can be made even if the impulsive aggressive outbursts occur in the context of an adjustment disorder.

Explanation: DSM-5 stipulates that for children ages 6–18 years, aggressive behavior that occurs as part of an adjustment disorder should not be considered for the diagnosis of IED.

15.10—Intermittent Explosive Disorder / diagnostic criteria; Diagnostic Features (pp. 466–467)

15.11 A 17-year-old boy with a history of bullying and initiating fights using bats and knives has also stolen from others, set fires, destroyed property, broken into homes, and "conned" others. This pattern of disturbed conduct covers all of the Criterion A behavior categories *except*

A. Aggression to people and animals.
B. Destruction of property.
C. Deceitfulness or theft.

D. Serious violations of rules.

E. Malevolent intent.

Correct Answer: D. Serious violations of rules.

Explanation: The essential feature of conduct disorder is a repetitive and persistent pattern of behavior in which the basic rights of others or major age-appropriate societal norms or rules are violated (Criterion A). These behaviors fall into four main groupings: aggressive conduct that causes or threatens physical harm to other people or animals (Criteria A1–A7); nonaggressive conduct that causes property loss or damage (Criteria A8–A9); deceitfulness or theft (Criteria A10–A12); and serious violations of rules (Criteria A13–A15). According to DSM-5, *serious violations of rules* include the following: often stays out at night despite parental prohibitions, beginning before age 13 years; has run away from home overnight at least twice while living in the parental or parental surrogate home, or once without returning for a lengthy period; and is often truant from school, beginning before age 13 years. "Malevolent intent" is not one of the conduct disorder criteria.

15.11—Conduct Disorder / Diagnostic Features (p. 472)

15.12 A 15-year-old girl with a history of cruelty to animals, stealing, school truancy, and running away from home shows no remorse when caught, or when she is confronted with how her behavior is affecting the rest of her family. She disregards the feelings of others and seems to not care that her conduct is compromising her school performance. The behavior has been present for over a year and in multiple relationships and settings. Which of the following components of the "With limited prosocial emotions" specifier is absent in this clinical picture?

A. Lack of remorse or guilt.

B. Callous—lack of empathy.

C. Lack of concern about performance.

D. Shallow or deficient affect.

E. The required time duration.

Correct Answer: D. Shallow or deficient affect.

Explanation: *Shallow or deficient affect* is defined in DSM-5 as "does not express feelings or show emotions to others, except in ways that seem shallow, insincere, or superficial (e.g., actions contradict the emotion displayed; can turn emotions 'on' or 'off' quickly) or when emotional expressions are used for gain (e.g., emotions displayed to manipulate or intimidate others)." Not enough information is given in this vignette to indicate whether this girl has shallow or deficient affect.

15.12—Conduct Disorder / diagnostic criteria (pp. 470–471)

15.13 Which of the following does *not* qualify as aggressive behavior under Criterion A definitions for the diagnosis of conduct disorder?

A. Cyberbullying.
B. Forcing someone into sexual activity.
C. Stealing while confronting a victim.
D. Being physically cruel to people.
E. Aggression in the context of a mood disorder.

Correct Answer: E. Aggression in the context of a mood disorder.

Explanation: Irritability, aggression, and conduct problems can occur in children or adolescents with a major depressive disorder, a bipolar disorder, or disruptive mood dysregulation disorder. The behavioral problems associated with these mood disorders can usually be distinguished from the pattern of conduct problems seen in conduct disorder based on their course. Specifically, persons with conduct disorder will display substantial levels of aggressive or nonaggressive conduct problems during periods in which there is no mood disturbance, either historically (i.e., a history of conduct problems predating the onset of the mood disturbance) or concurrently (i.e., display of some conduct problems that are premeditated and do not occur during periods of intense emotional arousal). In those cases in which criteria for conduct disorder and a mood disorder are met, both diagnoses can be given.

15.13—Conduct Disorder / Differential Diagnosis (p. 475)

15.14 In order to be considered a symptom of conduct disorder, running away must have occurred with what frequency?

A. At least three times.
B. At least five times.
C. Only once if the individual did not return for a lengthy period.
D. Twice, in response to physical or sexual abuse.
E. Six times over a 3-month period.

Correct Answer: C. Only once if the individual did not return for a lengthy period.

Explanation: DSM-5 specifies that running away can occur once if it is for a lengthy period, or at least twice otherwise. The running away cannot be in response to physical or sexual abuse.

15.14—Conduct Disorder / diagnostic criteria (p. 470)

15.15 Which of the following statements about childhood versus adolescent onset of conduct disorder (CD) is *true?*

A. Compared with individuals with adolescent-onset CD, those with childhood-onset CD are more often female and tend to get along better with peers.
B. Compared with individuals with adolescent-onset CD, those with childhood-onset CD are less aggressive and less likely to have oppositional defiant disorder (ODD) or attention-deficit/hyperactivity disorder (ADHD).
C. Compared with individuals with childhood-onset CD, those with adolescent-onset CD are more likely to have CD that persists into adulthood.
D. Compared with individuals with childhood-onset CD, those with adolescent-onset CD are more likely to display aggressive behaviors and to have disturbed peer relationships.
E. Compared with individuals with childhood-onset CD, those with adolescent-onset CD are less likely to have CD that persists into adulthood.

Correct Answer: E. Compared with individuals with childhood-onset CD, those with adolescent-onset CD are less likely to have CD that persists into adulthood.

Explanation: In childhood-onset CD, individuals are usually male, frequently display physical aggression toward others, have disturbed peer relationships, may have had ODD during early childhood, and usually have symptoms that meet full criteria for CD prior to puberty. Many children with this subtype also have concurrent ADHD or other neurodevelopmental difficulties. Individuals with childhood-onset type are more likely to have persistent CD into adulthood than are those with adolescent-onset CD. Compared with individuals with childhood-onset CD, individuals with adolescent-onset CD are less likely to display aggressive behaviors and tend to have more normative peer relationships (although they often display conduct problems in the company of others). These individuals are less likely to have CD that persists into adulthood. The ratio of males to females with CD is more balanced for the adolescent-onset type than for the childhood-onset type.

15.15—Conduct Disorder / Subtypes (p. 471)

15.16 Which of the following statements about individuals who qualify for the "With limited prosocial emotions" specifier for conduct disorder is *true?*

A. These individuals generally display personality features such as risk avoidance, fearfulness, and extreme sensitivity to punishment.
B. These individuals are less likely than other individuals with conduct disorder to engage in aggression that is planned for instrumental gain.

C. These individuals generally exert more effort in their activities compared with other individuals with conduct disorder, and consequently are more successful.
D. These individuals are more likely to have a severity specifier rating of mild.
E. These individuals are more likely to have the childhood-onset type of conduct disorder.

Correct Answer: E. These individuals are more likely to have the childhood-onset type of conduct disorder.

Explanation: To qualify for the "with limited prosocial emotions" specifier, an individual must have displayed at least two of the listed characteristics—lack of remorse or guilt, callousness/lack of empathy, unconcern about performance, and shallow or deficient affect—persistently over at least 12 months and in multiple relationships and settings. These characteristics must reflect the individual's typical pattern of interpersonal and emotional functioning over this period and not just occasional occurrences in some situations.

A minority of individuals with conduct disorder exhibit characteristics that qualify for this specifier. The indicators of this specifier are those that have often been labeled as callous and unemotional traits in research. Other personality features, such as thrill seeking, fearlessness, and insensitivity to punishment, may also distinguish those with characteristics described in the specifier. Individuals with characteristics described in this specifier may be more likely than other individuals with conduct disorder to engage in aggression that is planned for instrumental gain. Individuals with conduct disorder of any subtype or any level of severity can have characteristics that qualify for the specifier "with limited prosocial emotions," although individuals with the specifier are more likely to have childhood-onset type and a severity specifier rating of severe.

15.16—Conduct Disorder / diagnostic criteria; Specifiers (pp. 470–472)

15.17 Which of the following statements about the prevalence of conduct disorder is *true?*

A. One-year prevalence rates range from 5% to 15%, with a median of 7%.
B. The prevalence varies widely across countries that differ in race and ethnicity.
C. Prevalence rates are higher among males than among females.
D. Callous unemotional traits are present in more than half of individuals with conduct disorder.
E. Prevalence rates remain fairly constant from childhood to adolescence.

Correct Answer: C. Prevalence rates are higher among males than among females.

Explanation: According to DSM-5, 1-year prevalence rates range from 2% to more than 10%, with a median of 4%. The prevalence of conduct disorder appears to be relatively consistent across countries that differ in race and ethnicity. Only a minority of individuals with conduct disorder exhibit characteristics that qualify for the "with limited prosocial emotions" specifier. The course of conduct disorder after onset is variable. In a majority of individuals, the disorder remits by adulthood. Many individuals with conduct disorder—particularly those with adolescent-onset type and those with fewer and milder symptoms—achieve adequate social and occupational adjustment as adults. However, the early-onset type predicts a worse prognosis and an increased risk of criminal behavior, conduct disorder, and substance-related disorders in adulthood. Prevalence rates rise from childhood to adolescence and are higher among males than among females.

15.17—Conduct Disorder / Specifiers; Prevalence; Development and Course (pp. 471, 473)

15.18 Which of the following statements about the onset and developmental course of conduct disorder is *true?*

A. Onset may occur as early as the preschool years and is rare after age 16 years.
B. Onset typically occurs in adolescence.
C. Age at onset has no bearing on the developmental course of the disorder.
D. Oppositional defiant disorder is generally not a precursor to the childhood-onset type of conduct disorder.
E. Those with the adolescent-onset type of conduct disorder are less likely to adjust successfully as adults.

Correct Answer: A. Onset may occur as early as the preschool years and is rare after age 16 years.

Explanation: The onset of conduct disorder typically occurs in the period from middle childhood through middle adolescence, although symptoms may appear in the preschool years. Individuals with adolescent-onset type and those with fewer and milder symptoms tend to have a greater likelihood of being successful (from a social and occupational standpoint) as adults. Oppositional defiant disorder is a common precursor to the childhood-onset type of conduct disorder.

15.18—Conduct Disorder / Development and Course (p. 473)

15.19 Which of the following statements about risk factors in conduct disorder is *false?*

A. A difficult undercontrolled infant temperament and lower-than-average verbal IQ are risk factors for conduct disorder.
B. Family-based risk factors include parental rejection and neglect, inconsistent child-rearing practices, harsh discipline, physical or sexual abuse, lack of supervision, early institutional living, frequent changes of caregivers, large family size, and substance-related disorders.
C. Community-level risk factors include association with a delinquent peer group and neighborhood exposure to violence.
D. The risk of conduct disorder is increased in children who have a biological or adoptive parent or sibling with conduct disorder.
E. Parental history of attention-deficit/hyperactivity disorder (ADHD) does not constitute a risk factor for conduct disorder in offspring.

Correct Answer: E. Parental history of attention-deficit/hyperactivity disorder (ADHD) does not constitute a risk factor for conduct disorder in offspring.

Explanation: The risk for conduct disorder is increased in children with a biological or adoptive parent or a sibling with conduct disorder. The disorder also appears to be more common in children of biological parents with severe alcohol use disorder, depressive and bipolar disorders, or schizophrenia or biological parents who have a history of ADHD or conduct disorder.

15.19—Conduct Disorder / Risk and Prognostic Factors (p. 473–474)

15.20 Which of the following statements about risk and prognostic factors in conduct disorder (CD) is *false?*

A. Individuals with CD are at risk of later depressive and bipolar disorders, anxiety disorders, posttraumatic stress disorder, impulse control disorders, somatic symptom disorders, and substance-related disorders as adults.
B. Temperamental risk factors for CD include a difficult undercontrolled infant temperament and lower-than-average intelligence, particularly in regard to verbal IQ.
C. Structural and functional differences in brain areas associated with affect regulation and affect processing have been consistently noted in individuals with CD.
D. The risk that CD will persist into adulthood is increased by co-occurring attention-deficit/hyperactivity disorder and by substance abuse.
E. Increased autonomic fear conditioning, particularly high skin conductance, is well documented and diagnostic of CD.

Correct Answer: E. Increased autonomic fear conditioning, particularly high skin conductance, is well documented and diagnostic of CD.

Explanation: *Reduced* autonomic fear conditioning, particularly *low* skin conductance, is well documented in individuals with CD; however, this finding is not diagnostic of the disorder.

15.20—Conduct Disorder / Associated Features Supporting Diagnosis (pp. 472–473); Culture-Related Diagnostic Issues (p. 474); Comorbidity (p. 475)

15.21 Which of the following statements about the differential diagnosis of conduct disorder (CD) and oppositional defiant disorder (ODD) is *true?*

A. In both diagnoses, individuals tend to have conflict with authority figures.
B. In both diagnoses, individuals display significant emotional dysregulation.
C. In both diagnoses, individuals display aggression toward people or animals.
D. In both diagnoses, individuals destroy property, steal, or lie.
E. If criteria for CD are met, then an individual cannot also receive a diagnosis of ODD.

Correct Answer: A. In both diagnoses, individuals tend to have conflict with authority figures.

Explanation: Symptoms of significant emotional dysregulation are seen in ODD, not CD. Individuals with ODD do not typically display significant aggression toward people or animals, nor do they typically destroy property, steal, or lie. If criteria for ODD and CD are both met, then the individual can receive both diagnoses.

15.21—Conduct Disorder / Differential Diagnosis (pp. 474–475)

15.22 Which of the following comorbid disorders is associated with pyromania?

A. Antisocial personality disorder.
B. Substance use disorders.
C. Mood disorders.
D. Gambling disorder.
E. All of the above.

Correct Answer: E. All of the above.

Explanation: Pyromania appears to have high co-occurrence with all of the above psychiatric conditions. Juvenile fire setting may also be associated with conduct disorders or attention-deficit/hyperactivity disorder. Although fire setting in the United States among children and adolescents is a major problem, the actual diagnosis of pyromania is rare.

15.22—Pyromania / Differential Diagnosis (p. 477)

15.23 A 15-year-old male student in private school, without known psychiatric history, has been caught stealing other students' laptops and cell phones, even though he comes from a wealthy family and his parents continue to purchase the newest electronics for him in an effort to deter him from stealing. Which of the following would raise your clinical suspicion that he may have kleptomania?

    A. He demonstrates recurrent failure to resist impulses to steal objects that are not needed for personal use or for their monetary value.
    B. He demonstrates recurrent failure to resist impulses to steal objects during periods of detachment or boredom.
    C. He experiences increased tension before committing the theft but does not experience relief, pleasure, or gratification while committing the theft.
    D. He has a strong family history for antisocial personality disorder and conduct disorder.
    E. He has a strong family history for bipolar disorder.

Correct Answer: A. He demonstrates recurrent failure to resist impulses to steal objects that are not needed for personal use or for their monetary value.

Explanation: Kleptomania is defined by the recurrent failure to resist impulses to steal items even though the items are not needed for personal use or for monetary value. The individual experiences a rising sense of tension before the act and then derives pleasure or gratification when committing the theft. The act is not done in response to anger or vengeance, and the stealing that occurs in kleptomania "is not better explained by conduct disorder, a manic episode, or antisocial personality disorder" (Criterion E).

15.23—Kleptomania / diagnostic criteria (p. 478)

15.24 Which of the following statements about kleptomania is *false?*

    A. The prevalence of kleptomania in the general population is generally very low, and the disorder more frequent among females.
    B. First-degree relatives of individuals with kleptomania may have higher rates of obsessive-compulsive disorder and/or substance use disorders than the general population.
    C. Kleptomania is similar to ordinary theft in that the act of shoplifting, whether planned or impulsive, is deliberate and often motivated by the usefulness of the object.
    D. The age at onset is variable, but the disorder often begins in adolescence.
    E. Individuals with kleptomania generally do not preplan their thefts.

Correct Answer: C. Kleptomania is similar to ordinary theft in that the act of shoplifting, whether planned or impulsive, is deliberate and often motivated by the usefulness of the object.

Explanation: The key feature of kleptomania is recurrent failure to resist impulses to steal items even though they are not needed and the individual is aware that the act is senseless. Shoplifting, by contrast, is typically motivated by the perceived utility or monetary value of an object. In adolescents, shoplifting may also be the consequence of a dare.

15.24—Kleptomania / Diagnostic Features (p. 478)

CHAPTER 16

Substance-Related and Addictive Disorders

16.1 The diagnostic criteria for substance abuse, substance dependence, substance intoxication, and substance withdrawal were not equally applicable to all substances in DSM-IV. In DSM-5, this remains true, although *substance use disorder* now replaces the diagnoses of *substance abuse* and *substance dependence*. For which of the following substance classes is there adequate evidence to support diagnostic criteria in DSM-5 for the three major categories of *use disorder, intoxication,* and *withdrawal?*

A. Caffeine.
B. Cannabis.
C. Tobacco.
D. Hallucinogen.
E. Inhalant.

Correct Answer: B. Cannabis.

Explanation: Only cannabis has sufficient evidence to support all three categories of substance-related disorders. Cannabis withdrawal and caffeine withdrawal, neither of which was fully recognized in DSM-IV, are now included in DSM-5. Proposed criteria for caffeine use disorder are provided in the "Conditions for Further Study" chapter in DSM-5 Section III to encourage research in this area, but there is still insufficient evidence to support this diagnosis. Tobacco has no recognized clinically significant intoxication syndrome. Hallucinogens and inhalants have no consistent evidence of a clinically significant withdrawal syndrome.

16.1—Appendix / Highlights of Changes From DSM-IV to DSM-5 (p. 815)

16.2 Almost all of the possible physical and behavioral symptom criteria included in the DSM-IV definitions of *substance abuse* and *substance dependence* are included in the DSM-5 definition of *substance use disorder*. Which of the following possible criteria included in DSM-IV were intentionally *omitted* in DSM-5?

A. There is a persistent desire or unsuccessful efforts to cut down or control substance use.
B. The substance is often taken in larger amounts or over a longer period than was intended.

C. The recurrent substance use results in a failure to fulfill major role obligations at work, school, or home.

D. There is continued substance use despite having persistent or recurrent social or interpersonal problems caused or exacerbated by the effects of the substance.

E. There are recurrent substance-related legal problems.

Correct Answer: E. There are recurrent substance-related legal problems.

Explanation: The risk of detection and the legal consequences of the detection of use of a substance vary widely across and within cultures and geographic regions and may change over time. Research has shown that the presence of recurrent legal problems does not correlate with the diagnosis of substance abuse. Therefore, the DSM-5 definition of substance use disorder omits the DSM-IV substance abuse criterion of "recurrent substance-related legal problems."

16.2—Appendix / Highlights of Changes From DSM-IV to DSM-5 (p. 815)

16.3   Whereas in DSM-IV, there were 11 recognized substance classes, DSM-5 has only 10, because certain related substances have been combined into a single class. Which of the following pairs of drugs falls into a single class in DSM-5?

A. Cocaine and phencyclidine (PCP).

B. Cocaine and methamphetamine.

C. 3,4-Methylenedioxymethamphetamine (MDMA [Ecstasy]) and methamphetamine.

D. Lorazepam and alcohol.

E. Lorazepam and oxycodone.

Correct Answer: B. Cocaine and methamphetamine.

Explanation: In DSM-5, cocaine and amphetamines are no longer in separate classes but instead have been combined into a new class, stimulants. PCP is no longer a distinct class; it is now grouped with the hallucinogens. MDMA is chemically similar to methamphetamine, but its clinical manifestations are more similar to those of the hallucinogens, so it is included in that group. Alcohol and opioids remain in their own distinct classes, as do sedatives, hypnotics, and anxiolytics.

16.3—Stimulant Use Disorder / diagnostic criteria (p. 605)

16.4   Tolerance and withdrawal were each considered valid criteria for the diagnosis of substance dependence in DSM-IV, although neither was required. Which of the following statements about tolerance and withdrawal in the DSM-5 diagnosis of substance use disorder is *true?*

A. Tolerance and withdrawal are no longer considered to be valid diagnostic symptoms of substance use disorder.
B. The definitions of tolerance and withdrawal have been updated because the previous definitions had poor interrater reliability.
C. The presence of either tolerance or withdrawal is now required to make a diagnosis of substance use disorder.
D. The presence of either tolerance or withdrawal is now required to make a substance use disorder diagnosis for some but not all classes of substances.
E. Both tolerance and withdrawal are still listed as possible criteria, but if they occur during appropriate medically supervised treatment, they may not be counted toward the diagnosis of a substance use disorder.

Correct Answer: E. Both tolerance and withdrawal are still listed as possible criteria, but if they occur during appropriate medically supervised treatment, they may not be counted toward the diagnosis of a substance use disorder.

Explanation: In DSM-5, there is no change in how tolerance and withdrawal are defined, and either or both may be used to fulfill Criterion A for substance use disorder. Neither one is ever required, regardless of which substance is involved. Neither tolerance nor withdrawal may be counted toward a diagnosis when it occurs during appropriate medically supervised treatment (e.g., in a person taking opiates for pain, or stimulants for attention-deficit/hyperactivity disorder). A person receiving medically supervised treatment may still meet enough other criteria to be diagnosed with substance use disorder.

16.4—chapter intro: Substance Use Disorders / Features (p. 484)

16.5 Which of the following is *not* a recognized alcohol-related disorder in DSM-5?

A. Alcohol dependence.
B. Alcohol use disorder.
C. Alcohol intoxication.
D. Alcohol withdrawal.
E. Alcohol-induced sexual dysfunction.

Correct Answer: A. Alcohol dependence.

Explanation: For all substances including alcohol, the DSM-IV diagnoses of *substance abuse* and *substance dependence* have been replaced with a single diagnosis, *substance use disorder*. Substance intoxication and withdrawal remain from DSM-IV, with updated definitions. Substance/medication-induced sexual dysfunction is the DSM-5 diagnosis that replaced substance-induced sexual dysfunction from DSM-IV.

16.5—Appendix / Highlights of Changes From DSM-IV to DSM-5 (p. 815)

16.6   Which of the following statements about caffeine-related disorders is *true?*

A. Culturally appropriate levels of caffeine intake should be considered when making the diagnosis of caffeine intoxication.
B. In order to diagnose caffeine intoxication, at least one symptom must begin during caffeine use.
C. The diagnosis of caffeine withdrawal requires the preceding use of caffeine on a daily basis.
D. Caffeine withdrawal may be diagnosed even in the absence of clinically significant distress or impairment in social, occupational, or other important areas of functioning.
E. Extensive data are available regarding the prevalence of caffeine use disorder.

Correct Answer: C. The diagnosis of caffeine withdrawal requires the preceding use of caffeine on a daily basis.

Explanation: Criterion A of caffeine withdrawal is "prolonged daily use of caffeine." Caffeine intoxication may be diagnosed regardless of the individual's cultural background, and all symptoms may begin either during or shortly after caffeine use. In caffeine withdrawal, as in other substance withdrawal diagnoses, the symptoms must cause clinically significant distress or impairment in social, occupational, or other important areas of functioning. Currently there is insufficient evidence regarding the prevalence of the proposed diagnosis of caffeine use disorder, which is listed in the "Conditions for Further Study" chapter in DSM-5 Section III to encourage research.

16.6—Caffeine-Related Disorders (pp. 503–509)

16.7   Which of the following symptoms is a recognized consequence of the abrupt termination of daily or near-daily cannabis use?

A. Hallucinations.
B. Delusions.
C. Hunger.
D. Irritability.
E. Apathy.

Correct Answer: D. Irritability.

Explanation: Cannabis withdrawal is a newly recognized disorder in DSM-5. Common symptoms of cannabis withdrawal include irritability, anger, or aggression; nervousness or anxiety; sleep difficulty; decreased appetite or weight loss; restlessness; and depressed mood. Although typically not as severe as withdrawal from alcohol, sedative/hypnotics, or opioids, cannabis withdrawal can cause significant distress, contribute to difficulty quitting, and increase the risk of relapse.

16.7—Cannabis Withdrawal (pp. 517–519)

16.8 The Criterion A symptoms listed for *other hallucinogen use disorder* are the same as those listed for use disorders of most other substance classes, with one exception. Which of the following is *not* a recognized symptom associated with hallucinogen use?

·A. Withdrawal.
B. Tolerance.
C. A persistent desire or unsuccessful efforts to cut down or control use of the substance.
D. Recurrent use of the substance in situations in which it is physically hazardous.
E. Craving, or a strong desire or urge to use the substance.

Correct Answer: A. Withdrawal.

Explanation: The Criterion A symptoms listed for *other hallucinogen use disorder* are the same as those listed for use disorders of most other substance classes, with the exception of withdrawal. A clinically significant withdrawal syndrome associated with hallucinogens has not been consistently documented in humans, and therefore the diagnosis of *other hallucinogen withdrawal* is not included in DSM-5.

16.8—Other Hallucinogen Use Disorder (pp. 523–527)

16.9 To meet proposed criteria for the Section III condition *neurobehavioral disorder associated with prenatal alcohol exposure,* an individual's prenatal alcohol exposure must have been "more than minimal." How is "more than minimal" exposure defined, in terms of how much alcohol was used by the mother during gestation?

A. Fewer than 7 drinks per month, and no more than 1 drink per drinking occasion.
B. Fewer than 7 drinks per month, and no more than 2 drinks per drinking occasion.
C. Fewer than 7 drinks per month, and no more than 3 drinks per drinking occasion.
D. Fewer than 14 drinks per month, and no more than 1 drink per drinking occasion.
E. Fewer than 14 drinks per month, and no more than 2 drinks per drinking occasion.

Correct Answer: E. Fewer than 14 drinks per month, and no more than 2 drinks per drinking occasion.

Explanation: Proposed criteria for neurobehavioral disorder associated with prenatal alcohol exposure (ND-PAE) have been placed in DSM-5 Section III ("Conditions for Further Study") in order to encourage further research. Data suggest that a history of more than minimal gestational exposure (i.e., more than light drinking) prior to pregnancy recognition and/or following pregnancy recognition may be needed to significantly impact neurodevelopmental outcome. "Light drinking" is defined as 1–13 drinks per month during pregnancy with no more than 2 of these drinks consumed on any 1 drinking occasion. Confirmation of gestational exposure to alcohol may be obtained from maternal self-report of alcohol use in pregnancy, medical or other records, or clinical observation.

> 16.9—Conditions for Further Study (Section III) / Neurobehavioral Disorder Associated With Prenatal Alcohol Exposure diagnostic criteria / Diagnostic Features (pp. 798–799)

16.10 Which of the following is the only non-substance-related disorder to be included in the DSM-5 chapter "Substance-Related and Addictive Disorders"?

A. Gambling disorder.
B. Internet gaming disorder.
C. Electronic communication addiction disorder.
D. Compulsive computer use disorder.
E. Compulsive shopping.

Correct Answer: A. Gambling disorder.

Explanation: In addition to the substance-related disorders, the DSM-5 Substance-Related and Addictive Disorders chapter also includes gambling disorder, reflecting evidence that gambling behaviors activate reward systems similar to those activated by drugs of abuse and produce some behavioral symptoms that appear comparable to those produced by the substance use disorders. Other excessive behavioral patterns, such as Internet gaming, have also been described, but the research on these and other behavioral syndromes is less clear. (Proposed criteria for Internet gaming disorder have been placed in DSM-5 Section III ["Conditions for Further Study"] in order to encourage further research.) Thus, groups of repetitive behaviors, which some term *behavioral addictions*, with such subcategories as "sex addiction," "exercise addiction," or "shopping addiction," are not included because at this time there is insufficient peer-reviewed evidence to establish the diagnostic criteria and course descriptions needed to identify these behaviors as mental disorders.

> 16.10—chapter intro (p. 481)

16.11 In most substance/medication-induced mental disorders (with the exception of substance/medication-induced major or mild neurocognitive disorder and hallucinogen persisting perception disorder), if the person abstains from substance use, the disorder will eventually disappear or no longer be clinically relevant even without formal treatment. In what time frame is this likely to happen?

A. One hour.
B. One month.
C. Three months.
D. One year.
E. "Relatively quickly" but no specific period of time.

Correct Answer: B. One month.

Explanation: Although the symptoms of substance/medication-induced mental disorders can be identical to those of independent mental disorders (e.g., delusions, hallucinations, psychoses, major depressive episodes, anxiety syndromes), and although they can have the same severe consequences (e.g., suicide), most induced mental disorders are likely to improve relatively quickly with abstinence and are unlikely to remain clinically relevant for more than 1 month after complete cessation of use.

16.11—chapter intro: Substance-Induced Disorders / Substance/Medication-Induced Mental Disorders / Development and Course (p. 489)

16.12 Because opioid withdrawal and sedative, hypnotic, or anxiolytic withdrawal can involve very similar symptoms, distinguishing between the two can be difficult. Which of the following presenting symptoms would aid in making the correct diagnosis?

A. Nausea or vomiting.
B. Anxiety.
C. Yawning.
D. Restlessness or agitation.
E. Insomnia.

Correct Answer: C. Yawning.

Explanation: Opioid withdrawal is characterized by a pattern of signs and symptoms that are opposite to the acute agonist effects. The first of these are subjective and consist of complaints of anxiety, restlessness, and an "achy feeling" that is often located in the back and legs, along with irritability and increased sensitivity to pain. Three or more of the following must be present to make a diagnosis of opioid withdrawal: dysphoric mood; nausea or vomiting; muscle aches; lacrimation or rhinorrhea; pupillary dilation, piloerection, or increased sweating; diarrhea; yawning; fever; insomnia (Criterion B). Piloerection and fever are associated with more severe withdrawal and are not often seen in routine clinical practice because individuals with opioid use disorder usually obtain substances before withdrawal becomes that far advanced.

Sedative, hypnotic, or anxiolytic withdrawal also includes anxiety and psychomotor agitation among its DSM-5 symptom criteria. These are not criteria included in the DSM-5 definition of opioid withdrawal, but withdrawal from opioids is nonetheless often accompanied by anxiety and restlessness. Only opioid withdrawal presents with yawning, rhinorrhea or lacrimation, pupillary dilation, or muscle aches, any of which may be used to fulfill Criterion B for a withdrawal diagnosis.

> **16.12—Opioid Withdrawal / diagnostic criteria (pp. 547–548); Diagnostic Features (p. 548)**

16.13 In DSM-5, the sedative, hypnotic, or anxiolytic class contains all prescription sleeping medications and almost all prescription antianxiety medications. What is the reason that nonbenzodiazepine antianxiety agents (e.g., buspirone, gepirone) are *not* included in this class?

A. They are not generally available in nonparenteral (intravenous or intramuscular) formulations.
B. They do not appear to be associated with significant misuse.
C. They are not associated with illicit manufacturing or diversion (e.g., Schedule I–V drugs in the United States, or included in the list of psychotropic substances recognized by the International Narcotics Control Board and the United Nations).
D. They are not respiratory depressants.
E. They do not appear to be associated with cravings or tolerance.

Correct Answer: B. They do not appear to be associated with significant misuse.

Explanation: Sedative, hypnotic, or anxiolytic substances include benzodiazepines, benzodiazepine-like drugs (e.g., zolpidem, zaleplon), carbamates (e.g., glutethimide, meprobamate), barbiturates (e.g., secobarbital), and barbiturate-like hypnotics (e.g., glutethimide, methaqualone). This class of substances includes all prescription sleeping medications and almost all prescription antianxiety medications. Nonbenzodiazepine antianxiety agents (e.g., buspirone, gepirone) are not included in this class because they do not appear to be associated with significant misuse.

> **16.13—Sedative, Hypnotic, or Anxiolytic Use Disorder / Diagnostic Features (p. 596)**

16.14 Which of the following criteria for substance use disorder in DSM-5 was *not* one of the criteria for either substance abuse or substance dependence in DSM-IV?

A. Important social, occupational, or recreational activities are given up or reduced because of substance use.
B. The substance is often taken in larger amounts or over a longer period than was intended.
C. Craving, or a strong desire or urge to use the substance, is present.
D. Recurrent substance use results in a failure to fulfill major role obligations at work, school, or home.
E. A great deal of time is spent in activities necessary to obtain the substance, use the substance, or recover from its effects.

Correct Answer: C. Craving, or a strong desire or urge to use the substance, is present.

Explanation: *Craving,* defined as a strong desire or urge to use a substance, is a new addition to the symptoms listed under Criterion A for DSM-5 substance use disorder. Craving may occur at any time but is more likely when in an environment where the drug previously was obtained or used. Craving has also been shown to involve classical conditioning and is associated with activation of specific reward structures in the brain. Craving is queried by asking if there has ever been a time when they had such strong urges to take the drug that they could not think of anything else. Current craving is often used as a treatment outcome measure because it may be a signal of impending relapse.

16.14—chapter intro: Substance Use Disorders / Features (p. 483)

16.15 A 27-year-old woman presents for psychiatric evaluation after almost hitting someone with her car while driving under the influence of marijuana. She reports that she was prompted to seek treatment by her husband, with whom she has had several conflicts over the past year about her ongoing marijuana use. She has continued to smoke two joints daily and drive while under the influence of marijuana since this event. What is the appropriate diagnosis?

A. Cannabis abuse.
B. Cannabis dependence.
C. Cannabis intoxication.
D. Cannabis use disorder.
E. Unspecified cannabis-related disorder.

Correct Answer: D. Cannabis use disorder.

Explanation: The patient described in this vignette meets criteria for cannabis use disorder, which is manifested by recurrent cannabis use in situations in which it is physically hazardous and continued use despite having persistent interpersonal problems due to cannabis. Although this particular patient would have met DSM-IV criteria for cannabis abuse, in DSM-5 the separate diagnoses of cannabis abuse and cannabis dependence are subsumed under the diagnosis of cannabis use disorder. There is no information in the vignette to suggest that the patient is currently intoxicated. Because she meets criteria for a specific cannabis-related disorder, the diagnosis "unspecified cannabis-related disorder" would not be appropriate.

16.15—Appendix / Highlights of Changes From DSM-IV to DSM-5 (p. 815)

16.16 A 45-year-old man with a long-standing history of heavy alcohol use is referred for psychiatric evaluation after his recent admission to the hospital for acute hepatitis. The patient reports that he drank almost daily in college. Over the past 10 years, he has gradually increased his nightly alcohol intake from a single 6-pack to two 12-packs of beer, and this nightly drinking habit has resulted in his frequently oversleeping and missing work. He has tried to moderate his alcohol use on numerous occasions with little success, particularly after developing complications associated with alcoholic cirrhosis. The patient admits that he becomes anxious and gets hand tremors when he doesn't drink. This patient meets the criteria for which of the following diagnoses?

A. Alcohol abuse.
B. Alcohol dependence.
C. Alcohol use disorder, mild.
D. Alcohol use disorder, moderate.
E. Alcohol use disorder, severe.

Correct Answer: E. Alcohol use disorder, severe.

Explanation: Substance use disorders occur in a broad range of severity, from mild to severe, with severity based on the number of symptom criteria endorsed. As a general estimate of severity, a *mild* substance use disorder is suggested by the presence of two to three symptoms, *moderate* by four to five symptoms, and *severe* by six or more symptoms. Changing severity across time is also reflected by reductions or increases in the frequency and/or dose of substance use, as assessed by the individual's own report, report of knowledgeable others, clinician's observations, and biological testing. The patient described in this vignette meets criteria for alcohol use disorder, severe. Alcohol abuse and alcohol dependence are DSM-IV diagnoses that have been eliminated from DSM-5.

16.16—chapter intro: Substance Use Disorders / Severity and Specifiers (p. 484)

16.17 Which of the following statements about alcohol withdrawal is *true*?

A. Fewer than 10% of individuals undergoing alcohol withdrawal experience dramatic symptoms such as severe autonomic hyperactivity, tremors, or alcohol withdrawal delirium.
B. Delirium occurs in the majority of individuals who meet criteria for alcohol withdrawal.

C. Approximately 80% of all patients with alcohol use disorder will experience alcohol withdrawal.

D. Tonic-clonic seizures occur in about 15% of individuals who meet criteria for alcohol withdrawal.

E. Alcohol withdrawal symptoms typically begin between 24 and 48 hours after alcohol use has been stopped or reduced.

Correct Answer: A. Fewer than 10% of individuals undergoing alcohol withdrawal experience dramatic symptoms such as severe autonomic hyperactivity, tremors, or alcohol withdrawal delirium.

Explanation: It is estimated that approximately 50% of middle-class, highly functional individuals with alcohol use disorder have ever experienced a full alcohol withdrawal syndrome. Among individuals with alcohol use disorder who are hospitalized or homeless, the rate of alcohol withdrawal may be greater than 80%. Fewer than 10% of individuals who develop alcohol withdrawal will ever develop dramatic symptoms (e.g., severe autonomic hyperactivity, tremors, alcohol withdrawal delirium). Tonic-clonic seizures occur in fewer than 3% of individuals. Withdrawal symptoms typically begin when blood concentrations of alcohol decline sharply (i.e., within 4–12 hours) after alcohol use has been stopped or reduced.

16.17—Alcohol Withdrawal / Diagnostic Features; Prevalence (pp. 500, 501)

16.18 How many remission specifiers are included in the DSM-5 diagnostic criteria for substance use disorders?

A. One.
B. Two.
C. Three.
D. Four.
E. Five.

Correct Answer: B. Two.

Explanation: The DSM-5 diagnostic criteria for substance use disorder include two remission specifiers: "in early remission" and "in sustained remission." The "in early remission specifier" is used if, for at least 3 months but for less than 12 months, the individual does not meet any of the criteria for a substance use disorder (i.e., none of the criteria met except for Criterion 4, "Craving or a strong desire or urge to use a specific substance"). The "in sustained remission" specifier is used if none of the criteria for a substance use disorder have been met at any time during a period of 12 months or longer (i.e., none of the criteria met except for Criterion 4, "Craving or a strong desire or urge to use a specific substance").

These new remission specifiers replace the four remission specifiers included in the DSM-IV diagnostic criteria for substance dependence (early full remission, early partial remission, sustained full remission, and sustained partial remission).

16.18—Substance Use Disorders / Severity and Specifiers (p. 484); Appendix / Highlights of Changes From DSM-IV to DSM-5 (p. 815)

16.19 A 25-year-old woman is brought to the emergency department by her friends after a party. They report that the woman had been seen ingesting some unknown pills earlier in the evening. She became increasingly confused throughout the course of the night. She eventually had a witnessed seizure on the street, prompting activation of emergency medical services. Vital signs indicate that the patient is tachycardic and hypertensive. On evaluation, the patient is observed to be thin with dilated pupils. She is smiling to herself, is fidgety, and is oriented to self, place, and date. When queried about auditory hallucinations, the patient admits that she is hearing voices but is unconcerned, stating, "I only hear them while I'm partying, Doc." Which diagnosis best fits this clinical presentation?

A. Stimulant-induced manic episode.
B. Stimulant-induced psychotic disorder.
C. Stimulant intoxication, with perceptual disturbances.
D. Other hallucinogen-induced psychotic disorder.
E. Other hallucinogen intoxication.

Correct Answer: C. Stimulant intoxication, with perceptual disturbances.

Explanation: Although both *other hallucinogen intoxication* and *stimulant intoxication* can present with hallucinations, pupillary dilation, and tachycardia, only the stimulant intoxication criteria include development of confusion and seizures. The diagnosis of stimulant intoxication with perceptual disturbances is made when a person does not have delirium but has either hallucinations with intact reality testing—such as in this vignette—or auditory, visual, or tactile illusions.

16.19—multiple: diagnostic criteria for Substance/Medication-Induced Psychotic Disorder; Other Hallucinogen Intoxication; Stimulant Intoxication (pp. 110–111, 529, 567)

16.20 Which of the following substances is most likely to be associated with polydrug use?

A. Cannabis.
B. Tobacco.
C. 3,4-Methylenedioxymethamphetamine (MDMA [Ecstasy]).

D. Methamphetamine.

E. Alcohol.

Correct Answer: C. 3,4-Methylenedioxymethamphetamine (MDMA [Ecstasy]).

Explanation: Both adults and adolescents who use MDMA are more likely than those who use other drugs to be polydrug users and to have other substance use disorders.

16.20—Other Hallucinogen Use Disorder / Comorbidity (p. 527)

16.21 Alcohol intoxication, inhalant intoxication, and sedative, hypnotic, or anxiolytic intoxication have which of the following Criterion C signs/symptoms in common?

A. Depressed reflexes.

B. Generalized muscle weakness.

C. Blurred vision.

D. Impairment in attention or memory.

E. Nystagmus.

Correct Answer: E. Nystagmus.

Explanation: Nystagmus is a Criterion C sign of alcohol, inhalant, and sedative, hypnotic, or anxiolytic intoxication. Depressed reflexes, generalized muscle weakness, and blurred vision are Criterion C signs of inhalant intoxication but are not associated with either alcohol intoxication or sedative, hypnotic, or anxiolytic intoxication. Impairment in attention or memory is a Criterion C sign of both alcohol intoxication and of sedative, hypnotic, or anxiolytic intoxication but is not a diagnostic feature of inhalant intoxication.

16.21—multiple: diagnostic criteria for Alcohol Intoxication; Inhalant Intoxication; Sedative, Hypnotic, or Anxiolytic Intoxication (pp. 497, 538, 556)

16.22 In DSM-IV, caffeine withdrawal was included in Appendix B as a criteria set provided for further study. Which of the following statements correctly describes how caffeine withdrawal is classified in DSM-5?

A. Caffeine withdrawal is no longer considered a valid psychiatric diagnosis.

B. Caffeine withdrawal remains a proposed diagnosis in DSM-5 and is included in "Conditions for Further Study" in Section III.

C. Caffeine withdrawal is classified under *other (or unknown) substance withdrawal* in DSM-5.

D. Caffeine withdrawal is classified under *stimulant withdrawal* in DSM-5.

E. Caffeine withdrawal was moved to the main body of DSM-5 and is now included in the "Substance-Related and Addictive Disorders" chapter.

Correct Answer: E. Caffeine withdrawal was moved to the main body of DSM-5 and is now included in the "Substance-Related and Addictive Disorders" chapter.

Explanation: Caffeine withdrawal was moved from Appendix B, "Criteria Sets and Axes Provided for Further Study," in DSM-IV to the main body of DSM-5; it is now included among the Substance-Related and Addictive Disorders. While caffeine withdrawal can mimic other drug withdrawal states (e.g., from amphetamines, cocaine), caffeine withdrawal is considered distinct from stimulant withdrawal.

16.22—Caffeine Withdrawal (p. 508); Appendix / Highlights of Changes From DSM-IV to DSM-5 (p. 815)

16.23 A 25-year-old medical student presents to the student health service at 7 A.M. complaining of having a "panic attack." He reports that he stayed up all night studying for his final gross anatomy exam, which starts in an hour, but he feels too anxious to go. He reports vomiting twice. The patient is restless and appears flushed, with visible muscle twitching. He is urinating excessively, has tachycardia, and his electrocardiogram shows premature ventricular complexes. His thoughts and speech appear to be rambling in nature. His urine toxicology screen is negative. What is the most likely diagnosis?

A. Panic disorder.
B. Amphetamine intoxication, amphetamine-like substance.
C. Caffeine intoxication.
D. Cocaine intoxication.
E. Alcohol withdrawal.

Correct Answer: C. Caffeine intoxication.

Explanation: This patient is exhibiting signs of restlessness, flushed face, gastrointestinal disturbance, muscle twitching, diuresis, rambling flow of speech, and cardiac abnormalities, all of which are consistent with caffeine intoxication. While a panic episode might be associated with tachycardia or gastrointestinal distress, it would not cause muscle twitching or cardiac arrhythmias. Intoxication with stimulants such as amphetamine or cocaine would present very similarly with psychomotor agitation and cardiac arrhythmias, but these substances would not cause diuresis and would be expected to show up on a urine toxicology screen. Alcohol withdrawal could also present similarly but is typically characterized by tremor rather than muscle twitching, and it also does not cause diuresis.

16.23—Caffeine Intoxication / diagnostic criteria; Diagnostic Features (pp. 503–504)

16.24 Which substance use disorder of an illicit substance is the most prevalent in the United States?

A. Alcohol use disorder.
B. Caffeine use disorder.
C. Cannabis use disorder.
D. Opioid use disorder.
E. Stimulant use disorder.

Correct Answer: C. Cannabis use disorder.

Explanation: Cannabinoids are the most widely used illicit psychoactive substances in the United States. The 12-month prevalence of *cannabis use disorder* is approximately 3.4% among 12- to 17-year-olds and 1.5% among adults age 18 years or older. *Alcohol use disorder* is the most prevalent of all of the substance use disorders in the United States. The 12-month prevalence of *alcohol use disorder* is estimated to be 4.6% among 12- to 17-year-olds and 8.5% among adults age 18 years or older in the United States. Although caffeine is the most widely used behaviorally active substance in the world, there are insufficient data to determine the clinical significance of *caffeine use disorder* and its prevalence at this time. Thus, caffeine use disorder is not an officially recognized DSM-5 diagnosis but rather is included in "Conditions for Further Study" (Section III) as a proposed diagnostic set. The 12-month prevalence of *opioid use disorder* is approximately 0.37% among adults age 18 years or older in the community population. Regarding *stimulant use disorders,* the 12-month prevalence of cocaine use disorder in the United States is approximately 0.2% among 12- to 17-year-olds and 0.3% among adults age 18 years or older, and the 12-month prevalence of amphetamine-type stimulant use disorder in the United States is approximately 0.2% among 12- to 17-year-olds and 0.2% among adults age 18 years or older.

16.24—Cannabis Use Disorder / Prevalence (p. 512)

16.25 Which of the following laboratory tests can be used in combination with gamma-glutamyltransferase (GGT) to monitor abstinence from alcohol?

A. Alanine aminotransferase (ALT).
B. Alkaline phosphatase.
C. Carbohydrate-deficient transferrin (CDT).
D. Mean corpuscular volume (MCV).
E. Triglycerides.

Correct Answer: C. Carbohydrate-deficient transferrin (CDT).

Explanation: Elevation of GGT is a sensitive laboratory indicator of heavy drinking. At least 70% of individuals with a high GGT level are persistent heavy drinkers (i.e., consuming eight or more drinks daily on a regular basis). A second test with comparable or even higher levels of sensitivity and specificity is CDT, with levels of 20 units or higher useful in identifying individuals who regularly consume eight or more drinks daily. Since both GGT and CDT levels return toward normal within days to weeks of stopping drinking, both state markers are useful in monitoring abstinence, especially when the clinician observes increases, rather than decreases, in these values over time. The combination of CDT and GGT may have even higher levels of sensitivity and specificity than either test used alone. Although the MCV can be used to help identify those who drink heavily, it is a poor method of monitoring abstinence because of the long half-life of red blood cells. Liver function tests (e.g., ALT and alkaline phosphatase) can reveal liver injury that is a consequence of heavy drinking. Nonspecific elevations of lipid levels in the blood (e.g., triglycerides and lipoprotein cholesterol) may also be observed due to decreases in gluconeogenesis associated with heavy drinking.

16.25—Alcohol Use Disorder / Diagnostic Markers (p. 495)

16.26 Which substance or class of substances in the Substance-Related and Addictive Disorders chapter of DSM-5 is *not* associated with a substance use disorder?

A. Caffeine.
B. Hallucinogens.
C. Inhalants.
D. Stimulants.
E. Tobacco.

Correct Answer: A. Caffeine.

Explanation: Some caffeine users display symptoms consistent with problematic use, including tolerance and withdrawal. However, there are insufficient data to determine the clinical significance or prevalence of a caffeine use disorder.Therefore, caffeine use disorder does not appear in the Substance-Related and Addictive Disorders chapter of DSM-5 but instead is included as a proposed criteria set in the "Conditions for Further Study" chapter of DSM-5 Section III to encourage further research. In contrast, there is evidence that caffeine withdrawal and caffeine intoxication are clinically significant and sufficiently prevalent.

16.26—Conditions for Further Study (Section III) / Caffeine Use Disorder (pp. 792–795)

16.27 What is the hallmark feature of caffeine withdrawal?

A. Vomiting.
B. Drowsiness.
C. Flu-like symptoms.
D. Headache.
E. Dysphoria.

Correct Answer: D. Headache.

Explanation: Headache is the hallmark feature of caffeine withdrawal. The remaining options are also symptoms of caffeine withdrawal and could occur in absence of headache. Caffeine is the most widely consumed behaviorally active drug in the world. Because caffeine ingestion is often integrated into social customs and daily rituals (e.g., coffee break, tea time), some caffeine consumers may be unaware of their physical dependence on caffeine and thus withdrawal symptoms could be unexpected and misattributed to other causes (e.g., the flu, migraine). Caffeine withdrawal symptoms may occur when individuals are required to abstain from foods and beverages prior to medical procedures or when a usual caffeine dose is missed because of a change in routine (e.g., during travel, weekends).

16.27—Caffeine Withdrawal / Diagnostic Features (p. 506)

16.28 Which mental disorder or disorder class has the highest prevalence among individuals with cannabis use disorder?

A. Major depressive disorder.
B. Bipolar I disorder.
C. Anxiety disorders.
D. Schizophrenia spectrum and other psychotic disorders.
E. Conduct disorder.

Correct Answer: C. Anxiety disorders.

Explanation: Individuals with past-year or lifetime diagnoses of cannabis use disorder have high rates of concurrent mental disorders. Anxiety disorders are the most prevalent (24%), followed by bipolar I disorder (13%) and major depressive disorder (11%).

16.28—Cannabis Use Disorder / Comorbidity (p. 515)

16.29 Which personality disorder has the highest prevalence among individuals with cannabis use disorder?

A. Obsessive-compulsive personality disorder.
B. Paranoid personality disorder.
C. Schizotypal personality disorder.
D. Borderline personality disorder.
E. Antisocial personality disorder.

Correct Answer: E. Antisocial personality disorder.

Explanation: Antisocial personality disorder is the most prevalent (30%) personality disorder among individuals with cannabis use disorder, followed by obsessive-compulsive personality disorder (19%) and paranoid personality disorder (18%).

16.29—Cannabis Use Disorder / Comorbidity (p. 515)

16.30 What are the three main chemical classes of hallucinogens?

A. Ethnobotanical compounds, ergolines, and phenylalkylamines.
B. Ethnobotanical compounds, ergolines, and indoleamines.
C. Indoleamines, ergolines, and phenylalkylamines.
D. Tryptoamines, indoleamines, and ergolines.
E. Tryptoamines, phenylalkylamines, and hydrocarbons.

Correct Answer: C. Indoleamines, ergolines, and phenylalkylamines.

Explanation: Hallucinogens comprise a diverse group of substances that, despite having different chemical structures and possibly involving different molecular mechanisms, produce similar alterations of perception, mood, and cognition in users. Hallucinogens included are *phenylalkylamines* (e.g., mescaline, DOM [2,5-dimethoxy-4-methylamphetamine], and MDMA [3,4-methylenedioxymethamphetamine; also called Ecstasy]); the *indoleamines,* including psilocybin (i.e., psilocin) and dimethyltryptamine (DMT); and the *ergolines,* such as LSD (lysergic acid diethylamide) and morning glory seeds. In addition, miscellaneous other ethnobotanical compounds are classified as hallucinogens, of which *Salvia divinorum* and jimsonweed are two examples. Volatile hydrocarbons are included among the inhalants.

16.30—Other Hallucinogen Use Disorder / Diagnostic Features (p. 524)

16.31 Which of the following statements about 3,4-methylenedioxymethamphetamine (MDMA [Ecstasy]) is *false?*

A. Relative to use of other hallucinogenic drugs, use of MDMA increases the risk of developing a hallucinogen use disorder.
B. MDMA has both hallucinogenic and stimulant properties.

C. MDMA is more likely than other drugs in this class to be associated with withdrawal symptoms.
D. MDMA has a shorter half-life relative to other hallucinogens.
E. MDMA can be administered via inhalation and injection whereas most other hallucinogens are ingested orally and occasionally smoked.

Correct Answer: D. MDMA has a shorter half-life relative to other hallucinogens.

Explanation: MDMA has a long half-life and extended duration such that users may spend hours to days using and/or recovering from its effects. MDMA as a hallucinogen may have distinctive effects attributable to both its hallucinogenic and its stimulant properties. Whereas a clinically significant hallucinogen withdrawal syndrome has not been consistently documented in humans (hence the absence of a DSM diagnosis for hallucinogen withdrawal), there is evidence of withdrawal from MDMA, with endorsement of two or more withdrawal symptoms observed in 59%–98% in selected samples of Ecstasy users. Both psychological and physical problems have been commonly reported as withdrawal problems. There may be a disproportionate influence of use of specific hallucinogens on risk of developing other hallucinogen use disorder, with use of Ecstasy/MDMA increasing the risk of the disorder relative to use of other hallucinogens. Although hallucinogens are usually taken orally, some forms are smoked (e.g., dimethyltryptamine [DMT], *Salvia divinorum*) or—more rarely—taken intranasally or by injection (e.g., Ecstasy).

16.31—Other Hallucinogen Use Disorder / Diagnostic Features; Development and Course (pp. 525, 526)

16.32 Which of the following substance use disorders is more common among adolescent males than among adolescent females?

A. Other hallucinogen use disorder.
B. Inhalant use disorder.
C. Sedative, hypnotic, or anxiolytic use disorder.
D. Stimulant use disorder, cocaine subtype.
E. Stimulant use disorder, amphetamine-type substance subtype.

Correct Answer: D. Stimulant use disorder, cocaine subtype.

Explanation: Although for the majority of substances the prevalence of a substance use disorder is higher in adult men versus women, among adolescents there are a number of substances in which this trend is reversed. The 12-month prevalence of *stimulant use disorder, cocaine subtype* among 12- to 17-year-olds is greater in males (0.4%) relative to females (0.1%). The 12-month prevalence of *other hallucinogen use disorder* is slightly higher in adolescent females (0.6%) than in males (0.4%). For 12- to 17-year-olds, the rate of *sedative, hypnotic, or* *anxiolytic use disorder* in females (0.4%) exceeds that of males (0.2%). Among 12- to 17-year-olds, the rate of *stimulant use disorder, amphetamine-type substance subtype* in females (0.3%) is greater than the rate in males (0.1%). The *rate of inhalant use disorder* is 0.4% in both 12- to 17-year-old boys and girls. Of note, adolescent males are overall more likely than adolescent females to experiment with and use substances.

16.32—Stimulant Use Disorder / Prevalence (p. 564)

16.33 Which two groups of inhalant agents are *not* among the recognized substances qualifying for the DSM-5 inhalant use disorder diagnosis?

A. Butane lighters and toluene.
B. Xylene and butane.
C. Trichloroethane and hexane.
D. Nitrous oxide and nitrite gases.
E. Gasoline and cleaning compounds.

Correct Answer: D. Nitrous oxide and nitrite gases.

Explanation: The DSM-5 *inhalant use disorder* diagnosis is restricted to volatile hydrocarbons—toxic gases from glues, fuels, paints, and other volatile compounds. Disorders arising from inhalation of nitrous oxide or nitrite gases (amyl-, butyl-, or isobutylnitrite) are diagnosed as *other (or unknown) substance use disorder.*

16.33—Inhalant Use Disorder / Specifiers (p. 535); Other (or Unknown) Substance Use Disorder / Diagnostic Features; Associated Features Supporting Diagnosis (p. 579)

16.34 Match each of the following substances (A–E) with the population subgroup (i–v) most associated with its use, according to epidemiological data included in DSM-5.

A. Amphetamines.
B. *Salvia divinorum.*
C. Air fresheners and hair sprays.
D. Gasoline.
E. Cannabis.

i. 18- to 29-year-olds.
ii. 18- to 25-year-olds with risk-taking behaviors.
iii. Adolescent boys.
iv. Adolescent girls.
v. Adult males.

Correct Answer: A: i, B: ii, C: iv, D: iii, E. v.

Explanation: The prevalence of *amphetamine* use is greatest among 18- to 29-year-olds. Some of these individuals begin use in an attempt to control their weight or improve performance in school, work, or athletics. Others become introduced to these substances through the illegal market. Use of *Salvia divinorum* is prominent among individuals 18–25 years of age with other risk-taking behaviors and illegal activities. Calls to poison control centers for "intentional abuse" of inhalants concerning adolescent boys usually involve *gasoline,* whereas cases of teenage girls most often involve *air fresheners, hair sprays,* and nail polish or remover. The 12-month prevalence of *cannabis* use disorder is highest among 18- to 29-year-old adults, with rates of the disorder higher among adult males (2.2%) than adult females (0.8%).

16.34—multiple: Stimulant Use Disorder (p. 564); Other Hallucinogen Use Disorder (p. 526); Inhalant Use Disorder (p. 536); Cannabis Use Disorder (p. 512)

16.35 A 22-year-old university student presents to his primary care physician complaining of progressive worsening of numbness, tingling, and weakness in both of his legs over the past several weeks. His gait is unsteady, and he has difficulty grasping objects in his hands. He did not use any substances on the day of presentation but admits that over the past 3 months he has been consistently using one particular substance on a daily basis. Which substance use disorder most likely accounts for this patient's symptoms?

A. Cannabis use disorder.
B. Other hallucinogen use disorder.
C. Inhalant use disorder.
D. Opioid use disorder.
E. Other (or unknown) substance use disorder.

Correct Answer: E. Other (or unknown) substance use disorder.

Explanation: Because of increased access to nitrous oxide ("laughing gas"), membership in certain populations is associated with diagnosis of nitrous oxide use disorder. The role of this gas as an anesthetic agent leads to misuse by some medical and dental professionals. Its use as a propellant for commercial products (e.g., whipped cream dispensers) contributes to misuse by food service workers. With recent widespread availability of the substance in "whippet" cartridges for use in home whipped cream dispensers, nitrous oxide misuse by adolescents and young adults is significant, especially among those who also inhale volatile hydrocarbons. Some continuously using individuals, inhaling from as many as 240 whippets per day, may present with serious medical complications and mental conditions, including myeloneuropathy, spinal cord subacute combined degeneration (as seen in the patient in this vignette), peripheral neuropathy, and psychosis. These conditions are also associated with a diagnosis of nitrous oxide use disorder.

16.35—Inhalant Use Disorder / Associated Features Supporting Diagnosis (p. 579)

16.36 Which organ system or anatomical function is most commonly affected by chronic use of 3,4-methylenedioxymethamphetamine (MDMA [Ecstasy])?

A. Neurological.
B. Respiratory.
C. Cardiopulmonary.
D. Oral cavity.
E. Immunological/infectious.

Correct Answer: A. Neurological.

Explanation: There is significant evidence for *long-term neurotoxic effects* of MDMA use, including memory impairment, neuroendocrine function, sleep disturbance, psychological functioning, and serotonin system. Damage to brain microvasculature, white matter maturation, and axonal connections are included among neurotoxic events.

16.36—Other Hallucinogen Use Disorder / Functional Consequences of Other Hallucinogen Use Disorder (p. 527)

16.37 What percentage of individuals who undergo untreated sedative, hypnotic, or anxiolytic withdrawal experience a grand mal seizure?

A. 5%–10%.
B. 10%–20%.
C. 20%–30%.
D. 30%–40%.
E. 40%–50%.

Correct Answer: C. 20%–30%.

Explanation: A grand mal seizure may occur in as many as 20%–30% of individuals undergoing untreated withdrawal from sedative, hypnotic, or anxiolytic substances.

16.37—Sedative, Hypnotic, or Anxiolytic Withdrawal / Diagnostic Features (p. 558)

16.38 Which route of stimulant use is most prevalent among individuals who are in treatment for a stimulant use disorder?

A. Oral.
B. Intranasal.
C. Smoking.
D. Intravenous.
E. Mixed routes.

Correct Answer: C. Smoking.

Explanation: The smoked route of administration predominates among individuals in treatment: 66% of primary amphetamine-type stimulants admissions reported smoking, 18% reported injection, and 10% reported snorting. Stimulant use disorder can develop rapidly when the substance is used intravenously or smoked. Oral administration usually results in a slower progression from occasional use to a use disorder.

16.38—Stimulant Use Disorder / Development and Course (p. 565)

16.39 What is the most common co-occurring psychiatric diagnosis among individuals with a history of significant prenatal alcohol exposure?

A. Major depressive disorder.
B. Generalized anxiety disorder.
C. Attention-deficit/hyperactivity disorder.
D. Oppositional defiant disorder.
E. Substance use disorder.

Correct Answer: C. Attention-deficit/hyperactivity disorder.

Explanation: Mental health problems have been identified in more than 90% of individuals with histories of significant prenatal alcohol exposure. The most common co-occurring diagnosis is attention-deficit/hyperactivity disorder. Other high-probability co-occurring disorders include oppositional defiant disorder and conduct disorder. Mood symptoms have been described, including symptoms of bipolar disorder and depression. History of prenatal alcohol exposure is associated with an increased risk of later nicotine, alcohol, and drug misuse or dependence.

16.39—Conditions for Further Study (Section III) / Neurobehavioral Disorder Associated With Prenatal Alcohol Exposure / Comorbidity (pp. 800–801)

CHAPTER 17

Neurocognitive Disorders

17.1   The essential feature of the DSM-5 diagnosis of delirium is a disturbance in attention/awareness and in cognition that develops over a short period of time, represents a change from baseline, and tends to fluctuate in severity during the course of a day. Which of the following additional conditions must apply?

   A. There must be laboratory evidence of an evolving dementia.
   B. The disturbance must be associated with a disruption of the sleep-wake cycle.
   C. The disturbance must not occur in the context of a severely reduced level of arousal, such as coma.
   D. The disturbance must be a direct physiological consequence of a substance use disorder.
   E. The disturbance must not be superimposed on a preexisting neurocognitive disorder.

Correct Answer: C. The disturbance must not occur in the context of a severely reduced level of arousal, such as coma.

Explanation: The essential feature of delirium is a disturbance of attention or awareness (Criterion A) that is accompanied by a change in baseline cognition (Criterion C) that cannot be better explained by a preexisting or evolving neurocognitive disorder (Criterion D1). The ability to evaluate cognition to diagnose delirium depends on there being a level of arousal sufficient for response to verbal stimulation; hence, delirium should not be diagnosed in the context of coma (Criterion D2). The disturbance develops over a short period of time, usually hours to a few days, and tends to fluctuate during the course of the day (Criterion B). There is evidence from the history, physical examination, or laboratory findings that the disturbance is a physiological consequence of an underlying medical condition, substance intoxication or withdrawal, use of a medication, or a toxin exposure, or a combination of these factors (Criterion E).

Both major and mild neurocognitive disorders (NCDs) can increase the risk for delirium and complicate the course. The most common differential diagnostic issue when evaluating confusion in older adults is disentangling symptoms of delirium and dementia. The clinician must determine whether the individual has delirium; a delirium superimposed on a preexisting NCD, such as that due to Alzheimer's disease; or an NCD without delirium. The traditional distinction between delirium and dementia according to acuteness of onset and temporal course is particularly difficult in those elderly individuals who had a prior NCD that may not have been recognized, or who develop persistent cognitive impairment following an episode of delirium.

17.1—Delirium / diagnostic criteria (p. 596); Diagnostic Features (p. 599); Differential Diagnosis (p. 601)

17.2   Both major and mild neurocognitive disorders can increase the risk of delirium and complicate its course. Traditionally, delirium is distinguished from dementia on the basis of the key features of acute onset, impairment in attention, and which of the following?

A. Fluctuating course.
B. Steady course.
C. Presence of mania.
D. Presence of depression.
E. Cogwheeling movements.

Correct Answer: A. Fluctuating course.

Explanation: According to Criterion B for delirium, the disturbance develops over a short period of time, usually hours to a few days, and tends to fluctuate during the course of the day, often with worsening in the evening and night when external orienting stimuli decrease.

17.2—Delirium / Diagnostic Features (p. 599)

17.3   A 79-year-old woman with a history of depression is being evaluated at a nursing home for a suspected urinary tract infection. She is easily distracted, perseverates on answers to questions, asks the same question repeatedly, is unable to focus, and cannot answer questions regarding orientation. The mental status changes evolved over a single day. Her family reports that they thought she "wasn't herself" when they saw her the previous evening, but the nursing report this morning indicates that the patient was cordial and appropriate. What is the most likely diagnosis?

A. Major depressive disorder, recurrent episode.
B. Depressive disorder due to another medical condition.
C. Delirium.
D. Major depressive disorder, with anxious distress.
E. Obsessive-compulsive disorder.

Correct Answer: C. Delirium.

Explanation: This patient's symptoms are proximally related to the urinary tract infection: her mental status changes had a temporal, fluctuating course with disturbance in attention and cognition. These are the diagnostic features of delirium.

17.4   The diagnostic criteria for major or mild neurocognitive disorder with Lewy bodies (NCDLB) include fulfillment of criteria for major or mild neurocognitive disorder and presence of "a combination of core diagnostic features and suggested diagnostic features for either probable or possible neurocognitive disorder with Lewy bodies." Another feature necessary for the diagnosis is that "the disturbance is not better explained by cerebrovascular disease, another neurodegenerative disease, the effects of a substance, or another mental, neurological, or systemic disorder." Which of the following completes the list of features necessary for the diagnosis?

A. An acute onset and rapid progression.
B. An insidious onset and gradual progression.
C. An insidious onset and rapid progression.
D. A waxing and waning presentation.
E. A characteristic finding on ultrasound of the neck.

Correct Answer: B. An insidious onset and gradual progression.

Explanation: NCDLB includes not only progressive cognitive impairment (with early changes in complex attention and executive function rather than learning and memory) but also recurrent complex visual hallucinations; concurrent symptoms of rapid eye movement sleep behavior disorder (which can be a very early manifestation); as well as hallucinations in other sensory modalities, depression, and delusions. The symptoms fluctuate in a pattern that can resemble a delirium, but no adequate underlying cause can be found. The variable presentation of NCDLB symptoms reduces the likelihood of all symptoms being observed in a brief clinic visit and necessitates a thorough assessment of caregiver observations. The use of assessment scales specifically designed to assess fluctuation may aid in diagnosis. Another core feature is spontaneous parkinsonism, which must begin after the onset of cognitive decline; by convention, major cognitive deficits are observed *at least 1 year before* the motor symptoms. NCDLB is a gradually progressive disorder with insidious onset. However, there is often a prodromal history of confusional episodes (delirium) of acute onset, often precipitated by illness or surgery.

17.4—Major or Mild Neurocognitive Disorder With Lewy Bodies / diagnostic criteria (p. 618); Development and Course (p. 619)

17.5   Which of the following is *not* a diagnostic criterion, feature, or marker of major or mild neurocognitive disorder with Lewy bodies (NCDLB)?

A. Concurrent symptoms of rapid eye movement (REM) sleep behavior disorder.

B. High striatal dopamine transporter uptake in basal ganglia demonstrated by single-photon emission computed tomography (SPECT) or positron emission tomography (PET) imaging.
C. Low striatal dopamine transporter uptake in basal ganglia demonstrated by SPECT or PET imaging.
D. Severe neuroleptic sensitivity.
E. Insidious onset and gradual progression.

Correct Answer: B. High striatal dopamine transporter uptake in basal ganglia demonstrated by SPECT or PET imaging.

Explanation: The underlying neurodegenerative disease in NCDLB is primarily a synucleinopathy due to alpha-synuclein misfolding and aggregation. Cognitive testing beyond the use of a brief screening instrument may be necessary to define deficits clearly. Assessment scales developed to measure fluctuation can be useful. The associated condition REM sleep behavior disorder may be diagnosed through a formal sleep study or identified by questioning the patient or informant about relevant symptoms. Neuroleptic sensitivity (challenge) is not recommended as a diagnostic marker but raises suspicion of NCDLB if it occurs.

A diagnostically suggestive feature is *low* striatal dopamine transporter uptake on SPECT or PET scan. Other clinically useful markers potentially include relative preservation of medial temporal structures on computed tomography/magnetic resonance imaging brain scan; reduced striatal dopamine transporter uptake on SPECT/PET scan; generalized low uptake on SPECT/PET perfusion scan with reduced occipital activity; abnormal (low uptake) [123I]metaiodobenzylguanidine (123I-MIBG) myocardial scintigraphy suggesting sympathetic denervation; and prominent slow-wave activity on the electroencephalogram with temporal lobe transient waves.

17.5—Major or Mild Neurocognitive Disorder With Lewy Bodies / Diagnostic Markers (p. 620)

17.6 A 72-year-old man with no history of alcohol or other substance use disorders and no psychiatric history is brought to the emergency department (ED) because of transient episodes of unexplained loss of consciousness. His wife reports that he has experienced repeated falls and syncope over the past year, as well as auditory and visual hallucinations. A thorough workup for cardiac disease has found no evidence of structural heart disease or arrhythmias. In the ED, he is found to have severe autonomic dysfunction, including orthostatic hypotension and urinary incontinence. What is the best provisional diagnosis for this patient?

A. New-onset schizophrenia.
B. New-onset schizoaffective disorder.
C. Possible major or mild neurocognitive disorder with Lewy bodies.

D. Possible major or mild neurocognitive disorder due to Alzheimer's disease.

E. New-onset seizure disorder.

Correct Answer: C. Possible major or mild neurocognitive disorder with Lewy bodies.

Explanation: Further information on cognition, time frame, and other etiologies must be ascertained, but the best working diagnosis with the limited information available is neurocognitive disorder with Lewy bodies (NCDLB). Individuals with NCDLB frequently experience repeated falls and syncope and transient episodes of unexplained loss of consciousness. Severe autonomic dysfunction, such as orthostatic hypotension and urinary incontinence, may also be observed. Auditory and other nonvisual hallucinations are common, as are systematized delusions, delusional misidentification, and depression.

The patient has auditory and visual hallucinations but no other feature of schizophrenia or schizoaffective disorder, and the age at onset, along with the associated neurological symptoms, suggest a neurodegenerative disorder rather than schizophrenia or schizoaffective illness. Among neurocognitive disorders, the prominence of hallucinations, episodic loss of consciousness, and autonomic symptoms in the early course—rather than marked memory impairment—argue against a neurocognitive disorder due to Alzheimer's disease and in favor of NCDLB. The patient has one of the "core diagnostic features" of NCDLB, visual hallucinations, justifying a "possible" level of certainty for the diagnosis. A seizure disorder might cause episodic loss of consciousness but would not parsimoniously account for hallucinations and autonomic symptoms.

17.6—Major or Mild Neurocognitive Disorder With Lewy Bodies / Associated Features Supporting Diagnosis (p. 619)

17.7   The diagnostic criteria for neurocognitive disorder (NCD) due to HIV infection include fulfillment of criteria for major or mild NCD and documented infection with human immunodeficiency virus (as confirmed by established laboratory methods). Which of the following is a prominent feature of NCD due to HIV infection?

A. Impairment in executive functioning.

B. Conspicuous aphasia.

C. Significant delusions and hallucinations at onset of the disorder.

D. Marked difficulty with recall of learned information.

E. Rapid progression to profound neurocognitive impairment.

Correct Answer: A. Impairment in executive functioning.

Explanation: NCD associated with HIV infection generally shows a "subcortical pattern" with prominently impaired executive function, slowing of processing speed, problems with more demanding attentional tasks, and difficulty in learning new information, but fewer problems with recall of learned information. In major NCD, slowing may be prominent. Language difficulties, such as aphasia, are uncommon, although reductions in fluency may be observed. HIV pathogenic processes can affect any part of the brain; therefore, other patterns are possible. An NCD due to HIV infection can resolve, improve, slowly worsen, or have a fluctuating course. Rapid progression to profound neurocognitive impairment is uncommon in the context of currently available combination antiviral treatment; consequently, an abrupt change in mental status in an individual with HIV may prompt an evaluation of other medical sources for the cognitive change, including secondary infections.

17.7—Major or Mild Neurocognitive Disorder Due to HIV Infection / Diagnostic Features; Development and Course (pp. 632, 633)

17.8   In addition to documented infection with HIV and fulfillment of criteria for major or mild neurocognitive disorder (NCD), what other requirement must be met to qualify for a diagnosis of major or mild NCD due to HIV infection?

A. Presence of HIV in the cerebrospinal fluid.
B. A pattern of cognitive impairment characterized by early predominance of aphasia and impaired memory for previously learned information.
C. Presence of progressive multifocal leukoencephalopathy.
D. Inability to attribute the NCD to non-HIV conditions (including secondary brain diseases), another medical condition, or a mental disorder.
E. Presence of Kayser-Fleisher rings.

Correct Answer: D. Inability to attribute the NCD to non-HIV conditions (including secondary brain diseases), another medical condition, or a mental disorder.

Explanation: In addition to requiring fulfillment of criteria for major or mild NCD and documented infection with HIV, the diagnostic criteria for NCD due to HIV infection stipulate that the NCD is not better explained by non-HIV conditions, including secondary brain diseases such as progressive multifocal leukoencephalopathy or cryptococcal meningitis; and that it is not attributable to another medical condition and is not better explained by a mental disorder.

An NCD due to HIV infection generally shows a "subcortical pattern" with prominently impaired executive function, slowing of processing speed, problems with more demanding attentional tasks, and difficulty in learning new information, but fewer problems with recall of learned information. In major NCD, slowing may be prominent. Language difficulties, such as aphasia, are uncommon, although reductions in fluency may be observed. HIV pathogenic processes can affect any part of the brain; therefore, other patterns are possible. NCD due to HIV is more prevalent in individuals with high viral loads in the cerebrospinal fluid, but this is not a diagnostic criterion. Kayser-Fleisher rings are observed in Wilson's disease, not HIV.

17.8—Major or Mild Neurocognitive Disorder Due to HIV Infection / diagnostic criteria & Diagnostic Features (p. 632); Associated Features Supporting Diagnosis (p. 633)

17.9 Which of the following features characterizes alcohol-induced major or mild neurocognitive disorder, amnestic-confabulatory type?

A. Amnesia for new information and confabulation.
B. Seizures.
C. Amnesia for previously learned information and downward gaze paralysis.
D. Aphasia.
E. Anosognosia and apraxia.

Correct Answer: A. Amnesia for new information and confabulation.

Explanation: Neurocognitive disorder induced by alcohol frequently manifests with a combination of impairments in executive function and memory and learning domains. Features of alcohol-induced amnestic-confabulatory (Korsakoff's) neurocognitive disorder include prominent amnesia (severe difficulty learning new information with rapid forgetting) and a tendency to confabulate. These manifestations may co-occur with signs of thiamine encephalopathy (Wernicke's encephalopathy) with associated features such as nystagmus and ataxia. Ophthalmoplegia of Wernicke's encephalopathy is typically characterized by a lateral gaze paralysis.

17.9—Substance/Medication-Induced Major or Mild Neurocognitive Disorder / Diagnostic Features (p. 630)

17.10 Which of the following statements about the diagnosis of neurocognitive disorder due to Huntington's disease (NCDHD) is *true?*

A. NCDHD is a laboratory-based diagnosis/disorder.
B. NCDHD is a disorder that requires positive neuroimaging for diagnosis.
C. NCDHD is a clinical diagnosis based on abnormal physical findings and family history/genetic findings.
D. NCDHD is a diagnosis that is best defined as patients who have a pill-rolling tremor.
E. NCDHD is a diagnosis mostly based on radiological examination.

Correct Answer: C. NCDHD is a clinical diagnosis based on abnormal physical findings and family history/genetic findings.

Explanation: Genetic testing is the primary laboratory test for the determination of Huntington's disease, which is an autosomal dominant disorder with complete penetrance. A diagnosis of definite Huntington's disease is given in the presence of unequivocal extrapyramidal motor abnormalities in an individual with either a family history of Huntington's disease or genetic testing showing a CAG trinucleotide repeat expansion in the *HTT* gene, located on chromosome 4.

17.10—Major or Mild Neurocognitive Disorder Due to Huntington's Disease / Diagnostic Features (p. 639); Diagnostic Markers (p. 640)

17.11 Depression, irritability, anxiety, obsessive-compulsive symptoms, and apathy are frequently associated with Huntington's disease and often precede the onset of motor symptoms. Psychosis more rarely precedes the onset of motor symptoms. Which of the following is a core feature of major or mild neurocognitive disorder due to Huntington's disease?

A. Progressive cognitive impairment with early changes in executive function.
B. Prominent early memory impairment, mostly affecting short-term memory.
C. Psychosis in the early stages, with marked olfactory hallucinations.
D. Voluntary jerking movements.
E. Diminished hearing and smell.

Correct Answer: A. Progressive cognitive impairment with early changes in executive function.

Explanation: A core feature of Huntington's disease is progressive cognitive impairment with early changes in executive function (i.e., processing speed, organization, and planning) rather than learning and memory. Cognitive and associated behavioral changes often precede the emergence of the typical motor abnormalities of bradykinesia (i.e., slowing of voluntary movement) and chorea (i.e., involuntary jerking movements).

17.11—Major or Mild Neurocognitive Disorder Due to Huntington's Disease / Diagnostic Features; Associated Features Supporting Diagnosis (p. 639)

17.12 Genetic testing is the primary laboratory test for the determination of Huntington's disease. Which of the following best characterizes the genetic nature of Huntington's disease?

A. X-linked recessive inheritance with incomplete penetrance.
B. Autosomal recessive inheritance with complete penetrance.
C. Autosomal dominant inheritance with complete penetrance.
D. Random mutation.
E. X-linked dominant inheritance.

Correct Answer: C. Autosomal dominant inheritance with complete penetrance.

Explanation: The genetic basis of Huntington's disease is a fully penetrant autosomal dominant expansion of the CAG trinucleotide, often called a CAG repeat, in the huntingtin gene. A CAG repeat length of 36 or more is invariably associated with Huntington's disease, with longer repeat lengths associated with early age at onset.

17.12—Major or Mild Neurocognitive Disorder Due to Huntington's Disease / Risk and Prognostic Factors; Diagnostic Markers (p. 640)

17.13 Major or mild neurocognitive disorder (NCD) due to prion disease encompasses NCDs associated with a group of subacute spongiform encephalopathies caused by transmissible agents known as *prions*. What is the most common prion disease?

A. Creutzfeldt-Jakob disease.
B. Wernicke-Korsakoff syndrome.
C. Bovine spongiform encephalopathy.
D. Huntington's disease.
E. Neurosyphilis.

Correct Answer: A. Creutzfeldt-Jakob disease.

Explanation: Prion diseases include Creutzfeldt-Jakob disease, variant Creutzfeldt-Jakob disease, kuru, Gerstmann-Sträussler-Scheinker syndrome, and fatal insomnia. The most common type is sporadic Creutzfeldt-Jakob disease, typically referred to as Creutzfeldt-Jakob disease (CJD). (Variant CJD is much rarer and is associated with transmission of bovine spongiform encephalopathy, also called "mad cow disease.") Typically, individuals with CJD present with neurocognitive deficits, ataxia, and abnormal movements such as myoclonus, chorea, or dystonia; a startle reflex is also common. Typically, the history reveals rapid progression to major NCD over as little as 6 months, and thus the disorder is typically seen only at the major level. However, many individuals with the disorder may have atypical presentations, and the disease can be confirmed only by biopsy or at autopsy.

Wernicke-Korsakoff syndrome, neurosyphilis, and Huntington's disease are not prion diseases; rather, Wernicke-Korsakoff syndrome is secondary to thiamine deficiency, Huntington's disease is secondary to a genetic defect, and neurosyphilis is caused by a sexually transmitted infection.

17.13—Major or Mild Neurocognitive Disorder Due to Prion Disease / Diagnostic Features (p. 635)

17.14 Prion disease has been reported to occur in individuals of all ages, from the teenage years to late life. Which of the following best characterizes the time frame of disease progression?

A. Over a few months.
B. Over several days.
C. Over several weeks.
D. Over 5 years.
E. Over 10 years.

Correct Answer: A. Over a few months.

Explanation: Prion disease may develop at any age in adults—the peak age for sporadic Creutzfeldt-Jakob disease is approximately 67 years, although it has been reported to occur in individuals spanning the teenage years to late life. Prodromal symptoms of prion disease may include fatigue, anxiety, problems with appetite or sleeping, or difficulties with concentration. After several weeks, these symptoms may be followed by incoordination, altered vision, or abnormal gait or other movements that may be myoclonic, choreoathetoid, or ballistic, along with a rapidly progressive dementia. The disease typically progresses very rapidly to the major level of impairment over several months. More rarely, it can progress over 2 years and appear similar in its course to other neurocognitive disorders.

17.14—Major or Mild Neurocognitive Disorder Due to Prion Disease / Development and Course (p. 635)

17.15 Major and mild neurocognitive disorders (NCDs) exist on a spectrum of cognitive and functional impairment. Which of the following constitutes an important threshold differentiating the two diagnoses?

A. Whether or not the individual is concerned about the decline in cognitive function.
B. Whether or not there is impairment in cognitive performance as measured by standardized testing or clinical assessment.
C. Whether or not the cognitive impairment is sufficient to interfere with independent completion of activities of daily living.
D. Whether or not the cognitive deficits occur exclusively in the context of a delirium.
E. Whether or not the cognitive deficits are better explained by another mental disorder.

Correct Answer: C. Whether or not the cognitive impairment is sufficient to interfere with independent completion of activities of daily living.

Explanation: Criterion B for major or mild NCD relates to the individual's level of independence in everyday functioning. Individuals with *major* NCD will have impairment of sufficient severity to interfere with independence, such that others will have to take over tasks that the individuals were previously able to complete on their own. Individuals with *mild* NCD will have preserved independence, although there may be subtle interference with function or a report that tasks require more effort or take more time than previously. The distinction between major and mild NCD is inherently arbitrary, and the disorders exist along a continuum. Precise thresholds are therefore difficult to determine. Careful history taking, observation, and integration with other findings are required, and the implications of diagnosis should be considered when an individual's clinical manifestations lie at a boundary.

For both mild and major NCD, Criterion A requires evidence of a cognitive decline based on 1) concern on the part of the patient, a knowledgeable informant, or a clinician that there has been such a decline; and 2) impairment in cognitive performance as documented by standardized testing or other objective assessment. For major NCD, *significant* decline and *substantial* impairment are specified; for mild NCD, the words *modest* and *mild* are used.

Both disorders can occur with comorbid delirium, but they cannot be diagnosed if the cognitive impairment occurs only in the context of delirium (Criterion C). Both disorders can occur in patients with other significant disorders, but in order to make the diagnosis, the cognitive deficits must not be primarily attributable to another disorder (Criterion D).

17.15—Major and Mild Neurocognitive Disorders / diagnostic criteria (A and B) (pp. 602–603, 605); Diagnostic Features (p. 608)

17.16 Expressed as a percentile, what is the typical performance on neuropsychological testing of individuals with major neurocognitive disorder (NCD)?

A. Sixtieth percentile or below.
B. Fiftieth percentile or below.
C. Twenty-fifth percentile or below.
D. Sixteenth percentile or below.
E. Third percentile or below.

Correct Answer: E. Third percentile or below.

Explanation: Neuropsychological testing, with performance compared with norms appropriate to the patient's age, educational attainment, and cultural background, is part of the standard evaluation of NCDs. For major NCD, performance is typically 2 or more standard deviations below appropriate norms (3rd percentile or below). For mild NCD, performance typically lies in the 1–2 standard deviation range (between the 3rd and 16th percentiles).

17.16—Major and Mild Neurocognitive Disorders / Diagnostic Features (p. 607)

17.17 A 68-year-old semiretired cardiologist with responsibility for electrocardio-gram (ECG) interpretation at his community hospital is referred by the hospi-tal's Employee Assistance Program for clinical evaluation because of concerns expressed by other clinicians that he has been making many mistakes in his ECG interpretations over the past few months. The patient discloses symptoms of persistent sadness since the death of his wife 6 months prior to the evalua-tion, with frequent thoughts of death, trouble sleeping, and escalating usage of sedative-hypnotics and alcohol. He has some trouble concentrating, but he has been able to maintain his household, pay his bills, shop, and prepare meals by himself without difficulty. He scores 28/30 on the Mini-Mental State Examina-tion (MMSE). Which of the following would be the primary consideration in the differential diagnosis?

A. Major neurocognitive disorder (NCD).
B. Mild NCD.
C. Adjustment disorder.
D. Major depressive disorder.
E. No diagnosis.

Correct Answer: D. Major depressive disorder.

Explanation: Not enough information has been provided to know for certain whether this patient meets criteria for a specific mood disorder diagnosis—or for a substance use disorder diagnosis—but a major NCD can be ruled out. Al-though the patient's test score on the MMSE is within the normal range, he does meet Criterion A for major NCD, in that concerns about a decline in cog-nitive function have been raised due to his increased error rate in interpreting ECGs. Regarding Criterion B for major NCD, the patient does not demonstrate loss of ability to perform activities of daily living independently and so does not qualify for a diagnosis of major NCD. He does meet Criterion C, in that he is not demonstrating signs of delirium. The fact that his problems have become evident only in the context of mood issues strongly suggests that a depressive disorder and/or substance use may account for his work performance deficits; therefore, he likely will not meet Criterion D for NCD. Although he could meet Criterion B for mild NCD, a mood disorder would be the most prominent con-sideration in the differential diagnosis.

17.17—Major and Mild Neurocognitive Disorders / diagnostic criteria (pp. 602–603; 605)

17.18 A 69-year-old semiretired radiologist with responsibility for chest x-ray inter-pretation at his academic medical center has been referred by the hospital's Employee Assistance Program for clinical evaluation because of concerns ex-pressed by other clinicians that he has been making many mistakes in his x-ray interpretations over the past few months. Evaluation discloses a remote history of alcohol dependence with sobriety for the past 20 years, and a depressive ep-isode following the death of his wife 9 years before the current problem, treated with cognitive-behavioral therapy with full resolution of symptoms after 6 months and no recurrence. He acknowledges some trouble concentrating but no other symptoms, and he minimizes the alleged x-ray interpretation problems. He cannot state the correct date or day of the week and cannot recall the previous day's news events, but he can describe highlights of his long career in medicine in great detail. Collateral history from his children reveals that on several occasions in the past year neighbors in his apartment building had complained that he forgot to turn off his stove while cooking, resulting in a smoke-filled apartment. He scores 21/30 on the Mini-Mental State Examination. What diagnosis best fits this clinical picture?

A. Major neurocognitive disorder (NCD).
B. Mild NCD.
C. Adjustment disorder.
D. Major depressive disorder.
E. No diagnosis.

Correct Answer: A. Major NCD.

Explanation: Concern has been raised about cognitive decline affecting this patient's functioning, and his test performance is very abnormal, so he clearly meets Criterion A for major NCD. Forgetting to keep track of what is cooking on the stovetop, with the result that neighbors have to intervene because of a smoke condition, is a good example of inability to perform activities of daily living independently, so he meets Criterion B for major NCD, as opposed to mild NCD. He is not delirious, so he meets Criterion C. Neither his remote history of alcohol dependence nor his remote history of depression accounts for his cognitive problems, and there is no evidence of another mental disorder, so he probably also meets Criterion D.

17.18—Major and Mild Neurocognitive Disorders / diagnostic criteria (pp. 602–603; 605)

17.19 In a patient with *mild* neurocognitive disorder (NCD), which of the following would distinguish *probable* from *possible* Alzheimer's disease?

A. Evidence of a causative Alzheimer's disease genetic mutation from either genetic testing or family history.
B. Clear evidence of decline in memory and learning.
C. Steadily progressive, gradual decline in cognition, without extended plateaus.
D. No evidence of mixed etiology.
E. Onset after age 80.

Correct Answer: A. Evidence of a causative Alzheimer's disease genetic mutation from either genetic testing or family history.

Explanation: The only way that mild NCD due to *probable* Alzheimer's disease can be diagnosed is if there is evidence of a causative Alzheimer's disease genetic mutation from either genetic testing or family history. Mild NCD due to *possible* Alzheimer's disease is diagnosed on the basis of the presence of *all* of the clinical criteria described in options B–D above. Age at onset is not a diagnostic criterion.

17.19—Major or Mild Neurocognitive Disorder Due to Alzheimer's Disease / diagnostic criteria (p. 611)

17.20 In major or mild frontotemporal neurocognitive disorder, which of the following is a diagnostic feature of the language variant?

A. Severe semantic memory impairment.
B. Severe deficits in perceptual-motor function.
C. Receptive aphasia.
D. Grammar, word-finding, or word-generation difficulty.
E. Hyperorality.

Correct Answer: D. Grammar, word-finding, or word-generation difficulty.

Explanation: The language variant diagnosis specifically requires worsening in language function with at least relative sparing of learning and memory and perceptual-motor function. Hyperorality is a diagnostic feature of the behavioral deficit variant. Signs of either the language variant or behavior variant can also occur in patients in whom the other variant is predominant, but the diagnosis would be based on the predominant features.

17.20—Major or Mild Frontotemporal Neurocognitive Disorder / diagnostic criteria (pp. 614–615)

17.21 Which of the following neurocognitive disorders (NCDs) is especially characterized by deficits in domains such as speech production, word finding, object naming, or word comprehension, whereas episodic memory, perceptual-motor abilities, and executive function are relatively preserved?

A. Major or mild NCD due to Alzheimer's disease.
B. Major or mild NCD with Lewy bodies.
C. Major or mild vascular NCD.
D. Behavioral-variant major or mild frontotemporal NCD.
E. Language-variant major or mild frontotemporal NCD.

Correct Answer: E. Language-variant major or mild frontotemporal NCD.

Explanation: Major or mild frontotemporal NCD comprises a number of syndromic variants characterized by the progressive development of behavioral and personality change and/or language impairment. The behavioral variant and three language variants (semantic, agrammatic/nonfluent, and logopenic) exhibit distinct patterns of brain atrophy and some distinctive neuropathology. The criteria must be met for either the behavioral or the language variant to make the diagnosis, but many individuals present with features of both.

Individuals with language-variant major or mild frontotemporal NCD present with primary progressive aphasia with gradual onset, with three subtypes commonly described: semantic variant, agrammatic/nonfluent variant, and logopenic variant, and each variant has distinctive features and corresponding neuropathology.

Individuals with behavioral-variant major or mild frontotemporal NCD present with varying degrees of apathy or disinhibition. They may lose interest in socialization, self-care, and personal responsibilities, or display socially inappropriate behaviors. Insight is usually impaired, and this often delays medical consultation. The first referral is often to a psychiatrist. Individuals may develop changes in social style, and in religious and political beliefs, with repetitive movements, hoarding, changes in eating behavior, and hyperorality. In later stages, loss of sphincter control may occur. Cognitive decline is less prominent, and formal testing may show relatively few deficits in the early stages. Common neurocognitive symptoms are lack of planning and organization, distractibility, and poor judgment. Deficits in executive function, such as poor performance on tests of mental flexibility, abstract reasoning, and response inhibition, are present, but learning and memory are relatively spared, and perceptual motor abilities are almost always preserved in the early stages.

17.21—Major or Mild Frontotemporal Neurocognitive Disorder / Diagnostic Features (pp. 615–616)

17.22 Which of the following is a core feature of major or mild neurocognitive disorder with Lewy bodies?

A. Fluctuating cognition with pronounced variations in attention and alertness.
B. Recurrent auditory hallucinations.
C. Spontaneous features of parkinsonism, with onset at least 1 year prior to development of cognitive decline.
D. Fulfillment of criteria for rapid eye movement (REM) sleep behavior disorder.
E. Evidence of low striatal dopamine transporter uptake in basal ganglia as demonstrated by single photon emission computed tomography (SPECT) or positron emission tomography (PET) imaging.

Correct Answer: A. Fluctuating cognition with pronounced variations in attention and alertness.

Explanation: Recurrent well-formed *visual* hallucinations (not auditory hallucinations) and parkinsonism arising *after* (not earlier than) cognitive impairment are the other core features of major or mild neurocognitive disorder with Lewy bodies. REM sleep behavioral disorder and excessive sensitivity to neuroleptic agents are "suggestive diagnostic features"; low dopamine transporter uptake in basal ganglia is a diagnostic marker but is not included in the diagnostic criteria.

17.22—Major or Mild Neurocognitive Disorder With Lewy Bodies / diagnostic criteria; Diagnostic Markers (pp. 618, 620)

17.23 A previously healthy 67-year-old man, who is experiencing an acute change in mental status, is brought to the emergency department by his family. There is no evidence in the initial history, physical examination, and laboratory studies to indicate substance intoxication or withdrawal, or to suggest another medical problem as the cause of his altered mental state. Over the course of 1 hour of observation, his level of alertness varies from alert but distractible, with apparent auditory and visual hallucinations, to somnolent; he has difficulty sustaining attention to an examiner, and he cannot perform simple tasks such as serial subtractions or spelling words backwards. What is the most appropriate diagnosis?

A. Delirium.
B. Delirium due to another medical condition.
C. Delirium due to substance intoxication.
D. Delirium due to multiple etiologies.
E. Unspecified delirium.

Correct Answer: E. Unspecified delirium.

Explanation: This man meets criteria for some sort of delirium, but at this point in the course of his illness it cannot be determined what the cause is. The "unspecified delirium" category can be used when the clinician chooses not to specify a specific cause, when the diagnostic criteria for delirium are not entirely fulfilled, or when the specific diagnostic subtype of delirium cannot be ascertained.

17.23—Unspecified Delirium (p. 602)

17.24 A 35-year-old man brings his 60-year-old father for evaluation of cognitive and functional decline, stating that he thinks his father has dementia; the son is also worried about the possibility of a hereditary illness. The physician notes to herself that the patient has substantial cognitive impairment and features suggestive of the diagnosis of major neurocognitive disorder due to Huntington's disease, but she is not sure about the cause of the neurocognitive disorder. She also notes that the patient's son appears extremely anxious. She has a tight schedule and cannot provide a counseling session for the patient's son until the next day. What is the most appropriate diagnosis to record on the insurance claim form that the patient's son will submit on his father's behalf?

A. Unspecified central nervous system (CNS) disorder.
B. Unspecified neurocognitive disorder.
C. Unspecified mild neurocognitive disorder.
D. Huntington's disease.
E. Problem related to living alone (V code category reflecting other problems related to the social environment).

Correct Answer: B. Unspecified neurocognitive disorder.

Explanation: The category unspecified neurocognitive disorder applies to presentations in which symptoms characteristic of a neurocognitive disorder that cause clinically significant distress or impairment in social, occupational, or other important areas of functioning predominate but do not meet the full criteria for any of the disorders in the neurocognitive disorders diagnostic class. The unspecified neurocognitive disorder category is also used in situations in which the precise etiology cannot be determined with sufficient certainty to make an etiological attribution.

In this case, Huntington's disease is suspected but not established. "Unspecified CNS disorder" is not a DSM-5 diagnosis and would be inadequately specific to the patient's condition. The apparent severity of the deficits precludes a diagnosis of mild neurocognitive disorder or a V code designation of problem related to living alone.

17.24—Unspecified Neurocognitive Disorder (p. 643); Other Conditions That May Be a Focus of Clinical Attention (p. 724)

CHAPTER 18

Personality Disorders

18.1 Which of the following DSM-IV personality disorder diagnoses is no longer present in DSM-5?

A. Antisocial personality disorder.
B. Avoidant personality disorder.
C. Borderline personality disorder.
D. Personality disorder not otherwise specified (NOS).
E. Schizotypal personality disorder.

Correct Answer: D. Personality disorder not otherwise specified (NOS).

Explanation: Although the DSM-5 task force considered the possible elimination of several DSM-IV personality disorder diagnoses (including paranoid, schizoid, and histrionic personality disorders) based on their low prevalence and weak evidence for validity, the decision was made to keep all 10 DSM-IV personality disorders for DSM-5, with the exact same criteria. The NOS category has been removed, and instead two diagnoses have been introduced: other specified personality disorder and unspecified personality disorder.

18.1—Appendix / Highlights of Changes From DSM-IV to DSM-5 (p. 816)

18.2 While collaborating on a presentation to their customers, the members of a sales team become increasingly frustrated with their team leader. The leader insists that the members of the team adhere to his strict rules for developing the project. This involves approaching the task in sequential manner such that no new task can be begun until the prior one is perfected. When other members suggest alternative approaches, the leader becomes frustrated and insists that the team stick to his approach. Although the results are inarguably of high quality, the team is convinced that they will not finish in time for the scheduled presentation. When voicing these concerns to the leader, he suggests that the real problem is that the other members of the team simply don't share his high standards. Which of the following disorders would best explain the behavior of this team leader?

A. Narcissistic personality disorder.
B. Obsessive-compulsive disorder (OCD).
C. Avoidant personality disorder.
D. Obsessive-compulsive personality disorder (OCPD).
E. Unspecified personality disorder.

Correct Answer: D. Obsessive-compulsive personality disorder (OCPD).

Explanation: OCPD describes a series of enduring, maladaptive traits and behaviors characterized by excessive perfectionism, preoccupation with orderliness and detail, and need for control over one's emotions and environment. Although this borders on what might be considered a commendable work ethic, the frustration this leader causes among his team and the possibility that the project may not be completed in time raise the likelihood of a disorder. The differential diagnosis involves a number of other personality disorders, including narcissistic personality disorder and avoidant personality disorder. Whereas individuals with narcissistic personality disorder may profess a desire to strive for perfection, this is in the service of self-aggrandizement. Individuals with avoidant personality disorder may also wish for perfection, but they are highly self-critical. Neither of these disorders is characterized by the rigidity typical of OCPD. Despite the similarity in names, OCD is usually easily distinguished from OCPD by the presence of true obsessions and compulsions in OCD. When criteria for both OCPD and OCD are met, both diagnoses should be recorded.

18.2—Obsessive-Compulsive Personality Disorder / diagnostic criteria; Diagnostic Features (pp. 678–680); Differential Diagnosis (p. 681)

18.3   Individuals with obsessive-compulsive personality disorder are primarily motivated by a need for which of the following?

A. Efficiency.
B. Admiration.
C. Control.
D. Intimacy.
E. Autonomy.

Correct Answer: C. Control.

Explanation: Individuals with obsessive-compulsive personality disorder attempt to maintain a sense of control through a rigid preoccupation with order and detail. Unlike individuals with narcissistic personality disorder, their desire for perfection comes from this need for control rather than a need for admiration. The individual's rigidity and perfectionism can cause a debilitating degree of inefficiency. Individuals with this disorder may have difficulty expressing affection or tolerating expressions of affection from others and tend to avoid intimacy, but they do have the capacity for intimacy. They are sensitive to hierarchies and can be rigidly deferential to the authority figures they respect.

18.3—Obsessive-Compulsive Personality Disorder / Diagnostic Features (p. 679); Differential Diagnosis (p. 681)

18.4   Which of the following findings would rule out the diagnosis of obsessive-compulsive personality disorder (OCPD)?

A. A concurrent diagnosis of obsessive-compulsive disorder.
B. A concurrent diagnosis of antisocial personality disorder.
C. Evidence of psychotic symptoms.
D. Evidence that the behavioral patterns reflect culturally sanctioned interpersonal styles.
E. A concurrent diagnosis of cocaine use disorder.

Correct Answer: D. Evidence that the behavioral patterns reflect culturally sanctioned interpersonal styles.

Explanation: OCPD must be distinguished from behavior that remains within a normal range; for example, if an individual's OCPD-like behaviors are culturally sanctioned (e.g., they occur within the context of a culture that places substantial emphasis on work and productivity), then a personality disorder diagnosis would not be appropriate. OCPD can coexist with a number of other disorders. For example, OCPD can be comorbid with obsessive-compulsive disorder (OCD), and an OCD diagnosis carries an elevated risk for OCPD, even though the majority of those with OCD do not have OCPD. Substance use disorders can be comorbid with OCPD, and there may be an association between OCPD and depressive disorders, bipolar and related disorders, and eating disorders. Psychotic disorders may also coexist with OCPD.

18.4—Obsessive-Compulsive Personality Disorder / Culture-Related Diagnostic Issues; Differential Diagnosis (p. 681)

18.5   A 36-year-old woman is approached by her new boss, who has noticed that despite working for her employer for many years, she has not advanced beyond an entry level position. The boss hears that she is a good employee who works long hours. The woman explains that she has not asked for a promotion because she knows she's not as good as other employees and doesn't think she deserves it. She explains her long hours by saying that she is not very smart and has to check over all her work, because she's afraid that people will laugh at her if she makes any mistakes. On reviewing her past evaluations, her boss notes that there are only minor critiques and her overall evaluations have been very positive. Which of the following personality disorders would best explain this woman's lack of job advancement?

A. Narcissistic personality disorder.
B. Avoidant personality disorder.
C. Obsessive-compulsive personality disorder.
D. Schizoid personality disorder.
E. Borderline personality disorder.

Correct Answer: B. Avoidant personality disorder.

Explanation: Avoidant personality disorder is characterized by feelings of inadequacy, hypersensitivity to criticism, and a need for reassurance. As a result, a person with avoidant personality disorder tends to be reluctant to take risks or engage in challenging activities, which results in interpersonal and occupational impairment. People with narcissistic personality disorder or borderline personality disorder may also be highly sensitive to criticism, but a key feature of narcissistic disorder is grandiosity, and that of borderline personality disorder is an unstable self-image, rather than persistently low self-esteem. Long work hours and rechecking work can be seen with obsessive-compulsive personality disorder, but in that disorder the cause is a perfectionistic or rigid style of approach, not fear of criticism or humiliation. People with schizoid personality disorder are generally relatively indifferent to criticism from others.

18.5—Avoidant Personality Disorder / Differential Diagnosis (p. 674)

18.6 A cardiologist requests a psychiatric consultation for her patient, a 46-year-old man, because even though he is adherent to treatment, she is concerned that he "seems crazy." On evaluation, the patient makes poor eye contact, tends to ramble, and makes unusual word choices. He is modestly disheveled and wears clothes with mismatched colors. He expresses odd beliefs about supernatural phenomena, but these beliefs do not seem to be of delusional intensity. Collateral information from his sister elicits the observation that "He's always been like this—weird. He keeps to himself, and likes it that way." Which of the following conditions best explains this man's odd behaviors and beliefs?

A. Schizoid personality disorder.
B. Schizotypal personality disorder.
C. Paranoid personality disorder.
D. Delusional disorder.
E. Schizophrenia.

Correct Answer: B. Schizotypal personality disorder.

Explanation: Schizotypal personality disorder is characterized by pervasive social and interpersonal deficits, which include odd behaviors, odd beliefs and speech, and social withdrawal. The odd beliefs may include ideas of reference or even paranoid ideation, but true delusions and hallucinations are not present. Individuals with schizoid personality disorder or paranoid personality disorder may also be loners, and either of these disorders may coexist with schizotypal personality disorder. However, neither of those disorders is characterized by marked oddness or eccentricity.

18.6—Schizotypal Personality Disorder / Differential Diagnosis (p. 658)

18.7 Which of the following statements about the development, course, and prognosis of borderline personality disorder (BPD) is *true?*

A. The risk of suicide in individuals with BPD increases with age.
B. A childhood history of neglect, rather than abuse, is unusual in individuals with BPD.
C. Follow-up studies of individuals with BPD identified in outpatient clinics have shown that 10 years later, as many as half of these individuals no longer meet full criteria for the disorder.
D. Individuals with BPD have relatively low rates of improvement in social or occupational functioning.
E. There is little variability in the course of BPD.

Correct Answer: C. Follow-up studies of individuals with BPD identified in outpatient clinics have shown that 10 years later, as many as half of these individuals no longer meet full criteria for the disorder.

Explanation: The prognosis for symptomatic improvement in BPD is better than many clinicians realize, and there is considerable variability in the disorder's course. Individuals with BPD are at increased risk of suicide, but the risk is greatest during early adulthood and decreases with age. Also, a majority of individuals with BPD attain greater stability in their relationships and vocational functioning in their 30s and 40s. Individuals with BPD do have an increased incidence of childhood neglect as well as an increased incidence of childhood physical and sexual abuse.

> **18.7—Borderline Personality Disorder / Associated Features Supporting Diagnosis; Prevalence; Development and Course (p. 665)**

18.8   Which of the following is *not* a characteristic of narcissistic personality disorder (NPD)?

A. Excessive reference to others for self-definition and self-esteem regulation.
B. Impaired ability to recognize or identify with the feelings and needs of others.
C. Excessive attempts to attract and be the focus of the attention of others.
D. Persistence at tasks long after the behavior has ceased to be functional or effective.
E. Preoccupation with fantasies of unlimited success or power.

Correct Answer: D. Persistence at tasks long after the behavior has ceased to be functional or effective.

Explanation: Although individuals with NPD and those with obsessive-compulsive personality disorder (OCPD) may both profess a commitment to perfection, persistence at tasks long after the behavior has ceased to be functional is more characteristic of the perfectionism of individuals with OCPD rather than that of individuals with NPD. In contrast to the self-criticism of individuals with OCPD, individuals with NPD are more likely to believe that they have reached perfection. The other options are all characteristic traits of individuals with NPD.

18.9   Which of the following cognitive or perceptual disturbances are associated with borderline personality disorder?

A. Odd thinking and speech.
B. Ideas of reference.
C. Odd beliefs.
D. Transient, stress-related paranoid ideation.
E. Superstitiousness.

Correct Answer: D. Transient, stress-related paranoid ideation.

Explanation: In borderline personality disorder, transient paranoid ideation or dissociative symptoms (e.g., depersonalization) may occur during periods of extreme stress, but these are generally of insufficient severity or duration to warrant an additional diagnosis. These episodes occur most frequently in response to a real or imagined abandonment. Symptoms tend to be transient, lasting minutes or hours.

Odd thinking and speech, ideas of reference, odd beliefs, and superstitiousness are characteristic of schizotypal personality disorder rather than borderline personality disorder.

18.9—Borderline Personality Disorder / diagnostic criteria (p. 663); Diagnostic Features (p. 665); Schizotypal Personality Disorder / diagnostic criteria (p. 655)

18.10 A 43-year-old warehouse security guard comes to your office complaining of vague feelings of depression for the last few months. He denies any particular sense of fear or anxiety. As he gets older, he wonders if he should try harder to form relationships with other people. He feels little desire for this but notes that his coworkers seem happier than he, and they have many relationships. He has never felt comfortable with other people, not even with his own family. He has lived alone since early adulthood and has been self-sufficient. He almost always works night shifts to avoid interactions with others. He tries to remain low-key and undistinguished to discourage others from striking up conversations with him, as he does not understand what they want when they talk to him. Which personality disorder would best fit with this presentation?

A. Paranoid.
B. Schizoid.
C. Schizotypal.
D. Avoidant.
E. Dependent.

Correct Answer: B. Schizoid.

Explanation: His avoidance of others is not based on fears of being exploited, deceived, or harmed, as in paranoid personality disorder, nor is it based on a fear of being found inadequate, as might be seen in avoidant personality disorder. There is no mention of odd or eccentric behavior, and he even makes a deliberate effort not to appear unusual in any way. Individuals with dependent personality disorder often feel uncomfortable or helpless when alone, and constantly seek out nurturance and support from others.

18.10—Schizoid Personality Disorder / Differential Diagnosis (p. 654)

18.11 Which of the following behaviors or states would be highly unusual in an individual with schizoid personality disorder?

A. An angry outburst at a colleague who criticizes his work.
B. Turning down an invitation to a party.
C. Lacking desire for sexual experiences.
D. Drifting with regard to life goals.
E. Difficulty working in a collaborative work environment.

Correct Answer: A. An angry outburst at a colleague who criticizes his work.

Explanation: One of the hallmarks of schizoid personality disorder is the reduced expression of emotion in interpersonal settings, often making them appear indifferent to criticism from others. It is also typical of individuals with schizoid personality disorder to choose solitary experiences and avoid social events. They may have difficulty in collaborative work environments because of their lack of social skills, but can thrive in jobs with considerable social isolation, like a nighttime warehouse security guard.

18.11—Schizoid Personality Disorder / Diagnostic Features; Differential Diagnosis (p. 654)

18.12 What is the relationship between a history of conduct disorder before age 15 and the diagnosis of antisocial personality after age 18?

A. A history of some conduct disorder symptoms before age 15 is one of the required criteria for a diagnosis of antisocial personality disorder in adulthood.
B. All children with conduct disorder will go on to receive a diagnosis of antisocial personality disorder in adulthood.
C. Antisocial personality disorder diagnosis is independent of conduct disorder.
D. Conduct disorder is the same as antisocial personality disorder, except that financial irresponsibility is also a required feature of antisocial personality disorder.

E. Conduct disorder is the same as antisocial personality disorder except that remorse is present in conduct disorder.

Correct Answer: A. A history of some conduct disorder symptoms before age 15 is one of the required criteria for a diagnosis of antisocial personality disorder in adulthood.

Explanation: Criterion C for the diagnosis of antisocial personality disorder states, "there is evidence of conduct disorder with onset before age 15 years." Like antisocial personality disorder, conduct disorder involves a repetitive and persistent pattern of behavior in which the basic rights of others or major age-appropriate societal norms or rules are violated. The specific behaviors characteristic of conduct disorder fall into one of four categories: aggression to people and animals, destruction of property, deceitfulness or theft, or serious violation of rules. The likelihood of developing antisocial personality disorder in adult life is increased if the individual experienced childhood onset of conduct disorder (before age 10 years) and accompanying attention-deficit/hyperactivity disorder.

18.12—Antisocial Personality Disorder / diagnostic criteria (p. 659)

18.13 A 25-year-old man has a childhood history of repeated instances of torturing animals, setting fires, stealing, running away from home, and school truancy, beginning at the age of 9 years. As an adult he has a history of repeatedly lying to others; engaging in petty thefts, con games, and frequent fights (including episodes in which he used objects at hand—pipe wrenches, chairs, steak knives—to injure others); and using aliases to avoid paying child support. There is no history of manic, depressive, or psychotic symptoms. He is dressed in expensive clothing and displays an expensive wristwatch for which he demands admiration; he expresses feelings of specialness and entitlement; the belief that he deserves exemption from ordinary rules; feelings of anger that his special talents have not been adequately recognized by others; devaluation, contempt, and lack of empathy for others; and lack of remorse for his behavior. There is no sign of psychosis. What is the appropriate diagnosis?

A. Antisocial personality disorder.
B. Malignant narcissism.
C. Narcissistic personality disorder.
D. Antisocial personality disorder and narcissistic personality disorder.
E. Other specified personality disorder (mixed personality features).

Correct Answer: D. Antisocial personality disorder and narcissistic personality disorder.

Explanation: This individual's history indicates 1) a pervasive pattern of disregard for and violation of the rights of others, 2) age over 18 years, 3) features of conduct disorder beginning before age 15 years, and 4) no evidence of bipolar disorder or schizophrenia. Therefore, he meets the criteria for a diagnosis of antisocial personality disorder. In addition, he can be described as demonstrating grandiosity, feelings of specialness, need for admiration, and lack or empathy for the needs and feelings of others, suggesting that he also meets the criteria for a diagnosis of narcissistic personality disorder. Other personality disorders may be confused with antisocial personality disorder because they have certain features in common. It is therefore important to distinguish among these disorders based on differences in their characteristic features. If an individual has personality features that meet criteria for one or more personality disorders in addition to antisocial personality disorder, all can be diagnosed. Individuals with antisocial personality disorder and narcissistic personality disorder share a tendency to be tough-minded, glib, superficial, exploitative, and lack empathy; however, narcissistic personality disorder does not include characteristics of impulsivity, aggression, and deceit. In addition, individuals with antisocial personality disorder may not be as needy of the admiration and envy of others, and persons with narcissistic personality disorder usually lack the history of conduct disorder in childhood or criminal behavior in adulthood. Malignant narcissism is not a DSM-5 diagnostic term. The diagnosis of "other specified personality disorder" applies to presentations in which symptoms characteristic of a personality disorder that cause clinically significant distress or impairment in social, occupational, or other important areas of functioning predominate but do not meet the full criteria for any of the disorders in the personality disorders diagnostic class.

18.13—Antisocial Personality Disorder (p. 659); Narcissistic Personality Disorder (pp. 669–670)

18.14 Which of the following is one of the general criteria for a personality disorder in DSM-5?

A. An enduring pattern of inner experience that deviates markedly from the expectations of the individual's culture.
B. The pattern is flexible and confined to a single personal or social situation.
C. The pattern is fluctuating and of short duration.
D. The pattern leads to occasional mild distress.
E. The pattern's onset can be traced to a specific traumatic event in the individual's recent history.

Correct Answer: A. An enduring pattern of inner experience that deviates markedly from the expectations of the individual's culture.

Explanation: A personality disorder is an enduring pattern of inner experience and behavior that deviates markedly from the expectations of the individual's culture, is pervasive and inflexible, has an onset in adolescence or early adulthood, is stable over time, and leads to distress or impairment.

18.14—General Personality Disorder (pp. 646–647)

18.15 Which of the following presentations is characteristic of histrionic personality disorder?

A. A pattern of acute discomfort in close relationships, cognitive or perceptual distortions, and eccentricities of behavior.
B. A pattern of submissive and clinging behavior related to an excessive need to be taken care of.
C. A pattern of instability in interpersonal relationships, self-image, and affects, and marked impulsivity.
D. A pattern of grandiosity, need for admiration, and lack of empathy.
E. A pattern of excessive emotionality and attention seeking.

Correct Answer: E. A pattern of excessive emotionality and attention seeking

Explanation: The essential feature of histrionic personality disorder is pervasive and excessive emotionality and attention-seeking behavior. This pattern begins by early adulthood and is present in a variety of contexts. Individuals with histrionic personality disorder are uncomfortable or feel unappreciated when they are not the center of attention (Criterion 1). Often lively and dramatic, they tend to draw attention to themselves and may initially charm new acquaintances by their enthusiasm, apparent openness, or flirtatiousness.

18.15—Histrionic Personality Disorder / Diagnostic Features (p. 667)

18.16 Which of the following presentations is characteristic of borderline personality disorder?

A. A pattern of acute discomfort in close relationships, cognitive or perceptual distortions, and eccentricities of behavior.
B. A pattern of submissive and clinging behavior related to an excessive need to be taken care of.
C. A pattern of instability in interpersonal relationships, self-image, and affects, and marked impulsivity.
D. A pattern of grandiosity, need for admiration, and lack of empathy.
E. A pattern of excessive emotionality and attention seeking.

Correct Answer: C. A pattern of instability in interpersonal relationships, self-image, and affects, and marked impulsivity.

Explanation: The diagnostic criteria for borderline personality disorder require the presence of a pervasive pattern of instability of interpersonal relationships, self-image, and affects, and marked impulsivity, beginning by early adulthood and present in a variety of contexts. Individuals with borderline personality disorder make frantic efforts to avoid real or imagined abandonment (Criterion 1). The perception of impending separation or rejection, or the loss of external structure, can lead to profound changes in self-image, affect, cognition, and behavior.

18.16—Borderline Personality Disorder / Diagnostic Features (p. 663)

18.17 Which of the following presentations is characteristic of dependent personality disorder?

    A. A pattern of acute discomfort in close relationships, cognitive or perceptual distortions, and eccentricities of behavior.
    B. A pattern of submissive and clinging behavior related to an excessive need to be taken care of.
    C. A pattern of instability in interpersonal relationships, self-image, and affects, and marked impulsivity.
    D. A pattern of grandiosity, need for admiration, and lack of empathy.
    E. A pattern of social inhibition, feelings of inadequacy, and hypersensitivity to negative evaluation.

Correct Answer: B. A pattern of submission and clinging behavior related to an excessive need to be taken care of.

Explanation: The diagnostic criteria for dependent personality disorder require a pervasive and excessive need to be taken care of that leads to submissive and clinging behavior and fears of separation, beginning by early adulthood and presenting in a variety of contexts.

18.17—Dependent Personality Disorder / diagnostic criteria (p. 675)

18.18 Which of the following presentations is characteristic of avoidant personality disorder?

    A. A pattern of social inhibition, feelings of inadequacy, and hypersensitivity to negative evaluation.
    B. A pattern of acute discomfort in close relationships, cognitive or perceptual distortions, and eccentricities of behavior.
    C. A pattern of submissive and clinging behavior related to an excessive need to be taken care of.
    D. A pattern of instability in interpersonal relationships, self-image, and affects, and marked impulsivity.
    E. A pattern of grandiosity, need for admiration, and lack of empathy.

Correct Answer: A. A pattern of social inhibition, feelings of inadequacy, and hypersensitivity to negative evaluation.

Explanation: The essential feature of avoidant personality disorder is a pervasive pattern of social inhibition, feelings of inadequacy, and hypersensitivity to negative evaluation that begins by early adulthood and is present in a variety of contexts. Individuals with avoidant personality disorder avoid work activities that involve significant interpersonal contact because of fears of criticism, disapproval, or rejection.

18.18—Avoidant Personality Disorder / Diagnostic Features (p. 673)

18.19 Which of the following presentations is characteristic of schizotypal personality disorder?

A. A pattern of social inhibition, feelings of inadequacy, and hypersensitivity to negative evaluation.
B. A pattern of acute discomfort in close relationships, cognitive or perceptual distortions, and eccentricities of behavior.
C. A pattern of submissive and clinging behavior related to an excessive need to be taken care of.
D. A pattern of instability in interpersonal relationships, self-image, and affects, and marked impulsivity.
E. A pattern of grandiosity, need for admiration, and lack of empathy.

Correct Answer: B. A pattern of acute discomfort in close relationships, cognitive or perceptual distortions, and eccentricities of behavior.

Explanation: The essential feature of schizotypal personality disorder is a pervasive pattern of social and interpersonal deficits marked by acute discomfort with, and reduced capacity for, close relationships as well as by cognitive or perceptual distortions and eccentricities of behavior. This pattern begins by early adulthood and is present in a variety of contexts.

18.19—Schizotypal Personality Disorder / Diagnostic Features (p. 656)

18.20 Which of the following presentations is characteristic of paranoid personality disorder?

A. A pattern of social inhibition, feelings of inadequacy, and hypersensitivity to negative evaluation.
B. A pattern of distrust and suspiciousness such that others' motives are interpreted as malevolent.
C. A pattern of submissive and clinging behavior related to an excessive need to be taken care of.
D. A pattern of instability in interpersonal relationships, self-image, and affects, and marked impulsivity.
E. A pattern of grandiosity, need for admiration, and lack of empathy.

Correct Answer: B. A pattern of distrust and suspiciousness such that others' motives are interpreted as malevolent.

Explanation: The essential feature of paranoid personality disorder is a pattern of pervasive distrust and suspiciousness of others such that their motives are interpreted as malevolent. This pattern begins by early adulthood and is present in a variety of contexts. Individuals with this disorder assume that other people will exploit, harm, or deceive them, even if no evidence exists to support this expectation.

18.20—Paranoid Personality Disorder / Diagnostic Features (pp. 649–450)

18.21 Which of the following presentations is characteristic of narcissistic personality disorder?

    A. A pattern of social inhibition, feelings of inadequacy, and hypersensitivity to negative evaluation.

    B. A pattern of acute discomfort in close relationships, cognitive or perceptual distortions, and eccentricities of behavior.

    C. A pattern of submissive and clinging behavior related to an excessive need to be taken care of.

    D. A pattern of instability in interpersonal relationships, self-image, and affects, and marked impulsivity.

    E. A pattern of grandiosity, need for admiration, and lack of empathy.

Correct Answer: E. A pattern of grandiosity, need for admiration, and lack of empathy.

Explanation: The essential feature of narcissistic personality disorder is a pervasive pattern of grandiosity, need for admiration, and lack of empathy that begins by early adulthood and is present in a variety of contexts. Individuals with this disorder have a grandiose sense of self-importance.

18.21—Narcissistic Personality Disorder / Diagnostic Features (p. 669)

18.22 Which of the following presentations is characteristic of schizoid personality disorder?

    A. A pattern of social inhibition, feelings of inadequacy, and hypersensitivity to negative evaluation.

    B. A pattern of acute discomfort in close relationships, cognitive or perceptual distortions, and eccentricities of behavior.

    C. A pattern of detachment from social relationships and a restricted range of emotional expression.

    D. A pattern of instability in interpersonal relationships, self-image, and affects, and marked impulsivity.

    E. A pattern of grandiosity, need for admiration, and lack of empathy.

Correct Answer: C. A pattern of detachment from social relationships and a restricted range of emotional expression.

Explanation: The essential feature of schizoid personality disorder is a pervasive pattern of detachment from social relationships and a restricted range of expression of emotions in interpersonal settings. This pattern begins by early adulthood and is present in a variety of contexts. Individuals with schizoid personality disorder appear to lack a desire for intimacy, seem indifferent to opportunities to develop close relationships, and do not seem to derive much satisfaction from being part of a family or other social group.

18.22—Schizoid Personality Disorder / Diagnostic Features (p. 653)

18.23 Which of the following presentations is characteristic of antisocial personality disorder?

A. A pattern of preoccupation with orderliness, perfectionism, and control.
B. A pattern of detachment from social relationships and a restricted range of emotional expression.
C. A pattern of distrust and suspiciousness such that others' motives are interpreted as malevolent.
D. A pattern of disregard for, and violation of, the rights of others.
E. A pattern of social inhibition, feelings of inadequacy, and hypersensitivity to negative evaluation.

Correct Answer: D. A pattern of disregard for, and violation of, the rights of others.

Explanation: The essential feature of antisocial personality disorder is a pervasive pattern of disregard for, and violation of, the rights of others that begins in childhood or early adolescence and continues into adulthood. This pattern has also been referred to as psychopathy, sociopathy, or dyssocial personality disorder. Because deceit and manipulation are central features of antisocial personality disorder, it may be especially helpful to integrate information acquired from systematic clinical assessment with information collected from collateral sources. For this diagnosis to be given, the individual must be at least age 18 years (Criterion B) and must have had a history of some symptoms of conduct disorder before age 15 years.

18.23—Antisocial Personality Disorder / Diagnostic Features (p. 659)

18.24 Which of the following presentations is characteristic of obsessive-compulsive personality disorder?

A. A pattern of social inhibition, feelings of inadequacy, and hypersensitivity to negative evaluation.

B. A pattern of acute discomfort in close relationships, cognitive or perceptual distortions, and eccentricities of behavior.
C. A pattern of preoccupation with orderliness, perfectionism, and control.
D. A pattern of detachment from social relationships and a restricted range of emotional expression.
E. A pattern of grandiosity, need for admiration, and lack of empathy.

Correct Answer: C. A pattern of preoccupation with orderliness, perfectionism, and control.

Explanation: The essential feature of obsessive-compulsive personality disorder is a preoccupation with orderliness, perfectionism, and mental and interpersonal control, at the expense of flexibility, openness, and efficiency. This pattern begins by early adulthood and is present in a variety of contexts. Individuals with obsessive-compulsive personality disorder attempt to maintain a sense of control through painstaking attention to rules, trivial details, procedures, lists, schedules, or form to the extent that the major point of the activity is lost.

18.24—Obsessive-Compulsive Personality Disorder / Diagnostic Features (p. 679)

CHAPTER 19

Paraphilic Disorders

19.1 What changes were made to the diagnosis of paraphilias and paraphilic disorders in DSM-5?

A. A distinction has been made between paraphilias and paraphilic disorders.
B. Three specifiers have been added to paraphilic disorders: "in a controlled environment," 'in remission," and "benign."
C. Transvestic disorder has been eliminated.
D. To be diagnosed as a paraphilic disorder, a paraphilia must go beyond fantasy or urge to include behavior.
E. Paraphilic disorders are grouped in a chapter with sexual disorders.

Correct Answer: A. A distinction has been made between paraphilias and paraphilic disorders.

Explanation: In DSM-5, a distinction is made between paraphilias and paraphilic disorders. A paraphilic disorder is a paraphilia that is currently causing distress or impairment to the individual or a paraphilia whose satisfaction has entailed personal harm, or risk of harm, to others. A paraphilia is a necessary but not a sufficient condition for having a paraphilic disorder, and a paraphilia by itself does not automatically justify or require clinical intervention.

19.1—chapter intro (pp. 685–686)

19.2 Which of the following statements about paraphilias is *false?*

A. The presence of a paraphilia does not always justify clinical intervention.
B. Most paraphilias can be divided into those that involve an unusual activity and those that involve an unusual target.
C. Paraphilias may coexist with normophilic sexual interests.
D. It is rare for an individual to manifest more than one paraphilia.
E. The propensity to act on a paraphilia is difficult to assess "in a controlled environment."

Correct Answer: D. It is rare for an individual to manifest more than one paraphilia.

Explanation: It is not rare for an individual to manifest two or more paraphilias. In some cases, the paraphilic foci are closely related and the connection between the paraphilias is intuitively comprehensible. In other cases, the connection between the paraphilias is not so obvious, and the presence of multiple paraphilias may be coincidental or else related to some generalized vulnerability to anomalies of psychosexual development.

19.2—chapter intro (p. 686)

19.3   Which of the following is *not* a paraphilic disorder?

A. Sexual masochism disorder.
B. Transvestic disorder.
C. Transsexual disorder.
D. Voyeuristic disorder.
E. Fetishistic disorder.

Correct Answer: C. Transsexual disorder.

Explanation: Transsexualism is not a disorder and is not included in the DSM-5 Paraphilic Disorders chapter.

19.3—Gender Dysphoria chapter intro (p. 451); Paraphilic Disorders chapter intro (pp. 685–686)

19.4   Which of the following statements about pedophilic disorder is *true?*

A. Pedophilic disorder is found in 10%–12% of the male population.
B. There is no evidence that neurodevelopmental perturbation in utero increases the probability of development of a pedophilic orientation.
C. Adult males with pedophilia often report that they were sexually abused as children.
D. To meet criteria for the diagnosis, the individual must experience sexually arousing fantasies, sexual urges, or behaviors involving sexual activity with children age 8 years or younger.
E. To meet criteria for the diagnosis, the individual must be at least 8 years older than the victim(s).

Correct Answer: C. Adult males with pedophilia often report that they were sexually abused as children.

Explanation: Adult males with pedophilia often report that they were sexually abused as children. It is unclear, however, whether this correlation reflects a causal influence of childhood sexual abuse on adult pedophilia.

The population prevalence of pedophilic disorder is unknown. The highest possible prevalence for pedophilic disorder in the male population is approximately 3%–5%. The population prevalence of pedophilic disorder in females is even more uncertain, but it is likely a small fraction of the prevalence in males.

Since pedophilia is a necessary condition for pedophilic disorder, any factor that increases the probability of pedophilia also increases the risk of pedophilic disorder. There is some evidence that neurodevelopmental perturbation in utero increases the probability of development of a pedophilic orientation.

To meet criteria for the diagnosis of pedophilic disorder, an individual must have experienced or enacted—over a period of at least 6 months—recurrent, intense sexually arousing fantasies, sexual urges, or behaviors involving sexual activity with a prepubescent child or children (generally age 13 years or younger). The individual must be at least 16 years of age and at least 5 years older than the child or children victimized.

19.4—Pedophilic Disorder / diagnostic criteria (p. 697); Prevalence (p. 698); Development and Course (p. 699); Risk and Prognostic Factors (p. 699)

19.5   Which of the following statements about pedophilic disorder is *true?*

A. The extensive use of pornography depicting prepubescent or early pubescent children is not a useful diagnostic indicator of pedophilic disorder.
B. Pedophilic disorder is stable over the course of a lifetime.
C. There is an association between pedophilic disorder and antisocial personality disorder.
D. Although normophilic sexual interest declines with age, pedophilic sexual interest remains constant.
E. Vaginal plethysmography is a more reliable diagnostic instrument for pedophilia in women than is penile plethysmography for pedophilia in men.

Correct Answer: C. There is an association between pedophilic disorder and antisocial personality disorder.

Explanation: Pedophilia is associated with antisocial personality disorder. Pedophilic sexual interest may fluctuate over the course of a lifetime, and it generally declines with age, as does normophilic sexual interest. Because many pedophiles deny their interest, the extensive use of pornography depicting children can be a useful diagnostic indicator. Vaginal plethysmography is a less reliable diagnostic tool than is penile plethysmography.

19.5—Pedophilic Disorder (pp. 697–700)

19.6   A 35-year-old woman tells her therapist that she has recently become intensely aroused while watching movies in which people are tortured and that she regularly fantasizes about torturing people while masturbating. She is not distressed by these thoughts and denies ever having acted on these new fantasies, though she fantasizes about these activities several times a day. Which of the following best summarizes the diagnostic implications of this patient's presentation?

A. She meets all of the criteria for sexual sadism disorder.
B. She does not meet the criteria for sexual sadism disorder because the fantasies are not sexual in nature.

C. She does not meet the criteria for sexual sadism disorder because she has never acted on the fantasies.

D. She does not meet the criteria for sexual sadism disorder because the interest and arousal began after age 35.

E. She does not meet the criteria for sexual sadism disorder as the diagnosis is only made in men.

Correct Answer: C. She does not meet the criteria for sexual sadism disorder because she has never acted on the fantasies.

Explanation: Individuals who openly acknowledge intense sexual interest in the physical or psychological suffering of others are referred to as "admitting individuals." If these individuals also report psychosocial difficulties because of their sexual attractions or preferences for the physical or psychological suffering of another individual, they may be diagnosed with sexual sadism disorder. In contrast, if admitting individuals declare no distress, exemplified by anxiety, obsessions, guilt, or shame, about these paraphilic impulses, and are not hampered by them in pursuing other goals, and their self-reported, psychiatric, or legal histories indicate that they do not act on them, then they could be ascertained as having sadistic sexual interest but they would not meet criteria for sexual sadism disorder. There are no age or gender requirements in the diagnostic criteria.

19.6—Paraphilic Disorders / Sexual Sadism Disorder (pp. 695–697)

19.7 While intoxicated at a Mardi Gras celebration, a 19-year-old woman lifts her blouse and bra as a float goes by to get beads. The event appears on a cable news program watched by friends of her parents, who inform her parents. They insist that she get a psychiatric evaluation. She denies any other similar events in her life but admits that the experience was "sort of sexy." She is currently extremely anxious and distressed—to the point of being unable to focus on her work at college—about her parents' anger at her and their refusal to allow her to attend parties or go away on vacation. What is the most appropriate diagnosis?

A. Exhibitionistic disorder.
B. Frotteuristic disorder.
C. Voyeuristic disorder.
D. Adjustment disorder.
E. Antisocial personality disorder.

Correct Answer: D. Adjustment disorder.

Explanation: This woman's single episode of exposing herself while intoxicated does not qualify for a diagnosis of exhibitionistic disorder because she does not meet the diagnostic criteria—specifically, a 6-month history of "recurrent and intense sexual arousal from the exposure of one's genitals to an unsuspecting person, as manifested by fantasies, urges, or behaviors" (Criterion A). Exhibitionistic impulses appear to emerge in adolescence or early adulthood; very little is known about persistence over time. By definition, exhibitionistic disorder requires one or more contributing factors, which may change over time with or without treatment; subjective distress (e.g., guilt, shame, intense sexual frustration, loneliness), mental disorder comorbidity, hypersexuality, and sexual impulsivity; psychosocial impairment; and/or the propensity to act out sexually by exposing the genitals to unsuspecting persons. Exhibitionistic disorder is highly unusual in females, whereas single sexually arousing exhibitionistic acts might occur up to half as often among women compared with men.

This young woman's current distress is related not to the exhibitionistic act but rather to her parents' attitude and behavior. Because her distress interferes with her functioning, she meets criteria for an adjustment disorder.

19.7—Exhibitionistic Disorder / diagnostic criteria (p. 689); Development and Course (p. 690); Gender-Related Diagnostic Issues (p. 691); Differential Diagnosis (p. 691); Adjustment Disorders / diagnostic criteria (pp. 286–287)

CHAPTER 20

Assessment Measures (DSM-5 Section III)

20.1 Although the DSM classification represents a categorical approach to the diagnosis of mental disorders, such approaches have a number of shortcomings. Which of the following is *not* a limitation of categorical approaches as described in DSM-5?

A. Failure to find "zones of rarity" between diagnoses.
B. Need to create intermediate categories.
C. Low rates of comorbidity.
D. Frequent use of "not otherwise specified (NOS)" diagnoses.
E. Lack of treatment specificity for various diagnostic categories.

Correct Answer: C. Low rates of comorbidity.

Explanation: According to DSM-5, the limitations of a categorical diagnostic system include the failure to find zones of rarity between diagnoses (i.e., delineation of mental disorders from one another by natural boundaries), the need for intermediate categories like schizoaffective disorder, high rates of comorbidity, frequent use of NOS diagnoses, relative lack of utility in furthering the identification of unique antecedent validators for most mental disorders, and lack of treatment specificity for the various diagnostic categories.

20.1—chapter intro (p. 733)

20.2 Which of the following statements about the World Health Organization Disability Assessment Schedule, Version 2.0 (WHODAS 2.0), is *true*?

A. It is a clinician-administered scale.
B. It focuses only on disabilities due to psychiatric illness.
C. It assesses a patient's ability to perform activities in six functional areas.
D. It is available in both an adult self-rated version and a parent/guardian-rated version.
E. It primarily measures physical disability.

Correct Answer: C. It assesses a patient's ability to perform activities in six functional areas.

Explanation: The WHODAS 2.0 was developed to assess a patient's ability to perform activities in six areas: understanding and communicating; getting around; self-care; getting along with people; life activities (e.g., household, work/school); and participation in society. The scale corresponds to concepts contained in the WHO International Classification of Functioning, Disability and Health. This assessment can also be used over time to track changes in a patient's disabilities.

The *adult self-administered version* of WHODAS 2.0 was designed to be used in adults age 18 years and older with any medical disorder. If the adult individual is of impaired capacity and unable to complete the form (e.g., a patient with dementia), a knowledgeable informant may complete the *proxy-administered version* of the measure (available at www.psychiatry.org/dsm5).

20.2—chapter intro (p. 734); World Health Organization Disability Assessment Schedule 2.0 (p. 745)

20.3   Which of the following statements about the DSM-5 Level 1 Cross-Cutting Symptom Measure is *true?*

   A. It is intended to help clinicians assess a patient's ability to perform activities in six areas of daily life functioning.
   B. It asks about the presence and frequency of symptoms in 13 psychiatric domains.
   C. It focuses only on symptoms present *at the time of the interview.*
   D. It lacks validity data in clinical settings and is primarily intended as a research tool.
   E. Because it is self-rated, it cannot be used with patients who have communication or cognitive disorders.

Correct Answer: B. It asks about the presence and frequency of symptoms in 13 psychiatric domains.

Explanation: The DSM-5 Level 1 Cross-Cutting Symptom Measure is a patient- or informant-rated measure that assesses mental health domains that are important across psychiatric diagnoses. It is intended to help clinicians identify additional areas of inquiry that may have significant impact on the individual's treatment and prognosis. In addition, the measure may be used to track changes in the individual's symptom presentation over time.

The adult version of the self-rated DSM-5 Level 1 Cross-Cutting Symptom Measure consists of 23 questions that assess 13 psychiatric domains, including depression, anger, mania, anxiety, somatic symptoms, suicidal ideation, psychosis, sleep problems, memory, repetitive thoughts and behaviors, dissociation, personality functioning, and substance use. Each item inquires about how much (or how often) the individual has been bothered by the specific symptom during the past 2 weeks. If the individual is of impaired capacity and unable to complete the form (e.g., an individual with dementia), a knowledgeable adult informant may complete this measure. The measure was found to be clinically useful and to have good reliability in the DSM-5 field trials that were conducted in adult clinical samples across the United States and in Canada.

20.3—Cross-Cutting Symptom Measures / Level 1 Cross-Cutting Symptom Measure (p. 734)

20.4   In clinician review of item scores on the DSM-5 Level 1 Cross-Cutting Symptom Measure for an adult patient, a rating of "slight" would call for further inquiry if found for any item in which of the following domains?

A. Depression.
B. Mania.
C. Anger.
D. Psychosis.
E. Personality functioning.

Correct Answer: D. Psychosis.

Explanation: On the adult self-rated version of the DSM-5 Level 1 Cross-Cutting Symptom Measure, each item is rated on a 5-point scale (0=none or not at all; 1=slight or rare, less than a day or two; 2=mild or several days; 3=moderate or more than half the days; and 4=severe or nearly every day). Whereas for most domains, a rating of *mild* (i.e., 2) or greater for any item within the domain is the threshold to guide further inquiry, for the substance use, suicidal ideation, and psychosis domains, a rating of *slight* (i.e., 1) or greater is the threshold for pursuing additional inquiry and follow-up to determine if a more detailed assessment is needed (which may include the Level 2 cross-cutting symptom assessment for that domain).

20.4—Cross-Cutting Symptom Measures / Level 1 Cross-Cutting Symptom Measure; Table 1 [Adult DSM-5 Self-Rated Level 1 Cross-Cutting Symptom Measure: 13 domains, thresholds for further inquiry, and associated DSM-5 Level 2 measures] (pp. 734–735)

20.5   If a parent answers "I don't know" to the question "In the past TWO (2) WEEKS, has your child had an alcoholic beverage (beer, wine, liquor, etc.)?" in the parent/guardian-rated version of the DSM-5 Level 1 Cross-Cutting Symptom Measure, what is the appropriate clinician response?

A. Advise that the child be hospitalized before further workup proceeds.
B. Ask the child questions from the substance use domain of the child-rated Level 2 Cross-Cutting Symptom Measure.
C. Rely on other questions from the substance use domain and do not incorporate this answer into the final score.

D. Ask the parent to ask the child, and schedule a follow-up visit to readminister the questionnaire.

E. Consider reporting the parent to child protective services.

Correct Answer: B. Ask the child questions from the substance use domain of the child-rated Level 2 Cross-Cutting Symptom Measure.

Explanation: On the parent/guardian-rated version of the DSM-5 Level 1 Cross-Cutting Symptom Measure for children age 6–17, items in 2 of the 12 domains—suicidal ideation/attempts and substance use—are each rated on a "Yes, No, or Don't Know" scale. A parent or guardian's rating of "Don't Know" on the suicidal ideation, suicide attempt, and any of the substance use items, especially for children ages 11–17 years, would warrant additional probing of the issues with the child, including using the child-rated Level 2 Cross-Cutting Symptom Measure for the relevant domain (see Table 2).

> 20.5—Cross-Cutting Symptom Measures / Level 1 Cross-Cutting Symptom Measure; Table 2 [Parent/guardian-rated DSM-5 Level 1 Cross-Cutting Symptom Measure for child age 6–17: 12 domains, thresholds for further inquiry, and associated Level 2 measures] (pp. 735–736)

20.6 If a patient selects "mild/several days" in response to the question "During the past TWO (2) WEEKS, how much (or how often) have you been bothered by…Little interest or pleasure in doing things?" in the DSM-5 Self-Rated Level 1 Cross-Cutting Symptom Measure—Adult, what is the appropriate clinician response?

A. Continue asking additional questions from that domain and rely on the total score when assessing for depression.

B. Suggest that the patient begin treatment for depression and describe treatment options.

C. Follow up with a Level 2 assessment focusing on depressive symptoms.

D. Note the score and continue with the rest of the examination.

E. Immediately begin an assessment for suicidal ideation.

Correct Answer: C. Follow up with a Level 2 assessment focusing on depressive symptoms.

Explanation: A score of "mild" or worse on the depression domains of the DSM-5 Self-Rated Level 1 Cross-Cutting Symptom Measure—Adult should alert the clinician to the need for additional inquiry and follow-up to determine if a more detailed assessment is needed (which may include the Level 2 Cross-Cutting Symptom Measure for depression [see Table 1]).

20.7   When reviewing a patient's responses to items on the World Health Organization Disability Assessment Schedule 2.0 (WHODAS 2.0), the clinician asks the patient, "How much time did you spend on your health condition or its consequences?" The patient answers, "Hardly any." The clinician, who has treated the patient for several years, is surprised to hear this because she is quite certain that the patient spends most of the day dealing with health concerns. What is the appropriate action for this clinician?

A. Confront the patient about the clinician's concerns and ask the patient to reconsider.
B. Record the patient's response as is and score accordingly.
C. Indicate on the form that the clinician is making a correction and revise the score.
D. Attempt to obtain additional information from family members in order to clarify the discrepancy.
E. Take the average of the patient's and clinician's differing scores and use that for the final score.

Correct Answer: C. Indicate on the form that the clinician is making a correction and revise the score.

Explanation: The WHODAS 2.0 should be seen as a collaboration between the clinician and the patient, and the clinician should not blindly record patient responses to the various questions. If the clinician, using all available information and clinical judgment, believes an answer to be inaccurate, the clinician should record a correction to that item score and indicate the revised score in the raw item score box. The clinician is asked to review the individual's response on each item on the measure during the clinical interview and to indicate the self-reported score for each item in the section provided for "Clinician Use Only." If the clinician determines that the score on an item should be different based on the clinical interview and other information available, he or she may indicate a corrected score in the raw item score box.

20.8   The cross-cutting symptom measures in DSM-5 are modeled on which of the following?

A. The International Classification of Functioning, Disability, and Health.
B. The general medical review of systems.
C. The Brief Psychiatric Rating Scale.

D. The Clinical Global Impression Scale.

E. The DSM-IV Global Assessment of Functioning scale.

Correct Answer: B. The general medical review of systems.

Explanation: *Cross-cutting symptom measures* modeled on general medicine's review of systems can serve as an approach for reviewing critical psychopathological domains. The general medical review of systems is crucial to detecting subtle changes in different organ systems that can facilitate diagnosis and treatment. A similar review of various mental functions can aid in a more comprehensive mental status assessment by drawing attention to symptoms that may not fit neatly into the diagnostic criteria suggested by the individual's presenting symptoms, but may nonetheless be important to the individual's care.

20.8—chapter intro (p. 733)

20.9   Which of the following statements about severity measures in DSM-5 is *true?*

A. They are not related to specific disorders.

B. They are administered once in the course of diagnosis and treatment.

C. They are completed only by the clinician.

D. They have only a loose correspondence to diagnostic criteria.

E. They may be administered to patients who have a clinically significant syndrome that falls short of meeting full diagnostic criteria.

Correct Answer: E. They may be administered to patients who have a clinically significant syndrome that falls short of meeting full diagnostic criteria.

Explanation: *Severity measures* are disorder-specific, corresponding closely to the criteria that constitute the disorder definition. They may be administered to individuals who have received a diagnosis or who have a clinically significant syndrome that falls short of meeting full criteria for a diagnosis. Some of the assessments are self-completed by the individual, while others require a clinician to complete. As with the cross-cutting symptom measures, these measures were developed to be administered both at initial interview and over time to track the severity of the individual's disorder and response to treatment.

20.9—chapter intro (p. 733); Clinician-Rated Dimensions of Psychosis Symptom Severity (pp. 742–744)

CHAPTER 21

Cultural Formulation (DSM-5 Section III) and Glossary of Cultural Concepts of Distress (DSM-5 Appendix)

21.1   The DSM-5 Outline of Cultural Formulation is an update of the framework introduced in DSM-IV for assessing cultural features of a person's mental health presentation. Which of the following is *not* a category in the updated framework?

A. Cultural identity of the individual.
B. Cultural conceptualizations of distress.
C. Cultural stressors and cultural features of vulnerability and resilience.
D. Cultural preferences in leisure and entertainment choices.
E. Cultural features of the relationship between the individual and the clinician.

Correct Answer: D. Cultural preferences in leisure and entertainment choices.

Explanation: Although cultural aspects of leisure-time activity may have distal relevance to mental health, it is not a major category of the DSM-5 Outline for Cultural Formulation. *Cultural identity of the individual* includes aspects of ethnic, racial, linguistic, and cultural factors with which the individual identifies. *Cultural conceptualizations of distress* involve culturally specific ways of understanding and coping with distress. *Cultural stressors and cultural features of vulnerability and resilience* involve culturally specific stressors and social support systems and related concepts, as well as culturally bound conceptions of work and disability. Approaches to the patient-physician relationship may vary significantly across different cultures. It is essential to understand these differences if one is to establish a "helping" relationship.

21.1—Outline for Cultural Formulation (pp. 749–750)

21.2 *Cultural identity of the individual* is one of several categories in the DSM-5 Outline for Cultural Formulation. Which of the following is *not* a feature of cultural identity of the individual?

   A. Self-defined racial or ethnic reference group.
   B. For immigrants or minorities, the degree of involvement with both culture of origin and host culture.
   C. Language abilities and preferences.
   D. Political party affiliation.
   E. Sexual orientation.

Correct Answer: D. Political party affiliation.

Explanation: Political party affiliation is not generally part of the "cultural identity of the individual" category of the DSM-5 Outline for Cultural Formulation. Self-defined racial and/or ethnic reference group, degree of involvement with one's culture of origin and host culture, language ability and preferences, and sexual orientation are important aspects of identity that inform one's experience of mental health problems and approaches to treatment. Other clinically relevant aspects of identity may include religious affiliation, socioeconomic background, personal and family places of birth and growing up, and migrant status.

21.2—Outline for Cultural Formulation (pp. 749–750)

21.3 Which of the following statements about the Cultural Formulation Interview (CFI) is *true?*

   A. The CFI tests how well the patient is versed in the cultural heritage from which he or she originates.
   B. By determining the patient's culture of origin, the CFI helps the clinician predict the patient's attitudes toward the illness concept and the acceptability of treatments.
   C. The CFI is a carefully formulated, structured interview and should be followed closely to maintain the validity and accuracy of elicited responses.
   D. The CFI takes a person-centered approach to culture, focusing on an individual's beliefs and attitudes as well as those of others in the patient's social networks.
   E. Basic demographic information is elicited by the CFI, eliminating the need to obtain it separately.

Correct Answer: D. The CFI takes a person-centered approach to culture, focusing on an individual's beliefs and attitudes as well as those of others in the patient's social networks.

Explanation: The DSM-5 CFI is interested in the total experiential context in which an illness/distress experience occurs. This includes the cultural aspect of social networks to which the patient belongs, as well as the patient's personal differences from these norms. The CFI is not focused on how well versed an individual is in his or her culture, but rather the influence of the person's participation in that culture on health. Thus, knowing a patient's cultural membership (which may be one of many memberships) does not justify applying the norms of that one culture to this individual in a stereotyped fashion. The CFI is purposefully a loose set of suggested questions for probing cultural issues and not a formulaic and rigid cultural thermometer. The CFI assumes that basic demographic information is known, so it is best to obtain this information before administering the CFI, as part of the initial data of the psychiatric interview.

21.3—Cultural Formulation Interview (CFI) (pp. 750–751)

21.4 In which of the following clinical situations would the Cultural Formulation Interview (CFI) *not* be directly useful?

A. The clinician and the patient come from very different cultural backgrounds.
B. The clinician and patient have a shared belief system regarding the nature of the problem and the appropriate therapeutic approach.
C. The patient presents with a symptom complex that is distressing but does not fit any DSM-5 diagnosis.
D. The clinician is finding it difficult to get a sense of the severity of the patient's presenting problems.
E. The clinician and patient are having trouble agreeing on an approach to treatment.

Correct Answer: B. The clinician and patient have a shared belief system regarding the nature of the problem and the appropriate therapeutic approach.

Explanation: When the clinician and patient have a shared belief system regarding the nature of the problem and the appropriate therapeutic approach, there may be less of a need to administer the CFI—not because cultural factors are not playing a role, but because the clinician and patient are embedding these factors in their shared cultural assumptions and are therefore already addressing these issues even without a formal questionnaire. Note that this answer stresses a shared belief system and an agreed-upon approach to the current problem; however, one should not assume a shared belief system just because the patient is from the same ethnic or religious group. People may have multiple group identifications and individualized ways of incorporating these identifications, which is precisely what the CFI explores. Difficulty with problem description, questionable DSM-5 symptom fit, and disagreement on approach to treatment are all major reasons to administer the CFI as a means of clarifying what might be communication difficulties around cultural factors.

21.4—Cultural Formulation Interview (CFI) (p. 751)

21.5 The DSM-5 Cultural Formulation Interview (CFI) is intended not only as an adjunct to diagnosis but also as a holistic clinical approach to the patient. Which of the following clinician communications would be consistent with the spirit of the CFI?

A. "I want you to understand the medical approach to depression, so we can clarify any misunderstandings you may have."
B. "You need not worry, I have worked with many Latino patients who have been depressed, and I know how Latinos think about this."
C. "There is no need to feel ashamed—depression is an illness, like asthma, and it affects everybody in a similar way."
D. "How does your family view your illness?"
E. "The most important thing is to take medication regularly, and the depression will go away, just as an infection would disappear with antibiotics."

Correct Answer: D. "How does your family view your illness?"

Explanation: The CFI is a brief semistructured interview for systematically assessing cultural factors in the clinical encounter that may be used with any individual. The CFI focuses on the individual's experience and the social contexts of the clinical problem. As illustrated by the clinician communication in option D, the CFI follows a person-centered approach to cultural assessment by eliciting information from the individual about his or her own views and those of others in his or her social network. This approach is designed to avoid stereotyping, in that each individual's cultural knowledge affects how he or she interprets illness experience and guides how he or she seeks help. Because the CFI concerns the individual's personal views, there are no right or wrong answers to these questions.

The clinician communications in options A, B, C, and E involve imposing of the clinician's perspective onto the patient, who may have a very different context. Furthermore, some of these communications suggest—incorrectly—that all members of a group or of a diagnostic category have the same experience, as well as the same interpretation of the meaning of that experience.

21.5—Cultural Formulation / chapter intro (p. 749)

21.6 In DSM-5 the term *cultural concepts of distress* encompasses three main types of concepts. Which of the following options correctly lists these three subtypes?

A. Cultural syndromes, cultural idioms of distress, cultural explanations or perceived causes.
B. Cultural identity, culture-bound syndromes, cultural bias.
C. Cultural boundaries, cultural identity, cultural arts.
D. Culturally based sexuality, culture-based faith, cultural causes.
E. Culturally recognized etiologies, cultural grievances, cultural healers.

Correct Answer: A. Cultural syndromes, cultural idioms of distress, cultural explanations or perceived causes.

Explanation: *Cultural concepts of distress* refers to ways that cultural groups experience, understand, and communicate suffering, behavioral problems, or troubling thoughts and emotions. Three main types of cultural concepts may be distinguished. *Cultural syndromes* are clusters of symptoms and attributions that tend to co-occur among individuals in specific cultural groups, communities, or contexts and that are recognized locally as coherent patterns of experience. *Cultural idioms of distress* are ways of expressing distress that may not involve specific symptoms or syndromes, but that provide collective, shared ways of experiencing and talking about personal or social concerns. For example, everyday talk about "nerves" or "depression" may refer to widely varying forms of suffering without mapping onto a discrete set of symptoms, syndrome, or disorder. *Cultural explanations or perceived causes* are labels, attributions, or features of an explanatory model that indicate culturally recognized meaning or etiology for symptoms, illness, or distress.

21.6—Cultural Concepts of Distress (p. 758)

21.7   Information on cultural concepts to improve the comprehensiveness of clinical assessment is contained in various locations in DSM-5. Which of the following is *not* one of those locations?

A. The Cultural Formulation Interview (CFI) section of the "Cultural Formulation" chapter in Section III.
B. The "Glossary of Cultural Concepts of Distress" in the Appendix.
C. Culturally relevant information embedded in the DSM-5 criteria and text for specific disorders.
D. The Z and V codes in the "Other Conditions That May Be a Focus of Clinical Attention" chapter at the end of Section II.
E. The DSM-5 multiaxial diagnostic system.

Correct Answer. E. The DSM-5 multiaxial diagnostic system.

Explanation: The importance of culturally relevant assessment is reflected by the ubiquitous presence of cultural contextual data within DSM-5. In addition to the CFI and its supplementary modules, DSM-5 contains a variety of information and tools that may be useful when integrating cultural information in clinical practice. Text and criteria descriptions contain updates of diagnostic research that are culturally relevant, as do the Z and V codes. DSM-5 no longer has a multiaxial approach to diagnosis.

21.7—Cultural Concepts of Distress (p. 759)

21.8   Which of the following statements about *ataque de nervios* is *false?*

A. *Ataque* is a cultural syndrome as well as a cultural idiom of distress.
B. *Ataque* is related to panic disorder, other specified or unspecified dissociative disorder, conversion disorder (functional neurological symptom disorder), and other specified or unspecified trauma- and stressor-related disorder.
C. *Ataque* is most often associated with withdrawn and reserved behaviors and limited interaction.
D. *Ataque* often involves a sense of being out of control.
E. Community studies have found *ataque* to be associated with suicidal ideation, disability, and outpatient psychiatric service utilization.

Correct Answer: C. *Ataque* is most often associated with withdrawn and reserved behaviors and limited interaction.

Explanation: *Ataque* is often experienced with intense and outwardly expressed emotional upset representing a sense of being out of control, rather than withdrawn quiet internalization. *Ataque* is both a cultural syndrome (i.e., the cultures in which it occurs recognize it as a distinct syndrome) and a broader idiom of distress (i.e., the term *ataque de nervios* may also be used within the culture as a dimensional description of experienced distress rather than a defined syndromal category). Although no one-to-one correlation with a DSM-5 diagnosis exists, *ataque de nervios* is related to panic disorder, other specified or unspecified dissociative disorder, conversion disorder, and other specified or unspecified trauma- and stressor-related disorder, among others. Epidemiological research has established its association with suicidal ideation, disability, and outpatient psychiatric service utilization.

21.8—*Ataque de nervios* (Glossary of Cultural Concepts of Distress, DSM-5 Appendix, p. 833)

21.9   Which of the following statements about *dhat syndrome* is *false?*

A. It is a cultural syndrome found in South Asia.
B. It is related to widespread ideas regarding the harmful effects of loss of semen on sexual as well as general health.
C. The central feature of *dhat syndrome* is distress about loss of semen, to which is attributed diverse symptoms, including fatigue, weakness, and depressive mood.

D. The syndrome is most common among young men of lower socioeconomic status.

E. The estimated rate of *dhat syndrome* in men attending general medical clinics in Pakistan is 30%.

Correct Answer: A. *Dhat syndrome* is a cultural syndrome found in South Asia.

Explanation: Despite its name, *dhat syndrome* is not a discrete syndrome but rather a cultural explanation of distress for patients who attribute diverse symptoms—such as anxiety, fatigue, weakness, weight loss, impotence, other multiple somatic complaints, and depressive mood—to semen loss. The central feature of *dhat syndrome* is distress about the loss of *dhat* (semen) in the absence of any identifiable physiological dysfunction. *Dhat syndrome* is most commonly identified with young men from lower socioeconomic status backgrounds. Research in health care settings has yielded widely varying estimates of the syndrome's prevalence (e.g., 64% of men attending psychiatric clinics in India for sexual complaints; 30% of men attending general medical clinics in Pakistan).

> **21.9—*Dhat syndrome* (Glossary of Cultural Concepts of Distress, DSM-5 Appendix, pp. 833–834)**

21.10 A 22-year-old man from Zimbabwe presents to a clinic with a complaint of anxiety and pain in his chest. He tells the clinician that the cause of his symptoms is *kufungisisa,* or "thinking too much." Which of the following statements about *kufungisisa* is *true?*

A. In cultures in which *kufungisisa* is a shared concept, thinking a lot about troubling issues is considered to be a helpful way of dealing with them.

B. The term *kufungisisa* is used as both a cultural explanation and a cultural idiom of distress.

C. *Kufungisisa* involves concerns about bodily deformity.

D. *Kufungisisa* is related to schizophrenia.

E. B and C.

Correct Answer: B. The term *kufungisisa* is used as both a cultural explanation and a cultural idiom of distress.

Explanation: The term *kufungisisa* refers to both a cultural explanation and a cultural idiom of distress. It is believed to be caused by thinking too much, which is considered to be damaging to the mind and body. Because *kufungisisa* is associated with ruminations, it is possible that the concept of "thinking too much" refers to a cultural experience related to ruminations. It is not especially associated with schizophrenia.

> **21.10—*Kufungisisa* (Glossary of Cultural Concepts of Distress, DSM-5 Appendix, pp. 834–835)**

21.11 A young Haitian man from a prominent family becomes severely depressed after his first semester of university studies. The family brings the young man to a clinician and states that *maladi moun* has caused his problem. Which of the following statements about *maladi moun* is *false?*

A. It is similar to Mediterranean concepts of the "evil eye," in which a person's good fortune is envied by others who in turn cause misfortune to the individual.
B. It can present with a wide variety of symptoms, from anxiety to psychosis.
C. It is based on a shared social assumption that "rising tides lift all boats."
D. It is a Haitian cultural explanation for a diverse set of medical and emotional presentations.
E. It is also referred to as "sent sickness."

Correct Answer: C. It is based on a shared social assumption that "rising tides lift all boats."

Explanation: The cultural model of *maladi moun* is based on the idea that one's good fortune, or the flaunting of good fortune, can cause another to have jealous feelings that can be reflected back as actual negative health consequences. It therefore captures a sentiment opposite to that of "rising tides," which may also exist within the culture, as all cultures contain elements of competitive feelings (zero-sum games) and cooperative feelings (win-win games). *Maladi moun* is a cultural explanation of distress that can present in a wide variety of ways.

21.11—*Maladi moun* (Glossary of Cultural Concepts of Distress, DSM-5 Appendix, p. 835)

21.12 A 19-year-old man presents to the clinic complaining of headaches, irritability, emotional lability, and difficulty concentrating. He is accompanied by his mother, who tells you that her son has had *nervios* since childhood. Which of the following statements about *nervios* is *false?*

A. Unlike *ataque de nervios,* which is a syndrome, *nervios* is a cultural idiom of distress implying a state of vulnerability to stressful experiences.
B. The term *nervios* is used only when the individual has serious loss of functionality or intense symptoms.
C. *Nervios* can manifest with emotional symptoms, somatic disturbances, and an inability to function.
D. *Nervios* can be related to both trait characteristics of an individual and episodic psychiatric symptoms such as depression and dissociative episodes.
E. *Nervios* is a common term used by Latinos in the United States and Latin America.

Correct Answer: B. The term *nervios* is used only when the individual has serious loss of functionality or intense symptoms.

Explanation: *Nervios* is a cultural idiom of distress used by Latinos in the United States and Latin America to describe an individual with a general state of vulnerability to stressful experiences and difficult life circumstances. The symptoms of *nervios* range from very minor distress to severe incapacitation. Research studies indicate that individuals so labeled within the culture can manifest both characteristic trait features and discrete episodic symptoms.

21.12—*Ataque de nervios* (**Glossary of Cultural Concepts of Distress, DSM-5 Appendix, p. 833**)

21.13 Which of the following statements about *shenjing shuairuo* is *false?*

A. In the *Chinese Classification of Mental Disorders,* it is defined by a presentation of three out of five symptom clusters.
B. One of the psychosocial precipitants is an acute sense of failure.
C. It is related to traditional Chinese medicine concepts of depletion of *qi* (vital energy) and dysregulation of *jing* (bodily channels that convey vital forces).
D. Prominent psychotic symptoms must be present.
E. It is believed to be related in some cases to the inability to change a chronically frustrating and distressing situation.

Correct Answer: D. Prominent psychotic symptoms must be present.

Explanation: *Shenjing shuairuo* is a Mandarin Chinese term for a cultural syndrome that integrates conceptual categories of traditional Chinese medicine with the Western diagnosis of neurasthenia. Although well defined, it may not always correspond to DSM-5 disorders. It is believed to be precipitated by a sense of failure or loss of face. This includes situations in which someone feels incapable of changing an undesirable situation in which he or she is involved. *Shenjing shuairuo* has a proposed mechanism involving standard concepts in Chinese medicine such as *qi* and *jing* that involve the distribution of energy through the body.

21.13—*Shenjing shuairuo* (**Glossary of Cultural Concepts of Distress, DSM-5 Appendix, pp. 835–836**)

CHAPTER 22

Alternative DSM-5 Model for Personality Disorders (DSM-5 Section III)

22.1 Which of the following terms best describes the diagnostic approach proposed in the Alternative DSM-5 Model for Personality Disorders?

A. Categorical.
B. Dimensional.
C. Hybrid.
D. Polythetic.
E. Socratic.

Correct Answer: C. Hybrid.

Explanation: Shortly after the publication of DSM-III, debates about the relative merits of categorical versus dimensional approaches to personality disorder diagnoses arose. Critiques of a categorical approach included the arbitrary cutoff between "normal" and "disordered" as well as the use of polythetic (i.e., having many, but not all, properties in common) criteria, which resulted in heterogeneity among patients with the same diagnosis. Dimensional diagnoses, although having greater validity, make it difficult to distinguish between traits and disorders.

The transition from a categorical diagnostic system of individual disorders to one based on the relative distribution of personality traits has not been widely accepted. In DSM-5, the categorical personality disorders are virtually unchanged from the previous edition. However, an alternative "hybrid" model has been proposed in Section III to guide future research that separates interpersonal functioning assessments and the expression of pathological personality traits for six specific disorders. A more dimensional profile of personality trait expression is also proposed for a trait-specified approach.

22.1—Preface (p. xliii)

22.2 In addition to an assessment of pathological personality traits, a personality disorder diagnosis in the alternative DSM-5 model requires an assessment of which of the following?

A. Level of impairment in personality functioning.
B. Comorbidity with Axis I disorders.
C. Degree of introversion versus extroversion.
D. Stability of the personality traits over time.
E. Familial inheritance of specific traits.

Correct Answer: A. Level of impairment in personality functioning.

Explanation: In the Alternative DSM-5 Model for Personality Disorders, a diagnosis of a personality disorder requires two determinations: 1) an assessment of the level of impairment in personality functioning, which is needed for Criterion A, and 2) an evaluation of pathological personality traits, which is required for Criterion B. The impairments in personality functioning and personality trait expression are relatively inflexible and pervasive across a broad range of personal and social situations (Criterion C); relatively stable across time, with onsets that can be traced back to at least adolescence or early adulthood (Criterion D); not better explained by another mental disorder (Criterion E); not attributable to the effects of a substance or another medical condition (Criterion F); and not better understood as normal for an individual's developmental stage or sociocultural environment (Criterion G). All Section III personality disorders described by criteria sets, as well as personality disorder—trait specified (PD-TS), meet these general criteria, by definition.

22.2—General Criteria for Personality Disorder (p. 762)

22.3 Which of the following is a domain of the Alternative DSM-5 Model for Personality Disorders?

A. Neuroticism.
B. Extraversion.
C. Disinhibition.
D. Agreeableness.
E. Conscientiousness.

Correct Answer: C. Disinhibition.

Explanation: The personality trait system presented in the Alternative DSM-5 Model for Personality Disorders includes five broad domains of personality trait variation—Negative Affectivity (vs. Emotional Stability), Detachment (vs. Extraversion), Antagonism (vs. Agreeableness), Disinhibition (vs. Conscientiousness), and Psychoticism (vs. Lucidity)—comprising 25 specific personality trait facets. These five broad domains are maladaptive variants of the five domains of the extensively validated and replicated personality model known as the "Big Five," or Five Factor Model of personality (FFM), and are also similar to the domains of the Personality Psychopathology Five (PSY-5). The specific 25 facets represent a list of personality facets chosen for their clinical relevance.

22.3—The Personality Trait Model (p. 773); Table 3 [Definitions of DSM-5 personality disorder trait domains and facets] (pp. 779–781)

22.4 In addition to negative affectivity, which of the following maladaptive trait domains is most associated with avoidant personality disorder?

A. Detachment.
B. Antagonism.
C. Disinhibition.
D. Compulsivity.
E. Psychoticism.

Correct Answer: A. Detachment.

Explanation: Avoidant personality disorder is characterized by avoidance of social situations and inhibition in interpersonal relationships related to feelings of ineptitude and inadequacy, anxious preoccupation with negative evaluation and rejection, and fears of ridicule or embarrassment. In the Alternative DSM-5 Model for Personality Disorders, the specific maladaptive trait domains are Negative Affectivity and Detachment. In addition, characteristic difficulties are apparent in the personality functioning areas of identity, self-direction, empathy, and/or intimacy.

22.4—Avoidant Personality Disorder (pp. 765–766)

22.5 The diagnosis of personality disorder—trait specified in the Alternative DSM-5 Model of Personality Disorders differs from the DSM-IV diagnosis of personality disorder not otherwise specified in that the DSM-5 diagnosis includes personality trait domains based on which of the following?

A. The level of impairment.
B. Their resemblance to Axis I disorders.
C. The five-factor model of personality.
D. Cognitive theories of behavior.
E. Neurobiological correlates of behavior.

Correct Answer: C. The five-factor model of personality.

Explanation: The personality trait system presented in the Alternative DSM-5 Model for Personality Disorders includes five broad domains of personality trait variation—Negative Affectivity (vs. Emotional Stability), Detachment (vs. Extraversion), Antagonism (vs. Agreeableness), Disinhibition (vs. Conscientiousness), and Psychoticism (vs. Lucidity)—comprising 25 specific personality trait facets. These five broad domains are maladaptive variants of the five domains of the extensively validated and replicated personality model known as the "Big Five," or Five Factor Model of personality (FFM), and are also similar to the domains of the Personality Psychopathology Five (PSY-5).

22.5—The Personality Trait Model (p. 773)

22.6 In the Alternative DSM-5 Model for Personality Disorders, personality functioning includes both **self functioning** (involving *identity* and *self-direction*) and **interpersonal functioning** (involving *empathy* and *intimacy*). Which of the following is a characteristic of healthy self functioning?

A. Comprehension and appreciation of others' experiences and motivations.
B. Variability of self-esteem.
C. Tolerance of differing perspectives.
D. Fluctuating boundaries between self and others.
E. Experience of oneself as unique.

Correct Answer: E. Experience of oneself as unique.

Explanation: Disturbances in **self** and **interpersonal** functioning constitute the core of personality psychopathology, and in Criterion A of the Alternative DSM-5 Model for Personality Disorders, these aspects of personality functioning are evaluated on a continuum. The *identity* component of *self functioning* includes experience of oneself as unique, with clear boundaries between self and others; stability of self-esteem and accuracy of self-appraisal; and capacity for, and ability to regulate, a range of emotional experience. The *empathy* component of *interpersonal functioning* includes comprehension and appreciation of others' experiences and motivations; tolerance of differing perspectives; and understanding the effects of one's own behavior on others.

22.6—Criterion A: Level of Personality Functioning (p. 762)

22.7 Which of the following is *not* a personality disorder criterion in the Alternative DSM-5 Model for Personality Disorders?

A. The impairments in personality functioning and the individual's personality trait expression are relatively inflexible and pervasive across a broad range of personal and social situations.
B. The impairments in personality functioning and the individual's personality trait expression are relatively stable across time, with onsets that can be traced back to at least adolescence or early adulthood.
C. The impairments in personality functioning and the individual's personality trait expression are not solely attributable to the physiological effects of a substance or another medical condition (e.g., severe head trauma).
D. The impairments in personality functioning are not comorbid with another mental disorder.

E. The impairments in personality functioning and the individual's personality trait expression are not better understood as normal for an individual's developmental stage or sociocultural environment.

Correct Answer: D. The impairments in personality functioning are not comorbid with another mental disorder.

Explanation: In the Alternative DSM-5 Model for Personality Disorders, a diagnosis of a personality disorder requires two determinations: 1) an assessment of the level of impairment in personality functioning, which is needed for Criterion A, and 2) an evaluation of pathological personality traits, which is required for Criterion B. The impairments in personality functioning and personality trait expression are relatively inflexible and pervasive across a broad range of personal and social situations (Criterion C); relatively stable across time, with onsets that can be traced back to at least adolescence or early adulthood (Criterion D); not better explained by another mental disorder (Criterion E); not attributable to the effects of a substance or another medical condition (Criterion F); and not better understood as normal for an individual's developmental stage or sociocultural environment (Criterion G). Lack of comorbidity is not a criterion, and in fact, personality disorders are commonly comorbid with other mental disorders.

22.7—General Criteria for Personality Disorder (p. 761)

22.8 In order to meet the proposed diagnostic criteria for antisocial personality disorder (ASPD) in the Alternative DSM-5 Model for Personality Disorders, an individual must have maladaptive personality traits in which of the following domains?

A. Negative affectivity.
B. Detachment.
C. Antagonism.
D. Suicidality.
E. Psychoticism.

Correct Answer: C. Antagonism.

Explanation: ASPD is characterized by maladaptive traits in the domains of antagonism (especially manipulativeness, deceitfulness, callousness, and hostility) and disinhibition (especially irresponsibility, impulsivity, and risk taking). Negative affectivity is more characteristic of borderline personality disorder; detachment of schizotypal or avoidant personality disorders; and psychoticism of schizotypal personality disorder. Individuals with ASPD do not have a markedly increased incidence of suicidality (which is *not* a personality trait).

22.8—Antisocial Personality Disorder (pp. 764–765)

22.9   In the Alternative DSM-5 Model for Personality Disorders, which of the following is *not* an element used to assess level of impairment in personality functioning?

A. Identity.
B. Self-direction.
C. Empathy.
D. Work performance.
E. Intimacy.

Correct Answer: D. Work performance.

Explanation: Disturbances in *self* and *interpersonal* functioning constitute the core of personality psychopathology. Self functioning involves identity and self-direction; interpersonal functioning involves empathy and intimacy. Although work performance was used in the DSM-IV Global Assessment of Functioning Scale, it is not used for the assessment of personality functioning.

22.9—Criterion A: Level of Personality Functioning; Table 1 [Elements of personality functioning] (p. 762)

22.10 Which of the following statements about the relationship between severity of personality dysfunction—as rated on the Level of Personality Functioning Scale (LPFS)—and presence of a personality disorder is *false?*

A. A patient must have "some impairment" as rated on the LPFS in order to be diagnosed with a personality disorder.
B. "Moderate impairment" on the LPFS predicts the presence of a personality disorder.
C. "Severe impairment" on the LPFS predicts the presence of more than one personality disorder.
D. "Severe impairment" on the LPFS predicts the presence of one of the more severe personality disorders.
E. The LPFS does not take into account the level of impairment, merely the presence or absence of functional impairment.

Correct Answer: A. A patient must have "some impairment" as rated on the LPFS in order to be diagnosed with a personality disorder.

Explanation: The LPFS (see Table 2, DSM-5 pp. 775–778) uses the elements of self functioning (identity and self-direction) and interpersonal functioning (empathy and intimacy) to differentiate five levels of impairment, ranging from little or no impairment (i.e., healthy, adaptive functioning; Level 0) to some (Level 1), moderate (Level 2), severe (Level 3), and extreme (Level 4) impairment.

Impairment in personality functioning predicts the presence of a personality disorder, and the severity of impairment predicts whether an individual has more than one personality disorder or one of the more typically severe personality disorders. A moderate level of impairment in personality functioning is required for the diagnosis of a personality disorder; this threshold is based on empirical evidence that the moderate level of impairment maximizes the ability of clinicians to accurately and efficiently identify personality disorder pathology.

22.10—Criterion A: Level of Personality Functioning (p. 762); Table 2 [Level of Personality Functioning Scale] (pp. 775–778)

22.11 Which of the following statements about the Level of Personality Functioning Scale (LPFS) is *false?*

A. An assessment indicating "moderate impairment" as described by the LPFS is necessary for diagnosis of a personality disorder.
B. An assessment indicating "moderate impairment" as described by the LPFS is sufficient for diagnosis of a personality disorder.
C. The LPFS can be used without specification of a personality disorder diagnosis.
D. The LPFS can be used to describe individuals with personality characteristics that do not reach the threshold for a personality disorder diagnosis.
E. The LPFS can be used to describe a person's level of impairment at any given time.

Correct Answer: A. An assessment indicating "moderate impairment" as described by the LPFS is sufficient for diagnosis of a personality disorder.

Explanation: To use the LPFS, the clinician selects the level that most closely captures the individual's *current overall* level of impairment in personality functioning. The rating is necessary for the diagnosis of a personality disorder (moderate or greater impairment) and can be used to specify the severity of impairment present for an individual with any personality disorder at a given point in time. The LPFS may also be used as a global indicator of personality functioning without specification of a personality disorder diagnosis, or in the event that personality impairment is subthreshold for a disorder diagnosis.

22.11—Rating Level of Personality Functioning (p. 772); Table 2 [Level of Personality Functioning Scale] (pp. 775–778)

Glossary of Technical Terms (DSM-5 Appendix)

23.1 Match each term with the appropriate description.

   A. Affect.
   B. Alogia.
   C. Anhedonia.
   D. Autogynephilia
   E. Catalepsy.
   F. Cataplexy.
   G. Compulsion.
   H. Conversion symptom.
   I. Depressivity.
   J. Dissociation.
   K. Dysphoria.
   L. Euphoria.
   M. Flashback.
   N. Flight of ideas.
   O. Gender dysphoria.
   P. Hypervigilance.
   Q. Ideas of reference.
   R. Language pragmatics.
   S. Magical thinking.
   T. Mood.
   U. Panic attacks.
   V. Perseveration.
   W. Personality disorder—trait specified (PD-TS).
   X. Separation insecurity.
   Y. Subsyndromal.
   Z. Traumatic stressor.

   i. A condition in which a person experiences intense feelings of depression, discontent, and in some cases indifference to the world around them.
   ii. A pattern of observable behaviors that is the expression of a subjectively experienced feeling state (emotion). Examples include sadness, elation, and anger.

iii. Distress that accompanies the incongruence between one's experienced and expressed gender and one's assigned or natal gender.

iv. Below a specified level or threshold required to qualify for a particular condition. These conditions (formes frustes) are medical conditions that do not meet full criteria for a diagnosis—for example, because the symptoms are fewer or less severe than a defined syndrome—but that nevertheless can be identified and related to the "full-blown" syndrome.

v. In Section III "Alternative DSM-5 Model for Personality Disorders," a proposed diagnostic category for use when a personality disorder is considered present but the criteria for a specific disorder are not met.

vi. The splitting off of clusters of mental contents from conscious awareness. This mechanism is central to dissociative disorders. The term is also used to describe the separation of an idea from its emotional significance and affect, as seen in the inappropriate affect in schizophrenia.

vii. Sexual arousal of a natal male associated with the idea or image of being a woman.

viii. The feeling that casual incidents and external events have a particular and unusual meaning that is specific to the person.

ix. A mental and emotional condition in which a person experiences intense feelings of well-being, elation, happiness, excitement, and joy.

x. Passive induction of a posture held against gravity.

xi. Lack of enjoyment from, engagement in, or energy for life's experiences; deficits in the capacity to feel pleasure and take interest in things.

xii. Persistence at tasks or in particular way of doing things long after the behavior has ceased to be functional or effective; continuance of the same behavior despite repeated failures or clear reasons for stopping.

xiii. The erroneous belief that one's thoughts, words, or actions will cause or prevent a specific outcome in some way that defies commonly understood laws of cause and effect.

xiv. Repetitive behaviors (e.g., hand washing, ordering, checking) or mental acts (e.g., praying, counting, repeating words silently) that the individual feels driven to perform in response to an obsession, or according to rules that must be applied rigidly.

xv. A nearly continuous flow of accelerated speech with abrupt changes from topic to topic that are usually based on understandable associations, distracting stimuli, or plays on words. When the condition is severe, speech may be disorganized and incoherent.

xvi. Any event (or events) that may cause or threaten death, serious injury, or sexual violence to an individual, a close family member, or a close friend.

xvii. Fears of being alone due to rejection by and/or separation from significant others, based in a lack of confidence in one's ability to care for oneself, both physically and emotionally.

xviii. The understanding and use of language in a given context. For example, the warning "Watch your hands" when issued to a child who is dirty is intended not only to prompt the child to look at his or her hands but also to communicate the admonition "Don't get anything dirty."

xix. An enhanced state of sensory sensitivity accompanied by an exaggerated intensity of behaviors whose purpose is to detect threats. Other symptoms include abnormally increased arousal, a high responsiveness to stimuli, and a continual scanning of the environment for threats.

xx. A dissociative state during which aspects of a traumatic event are reexperienced as though they were occurring at that moment.

xxi. A loss of, or alteration in, voluntary motor or sensory functioning, with or without apparent impairment of consciousness. The symptom is not fully explained by a neurological or another medical condition or the direct effects of a substance and is not intentionally produced or feigned.

xxii. Episodes of sudden bilateral loss of muscle tone resulting in the individual collapsing, often occurring in association with intense emotions such as laughter, anger, fear, or surprise.

xxiii. A pervasive and sustained emotion that colors the perception of the world. Common examples include depression, elation, anger, and anxiety.

xxiv. An impoverishment in thinking that is inferred from observing speech and language behavior. There may be brief and concrete replies to questions and restriction in the amount of spontaneous speech (termed *poverty of speech*). Sometimes the speech is adequate in amount but conveys little information because it is overconcrete, overabstract, repetitive, or stereotyped (termed *poverty of content*).

xxv. Discrete periods of sudden onset of intense fear or terror, often associated with feelings of impending doom. During these events there are symptoms such as shortness of breath or smothering sensations; palpitations, pounding heart, or accelerated heart rate; chest pain or discomfort; choking; and fear of going crazy or losing control.

xxvi. Feelings of being intensely sad, miserable, and/or hopeless. Some patients describe an absence of feelings and/or dysphoria; difficulty recovering from such moods; pessimism about the future; pervasive shame and/or guilt; feelings of inferior self-worth; and thoughts of suicide and suicidal behavior.

Correct Answers: A: ii, B: xxiv, C: xi, D: vii, E: x, F: xxii, G: xiv, H: xxi, I: xxvi, J: vi, K: i, L: ix, M: xx, N: xv, O: iii, P: xix, Q: viii, R: xviii, S: xiii, T: xxiii, U: xxv, V: xii, W: v, X: xvii, Y: iv, Z: xvi.